Advances in Equine Dentistry

Editor

JACK EASLEY

VETERINARY CLINICS OF NORTH AMERICA: EQUINE PRACTICE

www.vetequine.theclinics.com

Consulting Editor
A. SIMON TURNER

August 2013 • Volume 29 • Number 2

ELSEVIER

1600 John F. Kennedy Boulevard • Suite 1800 • Philadelphia, Pennsylvania, 19103-2899

http://www.vetequine.theclinics.com

VETERINARY CLINICS OF NORTH AMERICA: EQUINE PRACTICE Volume 29, Number 2
August 2013 ISSN 0749-0739, ISBN-13: 978-0-323-18619-3

Editor: John Vassallo; j.vassallo@elsevier.com

Veterinary Clinics of North America: Equine Practice (ISSN 0749-0739) is published in April, August, and December by Elsevier Inc., 360 Park Avenue South, New York, NY 10010-1710. Business and Editorial Offices: 1600 John F. Kennedy Blvd., Suite 1800, Philadelphia, PA 19103-2899. Subscription prices are $267.00 per year (domestic individuals), $397.00 per year (domestic institutions), $126.00 per year (domestic students/residents), $299.00 per year (Canadian individuals), $496.00 per year (Canadian institutions), $346.00 per year (international individuals), $496.00 per year (international institutions), and $172.00 per year (international and Canadian students/residents). To receive student/resident rate, orders must be accompanied by name of affiliated institution, date of term, and the signature of program/residency coordinator on institution letterhead. Orders will be billed at individual rate until proof of status is received. Foreign air speed delivery is included in all *Clinics* subscription prices. All prices are subject to change without notice. **POSTMASTER:** Send address changes to *Veterinary Clinics of North America: Equine Practice*, 3251 Riverport Lane, Maryland Heights, MO 63043. Customer Service (orders, claims, online, change of address): Elsevier Health Sciences Division, Subscription Customer Service, 3251 Riverport Lane, Maryland Heights, MO 63043. Tel: 1-800-654-2452 (U.S. and Canada); 314-447-8871 (outside U.S. and Canada). Fax: 314-447-8029. E-mail: journalscustomer service-usa@elsevier.com (for print support); E-mail: journalsonlinesupport-usa@elsevier (for online support).

Reprints. For copies of 100 or more of articles in this publication, please contact the Commercial Reprints Department, Elsevier Inc., 360 Park Avenue South, New York, NY 10010-1710. Tel.: 212-633-3812; Fax: 212-462-1935; E-mail: reprints@elsevier.com.

Veterinary Clinics of North America: Equine Practice is covered in *MEDLINE/PubMed (Index Medicus), Excerpta Medica, Current Contents/Agriculture, Biology and Environmental Sciences*, and *ISI*.

Printed and bound by CPI Group (UK) Ltd, Croydon, CR0 4YY
Transferred to digital print 2013

Contributors

CONSULTING EDITOR

A. SIMON TURNER, BVSc, MS, DVSc
Diplomate, American College of Veterinary Surgeons; Professor Emeritus, Department of Clinical Sciences, College of Veterinary Medicine and Biomedical Sciences, Colorado State University, Fort Collins, Colorado

EDITOR

JACK EASLEY, DVM, MS
Diplomate, American Board of Veterinary Practitioners; Easley Equine Dentistry, Equine Veterinary Practice, LLC, Shelbyville, Kentucky

AUTHORS

ROBERT BARATT, DVM, FAVD, MS
Salem Valley Veterinary Clinic, Salem, Connecticut; Pieper Memorial Veterinary Center, Middletown, Connecticut; Part-time Resident (Dentistry), Cornell University Hospital for Animals, Ithaca, New York

MIRIAM CASEY, MVB, MSc, MRCVS
School of Veterinary Sciences, University of Bristol, Langford, Bristol, United Kingdom

PADRAIC M. DIXON, MVB, PhD, MRCVS
Division of Equine Veterinary Studies, The Royal (Dick) School of Veterinary Studies and Roslin Institute, The University of Edinburgh, Easter Bush Veterinary Centre, Midlothian, Scotland, United Kingdom

NICOLE DU TOIT, BVSc, MSc, CertEP, PhD, MRCVS
Equine Veterinary Dentistry, Tulbagh, Western Cape, South Africa

EDWARD EARLEY, DVM, FAVD (Equine)
Dentistry Resident, Cornell University Hospital for Animals, Ithaca, New York; Laurel Highland Veterinary Clinic, LLC, Williamsport, Pennsylvania

JACK EASLEY, DVM, MS
Diplomate, American Board of Veterinary Practitioners; Easley Equine Dentistry, Equine Veterinary Practice, LLC, Shelbyville, Kentucky

JEREMIAH T. EASLEY, DVM
Diplomate, American College of Veterinary Surgeons; Assistant Director, Surgical Research Laboratory, Department of Clinical Sciences, Colorado State University, Fort Collins, Colorado

DAVID L. FOSTER, VMD
Adjunct Assistant Professor, Department of Surgery, University of Pennsylvania School of Veterinary Medicine, New Bolton Center, Kennett Square, Pennsylvania; Private Practice, Morganville, New Jersey, Morganville, New Jersey

DAVID E. FREEMAN, MVB, PhD
Diplomate, American College of Veterinary Surgeons; Professor, Department of Clinical Sciences, College of Veterinary Medicine, University of Florida, Gainesville, Florida

STEPHEN S. GALLOWAY, DVM, FAVD (Equine)
Animal Care Hospital, Somerville, Tennessee

CLEET GRIFFIN, DVM
Diplomate, American Board of Veterinary Practitioners (Equine Practice); Clinical Assistant Professor, Equine Field Service, College of Veterinary Medicine and Biomedical Sciences, Texas A&M University, College Station, Texas

ROBERT MENZIES, BVSc
Diplomate, American Veterinary Dental College; Dentistry and Oral Surgery Service, Veterinary Teaching Hospital, University of Helsinki, Koetilantie, Finland

JENNIFER T. RAWLINSON, DVM
Diplomate, American Veterinary Dental College; Lecturer, Department of Clinical Sciences, College of Veterinary Medicine, Cornell University, Ithaca, New York

BAYARD A. RUCKER, DVM
Southwest Virginia Veterinary Services, Lebanon Virginia

KURT SELBERG, MS, DVM
Assistant Professor, Department of Biosciences and Diagnostic Imaging, University of Georgia, Athens, Georgia

CARSTEN STASZYK, Dr med vet
Professor, Institute for Veterinary Anatomy, Histology and Embryology, Faculty of Veterinary Medicine, Justus-Liebig-University Giessen, Gießen, Germany

HENRY TREMAINE, BVetMed, MPhi, Cert ES, MRVS
Diplomate, European College of Veterinary Surgeons; Department of Clinical Veterinary Science, University of Bristol, Langford, Bristol, United Kingdom

Contents

While there is currently insufficient scientific material of adequate quality to enable evidence-based medicine in equine dentistry, this by no means negates the clinician's responsibility to provide oral health care in a scientific and ethical manner. To do so requires that the clinician be knowledgable and skilled in dentistry and general medicine, that each case upholds the principles of scientific method, and that data is gathered and appraised in an objective, precise, consistent, uniform, and reliable manner.

have become more conservative, and extraction procedures more exacting. Periodontal and endodontic treatments are described to save teeth that would have succumbed to extraction in the past. Pathologic impacts on treatment decisions for equine odontoclastic tooth resorption and hypercementosis are significant, and veterinarians and owners need to be aware of treatment options and outcomes. Easy access to equid incisor and canine teeth offers a variety of therapeutic options, and this article reviews some of the practical procedures available.

The last decade has seen a number of studies that have illuminated our knowledge of hypsodont dental disease and re-examined some of the traditionally performed practices. In addition there has been a major interest in routine preventative dentistry and non-traumatic treatments. These have highlighted some potential risks of the use of modern tools when applied to traditional techniques. This has also led to a reflective review of equine dentistry with the emphasis on attempting to preserve and salvage dental and periodontal tissues, with minimal trauma. In addition, precise imaging and instrumentation have facilitated minimally invasive techniques in conscious sedated horses, and there is renewed interest in comparative dentistry leading to trials with restorative techniques that are practiced in other species.

The diagnosis and treatment of equine dental-related sinus disease is often challenging. Dental-related sinus disease is common and knowledge of these diseases is becoming increasingly important in veterinary medicine. Diagnostic capabilities are continually improving, leading to early diagnostic and therapeutic successes. With advanced imaging modalities, such as computed tomography and magnetic resonance imaging, understanding of the intimate anatomic relationship between teeth and the paranasal sinuses continues to progress. There are many therapeutic options available for the treatment of these common and challenging disorders. A complete understanding of the disease, therapeutic options, and potential complications is vital to overall successful resolution of clinical signs in equine dental-related sinus disorders.

Postpartum evaluation of the foal's head and mouth are performed to detect craniofacial malformations and other congenital defects. Detailed oral examination and diagnostic imaging can provide diagnostic and prognostic information about congenital abnormalities of the mouth or skull. Important abnormalities of foals include wry nose, cleft palate, overbite (parrot mouth), and underbite (monkey mouth, sow mouth). Tumors and cysts can be detected in young horses. In juvenile horses, primary dental care procedures include oral examination, management of sharp enamel points, management of deciduous teeth, and management of wolf teeth. Facial or jaw swellings are also important considerations.

This article discusses the primary odontogenic problems of the mature performance horse, including wolf teeth; hooks; overbite, overjet, underjet, and wry bite; equine odontoclastic tooth resorption and hypercementosis; infundibular caries; and secondary oral problems. It outlines the author's methods of taking the history, oral examination, and use of diagnostic nerve blocks.

Changes in normal equine dental anatomy with age result in dental disease specific to the geriatric horse. The culmination of dental disease throughout the life of a horse often results in advanced dental disease. Treatment of specific dental disease conditions has to be adapted for older horses to compensate for reduction in reserve crown and occlusal enamel. Ensuring oral comfort and maximizing masticatory ability are the mainstays of geriatric dental treatment. Recognition of dental disease common to older horses ensures that correct treatment is applied. Older patients often require long-term management changes, such as dietary modification, to manage dental disease effectively.

VETERINARY CLINICS OF
NORTH AMERICA: EQUINE PRACTICE

THE CLINICS ARE NOW AVAILABLE ONLINE!
Access your subscription at:
www.theclinics.com

Preface

Advances in Equine Dentistry

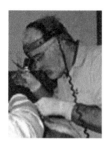

Jack Easley, DVM, MS
Editor

By the early 20th century, at least 3 American textbooks had been published on veterinary dentistry using the horse as the main focus. These texts were written to inform horsemen and very rudimentary trained veterinarians about basic dental anatomy and common forms of therapy for the most commonly diagnosed dental condition, "sharp enamel points." The same pathologic conditions seen today were recorded in early writings, but pathophysiology was poorly understood. Louis A. Merillat in his 1906 text, *Veterinary Surgery, Vol. 1, Animal Dentistry and Diseases of the Mouth,* wrote, "Human dentistry owes its existence to a single disease process, *caries,* while animal dentistry depends upon a single physical defect, *enamel points.*"

Human dentistry has advanced from the crude practices of John Hunter and survived the modern use of fluoridated drinking water. So too, has veterinary dentistry progressed from rasping enamel points from teeth. Ironically, one hundred years later, several current textbooks written about equine dentistry contain much of the same information and described techniques of the past without any scientific basis whatsoever for the recommendations of therapy. The notion, "it's been done successfully for over 100 years," is often used as justification for continuation of many unproven (and often damaging) practices and procedures.

Small animal dentistry involves diagnosing and treating diseases of brachydont dentition. Much of the *progress* in the field of small animal dentistry and the *delay* of progress in hyposodont (equine) dentistry is due to the application of human dental diagnostic and therapeutic techniques. Only recently has veterinary medicine come to better understand the dramatic differences in development, anatomy, physiology, and pathology between the brachydont omnivore and carnivore dentition and that of hyposodont herbivores. Much is left to understand about horses' teeth and even more about other domestic and wild species. Equine dentistry is a rich area for research over the next century. Evidence-based dentistry is still the goal, but much progress in basic and clinical research as well as properly constructed clinical field studies needs to be accomplished to push us toward the target.

Vet Clin Equine 29 (2013) xi–xii
http://dx.doi.org/10.1016/j.cveq.2013.05.001
0749-0739/13/$ – see front matter © 2013 Published by Elsevier Inc.

vetequine.theclinics.com

Ignorance in this area exists in the horse world, often rooted in superstition and myths of the past or well-intentioned horsemens' previous "experiences." The science of veterinary medicine, in this regard, contains misinformation about dental conditions and the relationship to mastication, digestion, musculoskeletal conformation, athletic performance, health, and comfort. The placebo effect is at work, and we, as professionals, must be on guard not to misinterpret one horse's perceived response to a treatment or manipulation as being evidence to continue a practice that may not be effective or even healthy for the patient. Such practices are often harmful to the animal and costly to owners.

As editor of this issue of *Veterinary Clinics of North America: Equine Practice*, I would like to thank friends and mentors. Simon Turner petitioned Elsevier to allow me to gather current equine dentistry information from colleagues and researchers. Equine dentistry brought a special person into my life 15+ years ago and we have been friends ever since—Paddy Dixon. His group at the Royal (Dick) School of Veterinary Studies, Edinburgh, Scotland, has been the frontrunner in performing valuable research for many years, setting the benchmark for evaluation, scientific studies, and published materials. A thank-you goes to equine dentistry authors, contributors, countless horses, clients, and veterinary colleagues that have allowed me to "practice" equine dentistry. It is my hope that the information contained in this issue will not only stimulate but also drive our profession toward the goal of practicing evidence-based equine dentistry.

What are the implications of current equine dental research on the future of equine health? I have attempted to recruit as authors the very best investigators and clinicians in the field of equine dentistry. Each author was asked not only to review the current knowledge on their topic but also to offer opinions on contentious issues and identify areas for future research. Thank you, authors, for your excellent contributions contained herein.

Special thanks to my friends and mentors, Eugene Schneider, Gordon Baker, Leon Scrutchfield, Jim Schumacher, Paddy Dixon, and many others, for keeping me on track as I reached each crossroad of my career. Finally, my heartfelt gratitude to my wife, Sydney, and our 3 children, who have allowed me to pursue this career as an equine practitioner and cultivate this often time-consuming and expensive hobby—equine dentistry.

Jack Easley, DVM, MS
Equine Veterinary Practice, LLC
P.O. Box 1075
Shelbyville, KY 40066, USA

E-mail address:
easleydvm@aol.com

A Fresh Look at the Anatomy and Physiology of Equine Mastication

Padraic M. Dixon, MVB, PhD, MRCVS[a],*,
Nicole du Toit, BVSc, MSc, CertEP, PhD[b], Carsten Staszyk, Dr med vet[c]

KEYWORDS

- Horse • Dentistry • Dental anatomy • Dentinal thickness • Equine • Pulp
- Periodontium

KEY POINTS

- Variation in cheek teeth occlusal angulation, with high angles (>30°) present in the caudal mandibular cheek teeth, is now accepted.
- The description of multiple (5–7) pulp horns in cheek teeth, and of their connections to each other and to the individual roots, is of major significance in endodontic therapy, as is the anatomical description of the shape of the single pulp horn in incisors.
- The description of the unique, continually remodeling collagen and vascular structures of equine periodontium (which allows prolonged dental eruption) is of great clinical interest.
- Equine dentine is very active because of prolonged dental eruption and the consequent need to prevent occlusal pulpar exposure, and a distinctive type of irregular secondary equine dentine has been described.

INTRODUCTION

Although dental anatomy is sometimes seen as a dry, uninteresting topic, there have been many significant and interesting developments in this field during the past 20 years that are of major clinical significance in helping us better understand the physiology of equine mastication, the etiopathogenesis of some dental disorders, and their safe treatment. Many important developments in this field are summarized in this article.

PERIPHERAL ENAMEL INFOLDING

Equine cheek teeth have evolved to become efficient at grinding tough fibrous food. Instead of having a single layer of enamel around the periphery of the cheek teeth

[a] Division of Equine Veterinary Studies, the Royal (Dick) School of Veterinary Studies and Roslin Institute, The University of Edinburgh, Easter Bush Veterinary Centre, Midlothian, EH25 9RG, Scotland, UK; [b] PO Box 210, Tulbagh 6820, South Africa; [c] Institute for Veterinary Anatomy, Histology and Embryology, Faculty of Veterinary Medicine, Justus-Liebig-University Giessen, Frankfurter Str. 98, Gießen D-35392, Germany
* Corresponding author.
E-mail address: p.m.dixon@ed.ac.uk

Vet Clin Equine 29 (2013) 257–272
http://dx.doi.org/10.1016/j.cveq.2013.04.006   vetequine.theclinics.com
0749-0739/13/$ – see front matter © 2013 Elsevier Inc. All rights reserved.

(like brachydont teeth), the lower cheek teeth in particular have extensive infolding of enamel, which increases the length of hard enamel folds on the occlusal surface and also protects the softer cementum and dentine from excessive wear. du Toit and colleagues[1] have shown that the ratio of peripheral enamel length to tooth perimeter in mandibular cheek teeth is 1.87 (indicating much infolding of enamel), compared with a value in maxillary cheek teeth of 1.48; however, the maxillary cheek teeth also have infundibular enamel folds, which compensates for their reduced peripheral enamel infolding. The degree of infolding present on the periphery of teeth decreases more apically. and thus with age, just a rim of peripheral enamel without infolding can be present in mandibular cheek teeth, which also become hollowed out. This anatomy eventually becomes a feature of most aged teeth and has been termed senile excavation (**Fig. 1**).

CHEEK TEETH INFUNDIBULAR ENAMEL

Normal infundibulae can be up to 10 cm long in young horses to as short as 2 mm in aged horses.[2] On average, infundibular length is a mean of 82% of the dental crown length; however, in individual cheek teeth and horses, they may be shorter.[2] Thus, with age (or occasionally in a young tooth), either one or both infundibulae can wear out (often in the 09 or 10 teeth), causing the adjacent unsupported primary and secondary dentine to wear fast and the tooth to become hollow, leading to senile excavation of the upper cheek teeth.

ENAMEL

Enamel is composed of 96% minerals, most of which is calcium hydroxyapatite crystals. The remaining organic 4% consists of proteins and water. This high mineral content makes enamel the hardest substance in the body but also makes it brittle. However, in brachydont species, the underlying layer of dentine, which has a more resilient matrix, maintains the integrity of enamel and thus helps prevent fractures. In horses, the thick external layer of peripheral cementum also greatly helps in this role (**Fig. 1**).[3]

The ultrastructural anatomy of enamel shows that it is composed of 2 components: prisms (rods), which are embedded in more homogeneous interprismatic enamel. Kilic

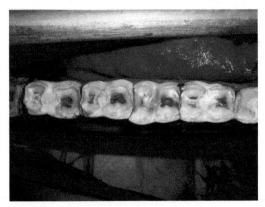

Fig. 1. Senile mandibular cheek teeth showing varying decreases in their peripheral enamel infolding, and with dental wear almost to root level in some teeth, and consequently, excessive occlusal wear.

and colleagues[4] described 3 different types of equine enamel based on the transverse appearance of their prisms and the amount and appearance of interprismatic enamel. Similar enamel types were identified in donkeys,[5] and it is most likely that all members of the Equidae family conform to these enamel types.

Equid type 1 enamel lies adjacent to the amelodentinal junction (more centrally in the tooth) and consists of rows of oval prisms that alternate with plates of interprismatic enamel (**Fig. 2**). This type of enamel is the hardest and is able to resist wear better, but it is more brittle and thus susceptible to shearing forces.[4] Kilic and colleagues[4] also found that the thickness of interprismatic enamel plates were similar to the diameter of enamel prisms adjacent to the amelodentinal junction, indicating similar wear resistance between prisms and plates.

Equine type 2 enamel is composed of bundles of keyhole-shaped or horseshoe-shaped prisms, with little or no interprismatic enamel present (**Fig. 3**).[4] This type of enamel usually lies adjacent to the amelocemental junction (more peripherally in the teeth). Equine type 2 enamel prisms also showed decussation (zones of prisms run in different orientations) (ie, prisms have an irregular, curving three-dimensional configuration, and this functions to increase their resistance to shearing forces).[6] Equine type 3 enamel is found infrequently at the amelodentinal or amelocemental junctions and consists of oval prisms surrounded by honeycomblike interprismatic enamel.[4]

Equine type 1 enamel is the predominant enamel type in the maxillary cheek teeth to enable better wear resistance.[4,5] Equine type 2 enamel is the predominant type of enamel found in equid incisors, so that they can resist shearing forces. This type 2 enamel was also more predominant than equine type 1 in mandibular cheek teeth. This finding indicates that maxillary and mandibular cheek teeth are subjected to different masticatory forces, with mandibular cheek teeth better able to accommodate shearing forces. Equine type 3 enamel is believed to be a transitional type of enamel and is found in low and varying amounts in cheek teeth and incisors.

At the end of enamel development, the apex of the equine tooth cannot be called a true root (by definition a root is an enamel-free area), but shortly after tooth eruption, much cemental deposition begins, and this continues over the life of the tooth to form the true roots, until the tooth becomes loose or is fully worn away. Histologic examination of undecalcified sections of equid (horses and donkeys) teeth has enabled the identification of microscopic features of enamel, in particular of the junctions of

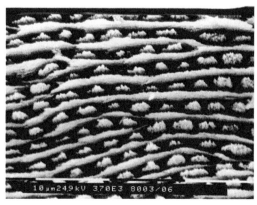

Fig. 2. Electron microscopic image of equine type 1 enamel, showing parallel plates of enamel prisms and plates. Although a hard type of enamel, it is susceptible to fracturing between these parallel structures.

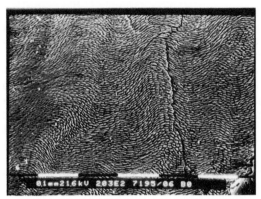

Fig. 3. Electron microscopic image of equine type 2 enamel. Note the absence of interprismatic enamel and that its prisms are oriented in 3 directions (decussation), which gives it great resistance to fracturing.

enamel with cementum and dentine. This factor has enabled the identification of features such as enamel spindles, which extend from dentine into the enamel.[5] Furthermore, the presence of enamel microfractures has been identified on undecalcified histology. These fractures were previously believed to be iatrogenic, because of a preparation artifact. In light of recent studies showing the common presence of enamel microfractures in cheek teeth when using oral endoscopy,[7,8] it may be that these microfractures are so common that they could be termed normal anatomic features.

DENTINE

Dentine is a softer dental tissue than enamel, containing 70% hydroxyapatite crystals and 30% organic fibers, mucopolysaccharides, and water. Dentine is sometimes referred to as 1 of the 2 components of the pulpodentine complex, because dentine and pulp are related embryologically, and remain intimately related anatomically and functionally throughout the life of the tooth. The modified classification of primary, secondary and tertiary dentine in equines by Dacre and colleagues[9] was supported by later histologic studies in donkey teeth.[5]

Using the standard brachydont dentinal classification, primary dentine in equids is histologically characterized by the presence of odontoblast processes surrounded by dentinal tubules that are filled with intratubular dentine. These dentinal tubules are in turn surrounded by intertubular dentine.[10,11] Secondary dentine consists of wider dentinal tubules without intratubular dentine (ie, only intertubular dentine is present). Secondary dentine is further divided into regular secondary dentine and irregular secondary dentine. Regular secondary dentine is continuous with primary dentine and is laid down throughout the life of the tooth, resulting in a gradual, lifelong narrowing of the pulp cavity.

Irregular secondary dentine was previously classified as tertiary dentine,[10,12] because it resembles brachydont tertiary dentine. However, Dacre and colleagues[9] and du Toit and colleagues[3] have all shown that irregular secondary dentine is laid down in response to normal attrition of the occlusal surface and prevents occlusal pulpar exposure of the most central part of the pulp horn. Irregular secondary dentine is now considered as a type of normal (physiologic) dentine (**Fig. 4**).

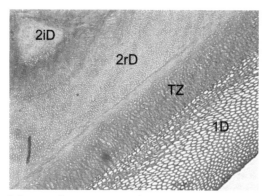

Fig. 4. This histologic image of an equine tooth shows primary dentine (1D) most peripherally, with a transition zone (TZ) between it and secondary regular dentine (2rD). Most centrally in the former pulp horn is secondary irregular dentine (2iD).

Tertiary dentine is a type of dentine that is laid down locally in response to a noxious stimulus and it may or may not contain dentinal tubules. Tertiary dentine has been identified as a separate entity to irregular secondary dentine in horse and donkey teeth.[5,9] Other anatomic variations of dentine that have been identified in equids include the presence of pulp stones (discrete calcified masses in the pulp) and of interglobular dentine (areas of hypocalcified dentine), neither of which is regarded as a pathologic entity.[5,9]

The presence of apparently open lumina of the dentinal tubules on the occlusal surface in horses was shown by Kilic and colleagues.[13] The remnants of odontoblast processes were later identified at this site.[5,10] The presence of an organic smear layer (pellicle; see later discussion) over the occlusal surface of equine teeth as observed on scanning electron microscopy may provide pulpar protection against descending bacterial or chemical insults.[13] The removal of this smear layer during dental rasping may make the teeth sensitive and possibly put the teeth at risk for descending bacterial infections. Deeper rasping, which that exposes sensitive dentine,[14] is even more likely to cause dental pain and quidding.

CEMENTUM

From an embryologic point of view, dental cementum is not a part of the tooth but part of the periodontium. During dental development, ectomesenchymal cells surrounding the developing tooth differentiate into cementoblasts. If the developing surfaces of both enamel (in the region of the entire crown) and dentine (in the region of the anatomic root) are covered by epithelial cells of the enamel organ or the epithelial root sheath, respectively, cementum production cannot occur. However, when the enamel organ and epithelial sheaths disappear, the denuded enamel and dentinal surfaces induce the cementoblasts to produce cementum. This process can also occur if denuded surfaces of enamel or dentin become exposed within the periodontal space (eg, because of trauma or odontoclastic lesions).

Cementum is the softest dental tissue, being composed of just 45% to 50% hydroxyapatite crystals. The remaining component contains collagen fibers (predominantly type 1) and water. Unlike in brachydont teeth, in which its main purpose is to act as an anchoring point for the periodontal ligaments (PDLs), equid peripheral cementum also forms a major structural component of the clinical crown.[3] Because of its high water and organic content, it also has a major role in preventing fractures of the adjacent (hard but brittle) enamel, which, as noted earlier, is infolded greatly into the peripheral cementum.[1,15]

Cemental thickness is greatest in the mandibular cheek teeth, where the deep peripheral enamel infoldings are filled with and surrounded by thick cementum. Peripheral cementum is formed subocclusally throughout the life of the tooth and can be deposited rapidly in response to various stimuli. For this reason, cementum is regarded as having reparative function, even filling defects in adjacent enamel. There is an increase in peripheral cementum deposition in the newly erupted clinical crown once it leaves the confining restrictions of the bony alveolus, and this deposition contributes to the size of the clinical crown.[1,5] Mitchell and colleagues[3] have also shown that this recently erupted cementum contains viable cementoblasts and cementocytes, with blood vessels running some millimeters from the PDLs into this recently deposited, supragingival, thick cementum. The PDL and gingiva provide the blood supply for peripheral cementum, therefore once it has erupted a few millimeters up onto the clinical crown, the cementum is inert.

Similarly, the main blood supply to the infundibular cementum comes from the dental sac (ie, from the occlusal aspect of the tooth) during dental development. This blood supply is lost at eruption and therefore infundibulae are mainly filled with inert cementum containing the central vascular channel, which once contained these blood vessels.[16] However, a recent study[2] has shown that there is an apical blood supply to some cheek teeth infundibulae for several years after eruption, which allows for continued infundibular cementum deposition during this time.

Not all cheek teeth infundibulae are completely filled with cementum. Scanning electron microscopy of equine teeth commonly identified the presence of cemental hypoplasia in apparently normal teeth.[16] Two different types of hypoplasia were identified, including, most commonly, central infundibular hypoplasia (at site of previous vasculature) and, less importantly, junctional cemental hypoplasia (at the amelocemental junction).[16] A later gross anatomic study of equine cheek teeth showed that complete cemental filling of infundibulae was rarely present (**Fig. 5**), being identified

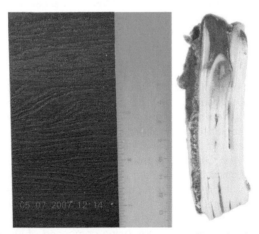

Fig. 5. The infundibulum of this young, 11-cm-long maxillary cheek tooth has a central cemental defect occlusally, with further cemental defects in its midsection and a bulbous apex, which is fully filled with cementum. The pink staining to the apex of this infundibulum is likely caused by an apical blood supply, but may also be partly caused by iatrogenic blood staining by the saw from blood in the adjacent pulp horns.

in only 15% of healthy equine maxillary cheek teeth. This finding may indicate that cemental hypoplasia is so common that it may even be considered as a normal anatomical variation.[2]

Inexplicably, the (maxillary) 09 position has more marked infundibular cemental hypoplasia than any other Triadan position, and this is the likely reason that the 09s commonly have severe infundibular caries and consequently develop fractures and apical infections. A recent computed tomographic study has confirmed Fitzgibbon and colleagues'[2] gross anatomic work, by showing that 90% of infundibulae have some cemental defects.[17]

Caries of maxillary cheek teeth infundibular cementum is common and often extensive.[2] Infundibular cementum can have a porous appearance in contrast to peripheral cementum, because of the presence of wide peripheral vascular channels connected to the central vascular channel. Moreover, infundibular cementum also has many wide lacunae, formerly occupied by cementocytes (**Fig. 6**). These defects allow ready access of food and saliva into the infundibulae, where there is then a suitable environment for microbial growth.

PULPAR ANATOMY
Rostral Teeth

Equine incisors have a Y-shaped pulp cavity, with 2 pulp horns, 1 lying labiomesial (rostromedial) and 1 labiodistal (rostrolateral) to the infundibulum. This configuration exists in both incisor arcades but is more pronounced in the upper incisors. The presence of 2 individual pulp horns is also reflected by the presence of 2 dental stars (areas of secondary dentine) in labiomesial and labiodistal positions adjacent to the infundibulum (**Fig. 7**).

In the upper incisors, the 2 pulp horns fuse at the level of the base of the infundibulum, but in the lower incisors, the 2 pulp horns fuse a few millimeters occlusal to this level. The endodontic cavity apical to the fused pulp horn lies within the reserve crown as well as the anatomic root. Therefore the term root canal, which is used for brachydont teeth, does not accurately describe this pulp compartment of the (hypsodont) equine incisor. Accordingly the term pulp canal is proposed for this structure. It has also been recently shown[18] that the shape of incisor pulp canals is not uniform but ranges from tubular to mesiodistally (laterally) flattened. These canals are usually unbranched in upper incisors, but small side branches are present in the apical half of the pulp canal of lower incisors.

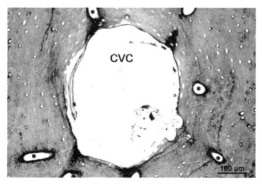

Fig. 6. Infundibular cementum. The central vascular channel (CVC) is surrounded by peripheral vascular channels (*asterisks*) in a radial fashion. There are also many large cementocyte lacunae present in this section.

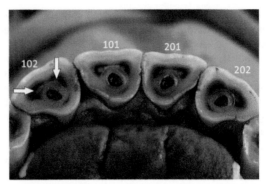

Fig. 7. Central (101, 201) and middle (102, 202) upper incisors of a 9-year-old horse. Arrows indicate the positions of 2 dental stars in a labiodistal and labiomesial position in tooth 102.

The equine canine (04s) and first premolars (05s) have a simple (unbranched) endodontic cavity, similar to brachydont teeth.

Cheek Teeth

Equine cheek teeth have a complex endodontic cavity, which is characterized by major age-related changes and individual variation. Up to a dental age (ie, after eruption age of the tooth) of 2 years, equine cheek teeth have a common pulp chamber in their apical aspect that divides into separate pulp horns toward the occlusal surface, such that each mature cheek tooth eventually has between 5 and 7 pulp horns.[9,19] When root formation occurs, the pulp cavity becomes completed by the development of root canals. On the occlusal surface, the dentine overlying each pulp horn appears as a dark brown area (regular secondary dentine) with a bright center (ie, a focal area of irregular secondary dentine). Thus, the positions of the individual pulp horns are clearly visible.

Cheek teeth 07 to 10 have 5 pulp horns each; the 06s and the lower 11s have 6 pulp horns, and the upper 11s have 7 pulp horns. An endodontic numbering system to aid in the identification of specific pulp horns during clinical examination[9] has been modified,[1] and this modified system is now in general use (**Fig. 8**).

The continued production of secondary dentine causes narrowing of the pulp cavities, the common pulp chamber eventually disappears, and the pulp system becomes divided into separate pulp compartments. A pulp compartment consists of at least 1 pulp horn and at least 1 root canal.[19] With increasing age, this pulp compartment segmentation becomes more pronounced. The resulting configuration of individual pulp compartments within a cheek tooth is more complex in maxillary than mandibular cheek teeth.[1,9,19,20]

The age-dependent changes and spatial configuration patterns of cheek teeth pulp compartments were recently described by Kopke and colleagues.[19] It is of great clinical significance that cheek teeth can contain several noncommunicating pulp compartments. Maxillary cheek teeth greater than 2 years dental age can have up to 4 individual pulp compartments, but in contrast, some of 9 years dental age can still have a single (common) pulp chamber. The number of pulp compartments is not statistically correlated with age and the connection of individual pulp horns to individual root canals can also vary greatly. Thus, the pulp compartment status of a maxillary cheek tooth is unpredictable, which makes effective endodontic restoration of these teeth problematic.[19]

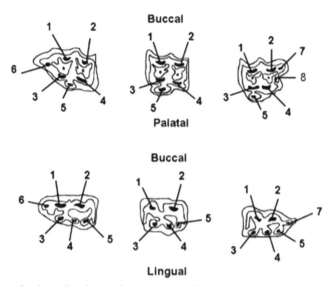

Fig. 8. Equine cheek teeth pulp numbering system of du Toit and colleagues. (*From* du Toit N, Kempson SA, Dixon PM. Donkey dental anatomy. Part 1: gross and computed axial tomography examinations. Vet J 2008;176:338–44; with permission.)

In contrast, mandibular cheek teeth 07 to 10 have a predictable pulp compartment pattern.[19] Whereas some mandibular cheek teeth of up to 15 years dental age can still have a common pulp chamber, most mandibular cheek teeth of more than 2 years dental age have 2 pulp compartments. The mesial (rostral) compartment comprises pulp horns 1 and 3 connected to the mesial (rostral) root canal and a distal (caudal) compartment comprising pulp horns 2 and 5 connected to the distal (caudal) root canals. The most variable component in this pattern is pulp horn 4, which can be part of either of the rostral or caudal compartment. Occasionally, pulp horn 4 is completely separate from the 2 pulp compartments above and therefore has no blood supply and is consequently nonvital. Mandibular 11 cheek teeth occasionally feature a third pulp compartment composed of pulp horn 7 and root canal III (**Fig. 9**).

Similar to brachydont teeth, continued deposition of secondary dentine circumferentially in the pulp horns results in narrowing and filling of the pulp horns in older horses.[9,20] In particular, equid teeth have deposition of regular secondary and irregular secondary dentine on the occlusal aspect of the pulp horns to prevent pulpar exposure as the teeth wear down (**Fig. 10**).[9] This subocclusal dentine layer does not become thicker with age,[21] as was traditionally believed, and many older teeth have a thinner layer of subocclusal secondary dentine than younger horses. It has also been shown that great variation can occur even in the individual pulps of a single cheek tooth, with some normal teeth having as little as 3 mm of subocclusal dentine. This feature is of major clinical significance when teeth are being floated (rasped); although high levels of enamel (inert tissue) overgrowths can be removed, great care must be taken in reducing dentine.

The distance of the pulp horn to the rostral (mesial) and caudal (distal) periphery of cheek teeth has been investigated by Bettiol and Dixon,[22] who showed similar small distances (3–5 mm) between pulp and tooth margin in some teeth and also great variation for this parameter in some teeth. Knowledge of this feature is of great clinical significance when performing diastema widening (to treat periodontal disease associated with cheek teeth diastemata) to avoid pulpar exposure.

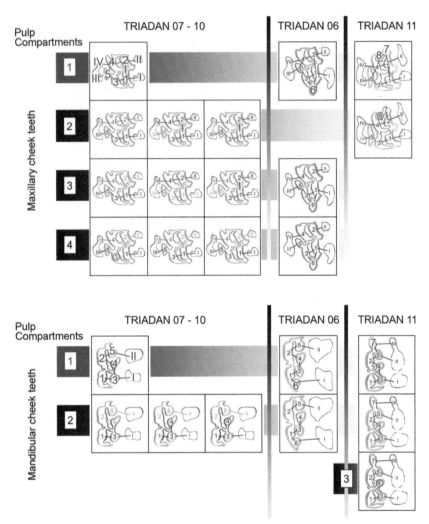

Fig. 9. Pulp configurations in equine maxillary and mandibular cheek teeth. Maxillary cheek teeth can have up to 4 separate pulp compartments, whereas mandibular cheek teeth can have up to 3. Pulp horns are labeled with Arabic numerals and root canals with Roman numerals. Connections are shown by straight lines. Encircled numerals represent either isolated pulp horns or pulp horns that are completely filled with secondary dentin. The diagrams of Triadan 06s and 11s show the connections of pulp horns 6, 7, and 8, respectively.

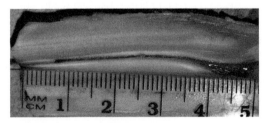

Fig. 10. This longitudinal section of a mandibular cheek tooth shows about 7 mm of subocclusal secondary dentine present in this plane.

The exposure of dentinal odontoblast processes on the occlusal surface is believed to play an important role in regulating the deposition of subocclusal secondary dentine.[14] This hypothesis has been recently supported by Marshall and Dixon,[23] who showed that overgrown cheek teeth often have less secondary dentine than adjacent normal teeth. This finding indicates that the absence of occlusal stimulus, which decreases dentinal deposition, outweighs the increased thickness because of reduced/absence of wear and the increased eruption present in poorly or unopposed teeth.

Cheek Teeth Occlusal Angle

Until recently, it was believed that the occlusal surface of all the cheek teeth had an angle of 15%, sloping in a medial to lateral (buccolingual; buccopalatal) direction. However, a recent study[24] has shown normal mandibular cheek teeth to have angles of circa 15° in the 06s that increase up to 32° in the 11s. In contrast, the maxillary cheek teeth have a higher angulation more rostrally (ie, vary from 19° in the 06's that decrease to about 9° in the 11s).[24] Consequently, it is inappropriate to mechanically alter all of the cheek teeth occlusal angles to an angle of 15° or to try to make the occlusal angles of rostral and caudal cheek teeth, or of the maxillary and mandibular cheek teeth, similar.

PELLICLE

The surfaces of mammalian teeth, including horses,[13] have an organic covering forming what is termed a pellicle. In other species, this pellicle has been shown to be composed mainly of mucopolysaccharides and glycoproteins from saliva, along with high numbers of oral bacteria. If this organic layer becomes thick (when it contains increased bacterial numbers), it can be termed dental plaque. It has been suggested that a value of 5 mm thickness should be used to differentiate between pellicle and plaque in the horse.[25] In the normal horse, the ingestion and mastication of coarse forage (which is also is low in soluble carbohydrates) for prolonged periods acts as effective tooth-brushing, and therefore, plaque is not normally present on normal equine teeth, except in the interdental areas that are not exposed to this mechanical effect, as recently shown by Cox and colleagues.[26]

PERIODONTIUM

The equine periodontium is a complex arrangement of 4 constituents: alveolar bone, dental cementum, gingival, and PDL. The PDL is interposed between the alveolar bone and the dental cementum, and its collagen fiber apparatus anchors the tooth to the alveolar bone. The periodontium, especially the PDL, provides tooth support and withstands masticatory forces. Moreover, normal occlusal wear of 3 to 4 mm per year has to be compensated by continuous eruption of the tooth, which requires remodeling of the periodontal tissues at a high rate.[27] Over the last few years, several histologic characteristics of equine periodontium have been identified, outlining its unique functional, remodeling, and regenerative capacity.

Periodontal Collagen Fiber Apparatus and Vasculature

The functional requirements of tooth support are met by the spatial arrangement of the periodontal collagen fiber apparatus along with its extensive vascular system.[28,29] The anchoring collagen fiber bundles are aligned in multidirectional arrangements,[6] which ensures transmission and dissemination of masticatory loads during all phases of the complex equine chewing cycle.[29] The periodontal vasculature supplements the collagen fiber apparatus (**Fig. 11**) and consists of an inner capillary layer (near the cementum), and an outer venous layer, near the alveolar bone.[28] The outer venous

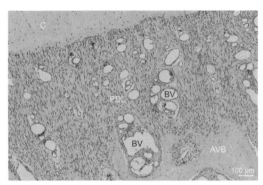

Fig. 11. Horizontal section through the periodontium. At midtooth level, of a 409 in 20-year-old horse. The cementum (C) and the alveolar bone (AVB) are connected by collagen fiber bundles of the PDL. The extensive periodontal vascular system is represented by groups of longitudinally arranged blood vessels (BV).

layer has unusual vascular structures (ie, blind ending vessels and large ampullae), but no venous valves, and these features are likely to be functional adaptions to facilitate shock absorption.[30]

This structural combination of collagen fibers and blood vessels also enhances the dissemination of masticatory forces within the equine PDL.[31,32] In a so-called type I arrangement, a sheath of collagen fibers and fibroblastic cells protects the blood vessels from deformations occurring in the surrounding tissues. In a type II arrangement, tensile forces in collagen fibers are transferred to compress adjacent blood vessels (by a lateral compression mechanism); in a type III arrangement, wide venules are believed to act as a hemodynamic cushion, with collagen fibers preventing the vasculature from moving. Overall, the physical properties of the collagen fibers and the intravascular blood content combine to form an effective viscoelastic shock-absorbing system.

Although the mechanism of dental eruption is not fully understood, it is generally believed that the periodontal vasculature facilitates an intravascular-extravascular shift of fluids, thus generating increased hydrostatic pressures within the PDL extracellular matrix.[33–35] However, as eruption continues for life in most equine teeth, the anchoring collagen fibers of the PDL must be degraded and remodeled continuously. Collagen fiber degradation in the equine PDL is initiated by matrix metalloproteinase 1 and occurs in a coordinated, mosaic spatial pattern,[36] allowing dental support to be maintained while the collagen apparatus remodels and adjusts to a changing morphologic and biomechanical environment.

The periodontal cells play a pivotal role in regulating PDL remodeling and tissue repair. This role is reflected by an exceptionally high rate of cell proliferation in the equine PDL compared with other species.[27] In addition, the equine PDL contains a population of multipotent mesenchymal stromal cells, which are capable of differentiation into all of the cell lineages, including fibroblasts, osteoblasts, and cementoblasts, that are needed to remodel and repair the periodontal tissues.[37,38]

The PDL is able to meet the biomechanical requirements of mastication in later life, even although the tooth becomes shorter and the surface area for the insertion of the collagen fibers is greatly reduced. This loss of attachment area is compensated for by an increasing bundling and thickness of the remaining collagen fibers, together with an adjustment of the attachment angle between the collagen fiber and the dental cementum.[29] These histologic observations were recently supported by biomechanical studies investigating dental movement within the bony alveolus.[39,40]

Periodontal Biomechanics

By performing finite element simulations of the equine masticatory cycle, it has been shown that the mechanical load within the PDL markedly increases with decreasing tooth length (ie, increasing dental age).[40] In horses older than 15 years, simulated loads on the PDL near the alveolar crest reached levels that cause collagen fiber disruption and local inflammation in the human PDL.[41] This finding might help to explain the high prevalence of diastemata and periodontal disorders in aged equids.[42,43] It has also been shown that high loads occur in the PDL near the apex of the roots. In nonequine species, such a concentration of forces in apical regions can cause tissue necrosis,[44] which can predispose to the settlement of microorganisms.[45] These results support the proposal that a high percentage of equine periapical infections are caused by a hematogenous spread and settlement of microorganisms (ie, anachoresis).[46–48] Therefore, it has been hypothesized that biomechanical imbalances contribute to the development of periapical diseases in the horse.[40] It was shown earlier that finite element simulations derived from human orthodontics are applicable for equine dental and periodontal research. This technique may also be useful to help develop innovative therapies.[39,49]

Periodontal Disorders, Repair, and Regeneration

Although equine periodontal disease is a common and painful condition,[4] its histo-pathologic characteristics are poorly understood. Cox and colleagues[26] found a large overlap in histologic findings between physiologic and likely pathologic equine periodontal tissues. In particular, the gingival epithelium (**Fig. 12**) and its underlying lamina

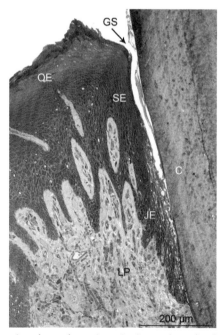

Fig. 12. Longitudinal section through equine gingiva and tooth. The junctional epithelium (JE) attaches the gingiva to the tooth and allows transmigration of leukocytes into the gingival sulcus (GS). C, dental cementum; LP, lamina propria; OE, oral epithelium; SE, sulcular epithelium.

propria commonly showed eosinophilic infiltration and hyperplasia, and the presence of these features was poorly associated with clinical periodontal disease. These results reflect a unique and specific characteristic of the equine periodontium. To remain functional, the equine PDL must, as noted earlier, remodel at a high rate and therefore mild hyperplasia and the presence of eosinophils might be transient expressions of remodeling processes rather than pathologic changes.[26] Cox and colleagues[26] reported that even periodontal disorders that were classified as severely diseased had a reversible character. These results support previous findings showing the presence of regenerative cells within the equine periodontium,[38] which may allow the development of regenerative therapies for equine periodontal diseases. However, more investigations are needed to understand the normal equine periodontium, the etiopathogenesis of its disorders, and its inherent regenerative capacities.

REFERENCES

1. du Toit N, Kempson SA, Dixon PM. Donkey dental anatomy. Part 1: gross and computed axial tomography examinations. Vet J 2008;176:338–44.
2. Fitzgibbon CM, du Toit N, Dixon PM. Anatomical studies of maxillary cheek teeth infundibula in clinically normal horses. Equine Vet J 2010;42:37–42.
3. Mitchell SR, Kempson SA, Dixon PM. Structure of peripheral cementum of normal equine cheek teeth. J Vet Dent 2003;20:199–208.
4. Kilic S, Dixon PM, Kempson SA. A light microscopic and ultrastructural examination of calcified dental tissues of horses: 2. Ultrastructural enamel findings. Equine Vet J 1997;29:198–205.
5. du Toit N, Kempson SA, Dixon PM. Donkey dental anatomy. Part 2: histological and scanning electron microscopic examinations. Vet J 2008;176:345–53.
6. Fortelius M. Ungulate cheek teeth: developmental, functional, and evolutionary interrelations. Acta Zoolog Fennica 1985;180:1–76.
7. Simhofer H, Griss R, Zetner K. The use of oral endoscopy for the detection of cheek teeth abnormalities in 300 horses. Vet J 2008;178:396–404.
8. Ramzan PH, Palmer L. Occlusal fissures of the equine cheek tooth: prevalence, location and association with disease in 91 horses referred for dental investigation. Equine Vet J 2010;42:124–8.
9. Dacre IT, Kempson S, Dixon PM. Pathological studies of cheek teeth apical infections in the horse: part 1 normal endodontic anatomy and dentinal structure of cheek teeth. Vet J 2008;178:311–20.
10. Kilic S, Dixon PM, Kempson SA. A light microscopic and ultrastructural examination of calcified dental tissues of horses: 3. Dentine. Equine Vet J 1997;29:206–12.
11. Muylle S, Simoens P, Lauwers H. The distribution of intratubular dentine in equine incisors: a scanning electron microscopic study. Equine Vet J 2001;33:65–9.
12. Muylle S, Simoens P, Lauwers H. A study of the ultrastructure and staining characteristics of the 'dental star' of equine incisors. Equine Vet J 2002;34:230–4.
13. Kilic S, Dixon PM, Kempson SA. A light microscopic and ultrastructural examination of calcified dental tissues of horses: 1. The occlusal surface and enamel thickness. Equine Vet J 1997;29:190–7.
14. Kempson SA, Davidson ME, Dacre IT. The effect of three types of rasps on the occlusal surface of equine cheek teeth: a scanning electron microscopic study. J Vet Dent 2003;20:19–27.
15. Dixon PM. The gross, histological, and ultrastructural anatomy of equine teeth and their relationship to disease. In: Proceedings of the 48th AAEP Annual Convention. Orlando (FL): 2002. p. 421–37.

16. Kilic S, Dixon PM, Kempson SA. A light microscopic and ultrastructural examination of calcified dental tissues on horses: 4. Cement and the amelocemental junction. Equine Vet J 1997;29:213–9.
17. Windley Z, Weller R, Tremaine WH, et al. Two- and three-dimensional computed tomographic anatomy of the enamel, infundibulae and pulp of 126 equine cheek teeth. Part 1: findings in teeth without macroscopic occlusal or computed tomographic lesions. Equine Vet J 2009;41:441–7.
18. Schrock P, Lüpke M, Seifert H, et al. Finite element analysis in equine incisors: morphological basics, tooth movements and periodontal stresses 10. Jahrestagung der Internationalen Gesellschaft zur Funktionsverbesserung der Pferdezähne. IGFP e.V. Proceedings. 2012. ISBN 978-3-00-037535-4.
19. Kopke S, Angrisani N, Staszyk C. The dental cavities of equine cheek teeth: three-dimensional reconstructions based on high resolution micro-computed tomography. BMC Vet Res 2012;8:173.
20. Windley Z, Weller R, Tremaine WH, et al. Two- and three-dimensional computed tomographic anatomy of the enamel, infundibulae and pulp of 126 equine cheek teeth. Part 2: findings in teeth with macroscopic occlusal or computed tomographic lesions. Equine Vet J 2009;41:441–7.
21. White C, Dixon PM. A study of the thickness of cheek teeth subocclusal secondary dentine in horses of different ages. Equine Vet J 2010;42:119–23.
22. Bettiol N, Dixon PM. An anatomical study to evaluate the risk of pulpar exposure during mechanical widening of equine cheek teeth diastemata and 'bit seating'. Equine Vet J 2011;43:163–9.
23. Marshall R, Dixon PM. A study of the thickness of subocclusal secondary dentine in overgrown equine cheek teeth. Vet J 2012;193:53–7.
24. Brown S, Arkins S, Shaw DJ, et al. The occlusal angles of cheek teeth in normal horses and horses with dental disease. Vet Rec 2008;162:807–10.
25. Erridge ME, Cox AL, Dixon PM. A histological study of peripheral dental caries of equine cheek teeth. J Vet Dent 2011;29:150–6.
26. Cox A, Dixon PM, Smith S. Histopathological lesions associated with equine periodontal disease. Vet J 2012;194:386–91.
27. Warhonowicz M, Staszyk C, Rohn K, et al. The equine periodontium as a continuously remodeling system: morphometrical analysis of cell proliferation. Arch Oral Biol 2006;51:1141–9.
28. Masset A, Staszyk C, Gasse H. The blood vessel system in the periodontal ligament of the equine cheek teeth–part I: the spatial arrangement in layers. Ann Anat 2006;188:529–33.
29. Staszyk C, Wulff W, Jacob HG, et al. The periodontal ligament of equine cheek teeth: the architecture of its collagen fiber apparatus. J Vet Dent 2006;23:143–7.
30. Masset A, Staszyk C, Gasse H. The blood vessel system in the periodontal ligament of the equine cheek teeth–part II: the micro-architecture and its functional implications in a constantly remodelling system. Ann Anat 2006;188:535–9.
31. Staszyk C, Gasse H. Oxytalan fibres in the periodontal ligament of equine molar cheek teeth. Anat Histol Embryol 2004;33:17–22.
32. Staszyk C, Gasse H. Distinct fibro-vascular arrangements in the periodontal ligament of the horse. Arch Oral Biol 2005;50:439–47.
33. Moxham BJ, Shore RC, Berkovitz BK. Fenestrated capillaries in the periodontal ligaments of the erupting and erupted rat molar. Arch Oral Biol 1987;32:477–81.
34. Berkovitz BK. The structure of the periodontal ligament: an update. Eur J Orthod 1990;12:51–76.

35. Burn-Murdoch R. The role of the vasculature in tooth eruption. Eur J Orthod 1990; 12:101–8.
36. Warhonowicz M, Staszyk C, Gasse H. Immunohistochemical detection of matrix metalloproteinase-1 in the periodontal ligament of equine cheek teeth. Tissue Cell 2007;39:369–76.
37. Staszyk C, Gasse H. Primary culture of fibroblasts and cementoblasts of the equine periodontium. Res Vet Sci 2007;82:150–7.
38. Mensing N, Gasse H, Hambruch N, et al. Isolation and characterization of multi-potent mesenchymal stromal cells from the gingiva and the periodontal ligament of the horse. BMC Vet Res 2011;7:42.
39. Cordes V, Gardemin M, Lüpke M, et al. Finite element analysis in 3-D models of equine cheek teeth. Vet J 2012;193:391–6.
40. Cordes V, Lüpke M, Gardemin M, et al. Periodontal biomechanics: finite element simulations of closing stroke and power stroke in equine cheek teeth. BMC Vet Res 2012;8:60.
41. Atkinson HF, Ralph WJ. In vitro strength of the human periodontal ligament. J Dent Res 1977;56:48–52.
42. Crabill MR, Schumacher J. Pathophysiology of acquired dental diseases of the horse. Vet Clin North Am Equine Pract 1998;14:291–307.
43. Dixon PM, Dacre I. A review of equine dental disorders. Vet J 2005;169:165–87.
44. Brudvik P, Rygh P. Non-clast cells start orthodontic root resorption in the periphery of hyalinized zones. Eur J Orthod 1993;15:467–80.
45. Bender IB, Bender A. Diabetes mellitus and the dental pulp. J Endod 2003;29: 383–9.
46. van den Enden MS, Dixon PM. Prevalence of occlusal pulpar exposure in 110 equine cheek teeth with apical infections and idiopathic fractures. Vet J 2008; 178:364–71.
47. Dacre IT, Kempson S, Dixon PM. Pathological studies of cheek teeth apical infections in the horse: 4. Aetiopathological findings in 41 apically infected mandibular cheek teeth. Vet J 2008;178:341–51.
48. Dacre IT, Kempson S, Dixon PM. Pathological studies of cheek teeth apical infections in the horse: 5. Aetiopathological findings in 57 apically infected maxillary cheek teeth and histological and ultrastructural findings. Vet J 2008;178: 352–63.
49. Lüpke M, Gardemin M, Kopke S, et al. Finite element analysis of the equine periodontal ligament under masticatory loading. Wiener Tierärztliche Monatsschrift/ Veterinary Medicine Austria 2010;97:101–6.

A New Understanding of Oral and Dental Disorders of the Equine Incisor and Canine Teeth

Edward Earley, DVM, Fellow EQ AVD[a,b,*], Jennifer T. Rawlinson, DVM[c]

KEYWORDS

- Equine • Fracture • Tooth resorption • Hypercementosis • Avulsion
- Apical infection • Periodontal • Gemination

KEY POINTS

- Equine pulp is more cellular than brachyodont pulp, which may explain the regenerative properties of equine teeth and how they respond to dental insult and disorders.
- Accurate clinical and radiographic evaluations of a dental fracture are necessary to understand and select an appropriate treatment option.
- A diagonal incisor malocclusion is commonly associated with skull asymmetry. The asymmetry usually includes the premolars and molars. Equalizing the incisor and cheek teeth arcades is not usually indicated.
- Repair of an incisor avulsion associated with an incisive bone fracture may be indicated if there is no evidence of a complicated (pulp/root canal exposure) tooth fracture involving the reserve crown or root.
- Canine odontoplasty causing chronic pulp exposure may lead to endodontic infection and resorption. This decay process can proceed over 1 to 2 years or take up to 15 to 20 years before clinical signs are evident.
- Excessive plaque and calculus of the lower canines could lead to periodontal disease and infection.
- The use of intraoral radiography is essential for the evaluation of disorders that involve the canine and incisor teeth.

INTRODUCTION

Disorders associated with equid incisor and canine teeth can significantly affect prehension, function, comfort, and/or aesthetics of an animal. The location of the incisors and canine teeth make it easier for owners and veterinarians to detect, examine,

[a] Dentistry Department, Cornell University Hospital for Animals, Ithaca, NY, USA; [b] Laurel Highland Veterinary Clinic, LLC, 2586 Northway Road Extension, Williamsport, PA 17701, USA; [c] Department of Clinical Sciences, College of Veterinary Medicine, Cornell University, Ithaca, NY 14850, USA
* Corresponding author. Laurel Highland Farm and Equine Services, LLC, 2586 Northway Road Extension, Williamsport, PA 17701.
E-mail address: etearley@laurelhighland.com

Vet Clin Equine 29 (2013) 273–300
http://dx.doi.org/10.1016/j.cveq.2013.04.011
0749-0739/13/$ – see front matter © 2013 Elsevier Inc. All rights reserved.

diagnose, and treat disorders in this region. It has been shown that incisor disorders are less common than cheek tooth disorders, which comprise roughly 11% of diagnosed dental disorders.[1] Presenting clinical history and signs can include direct observation of disorders by the owner, facial swelling, quidding, masticatory abnormalities, weight loss, halitosis, resistance to bitting, abnormal head carriage, or no clinical signs. The most commonly reported incisor abnormalities were dental fracture with or without damage to supporting bones/structures, developmental displacement caused by retained deciduous and supernumerary incisors, mandibular brachygnathia (parrot mouth), mandibular prognathism (sow mouth), apical infection, periodontal disease, abnormalities of wear, diastemata, dental dysplasia, and oral mass.[2,3] Disorders associated with the canine teeth include calculus deposition, periodontal disease, dental fracture, apical infection, developmental anomalies, maleruption, and idiopathic pulp exposure.[3,4] An emerging disease process leading to tooth resorption and hypercementosis of both incisor and canine teeth is described in the literature, and continuing research is being published regarding the causes, pathophysiology, and histopathology of this disease.[5] This article reviews new developments in the recognition, recording, diagnosing, and/or understanding of some of the aforementioned disorders in which changes have occurred in the last 10 years; therefore, disorders discussed in this article include dental fracture, trauma to the rostral maxilla and mandible, diagonal incisor malocclusion, tooth resorption and hypercementosis, periodontal-endodontic infection, and gemination. The Modified Triadan system is used for numbering equine dentition in this article.[6]

To recognize, appreciate, and treat incisor and canine disorders, a solid understanding of the anatomy and physiology of these teeth is necessary. This article discusses the basic anatomy of these teeth and their use during mastication. Excellent resources are available for further reading and information regarding the gross anatomic structure of these teeth.[7,8] Beyond gross anatomy is the important topic of physiology of equine teeth. How these teeth physiologically respond to normal wear and a traumatic event is critical to determining normal dental aging, the development and progression of disorders, response to treatment, and reasonable prognoses. The structure and function of the pulp play a key role in how the tooth responds to normal attrition, abrasion, and pathologic insults (such as apical infections and tooth fracture). When the structural integrity of a tooth is challenged, the pulpodentinal complex is stimulated through the dentinal tubules, which house cytoplasmic extensions of odontoblasts called odontoblastic processes. The pulpodentinal complex refers to the complex union of dentin and odontoblasts with the soft tissue structures of the pulp, and odontoblasts are the cells that create dentin.[9] Dental pulp possesses many characteristics of early embryonic connective tissue. Even a mature pulp is rich with components such as nerve axons, vascular tissue, connective tissue fibers, ground substance, interstitial fluid, odontoblasts, fibroblasts, immunocompetent cells, and other cellular components.[10]

The junction between the pulp and dentin contains several morphologic zones that have been well described for the brachydont. These zones from pulp to dentin include a cell-rich zone, a narrow cell-poor zone, an odontoblastic layer, and predentin (**Fig. 1**A).[11,12] The significance of the pulpodentinal junction is that it allows for repair and regeneration of damaged odontoblasts. Cells migrating peripherally from the central region of the pulp create the cell-rich zone, and it has been shown that the rate of mitosis greatly increases within this layer with death of odontoblasts.[13] This increase in activity within the cell-rich zone represents the stimulation and response of the pulp to odontoblastic injury, and is most likely the first step in the formation of a new odontoblastic layer.[11] In very active brachydont pulp, the pulp of young teeth or older teeth

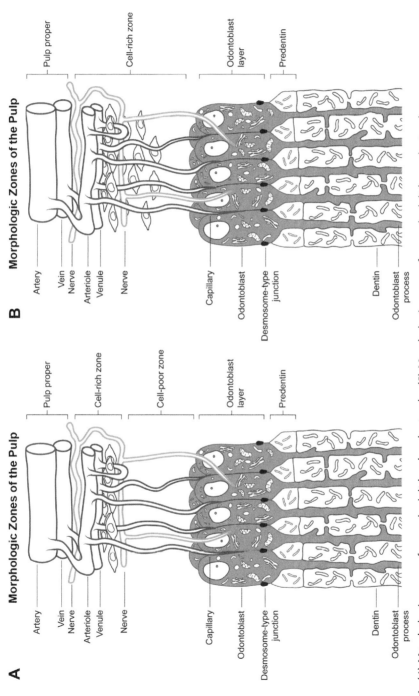

Fig. 1. (A) Morphologic zones of normal adult brachyodont pulp. (B) Morphologic zones of normal adult hypsodont pulp.

undergoing a reparative process, it has been shown that the cell-poor zone does not exist.[12] The pulpodentinal complex of equine hypsodont teeth is continuously stimulated by normal wear of the tooth and needs to have a robust reparative capacity to produce normal secondary regular and irregular dentin.[14–16] The main difference between the morphologic zones of brachydont and equine hypsodont teeth is that the hypsodont does not have a cell-poor zone; instead, there is a high degree of cellularity from the pulp proper to the odontoblastic layer (see **Fig. 1**B)[17] (Carsten Staszyk, personal communication, 2013). The absence of a cell-poor zone in the equine pulpodentinal complex is similar to what is seen in the very active pulp of young developing and old reparative brachydont teeth. This difference in normal pulpodentinal histologic structure may partially explain the more regenerative/reparative response to insult within equine as opposed to brachydont teeth, although no study currently exists to support this theory. The implication of such an exuberant response to insult is that the horse may be better equipped to respond to dental injuries that would be terminal for brachydont teeth.

Evaluating dental disorders requires a complete maxillofacial-oral examination and supplemental radiographs. These two steps are critical to making an accurate diagnosis and formulating a treatment plan. The importance of these two steps should not be underestimated because the internal reparative process of a tooth and surrounding tissue cannot be evaluated and monitored solely based on a passing glance. In addition, radiographs are sometimes necessary to accurately identify which incisors are involved in a pathologic process, greatly affecting recommendations for treatment. Examination and radiographic techniques are discussed elsewhere in this issue, and practitioners should strive to become proficient in these two procedures. Although most forms of incisor and canine disorder require some type of management, not all abnormalities require medical or surgical treatments. Considering the robust reparative potential of equine teeth, it may be more appropriate to conservatively manage and monitor some disorders with frequently scheduled clinical and radiographic reexaminations.

DENTAL FRACTURE AND REGIONAL TRAUMA

Fracture of incisor and canine teeth can result from trauma to the region or from a singular unidentified event in a horse of any age. The most commonly indentified incisor abnormality in one study was transversely fractured teeth with or without fracture of the supporting bones; this was particularly true of young horses (2 years).[1] Fractures may be to a singular tooth, multiple teeth, and/or include supporting structures to the tooth. Teeth may become avulsed because of trauma, or a bony fracture may include deciduous teeth and permanent tooth buds. No matter the cause or presentation, a fractured tooth or fractured bones supporting dentition warrants a complete oral examination and radiographs of the surrounding structures to fully determine the extent of regional damage and reveal any additional lesions.

Considerations for Evaluation of Dental Fracture

When evaluating a dental fracture it is important to consider tooth age, time interval between trauma and evaluation, fracture severity, and radiographic appearance before shaping a treatment plan. Age of the patient and of the tooth greatly affects capacity for injury and healing response. Young developing teeth have a large apical foramen with ample blood supply that encourages dental healing. The robust vascularity of the pulp supports an active cell-rich zone, and the open foramen accommodates greater amounts of swelling and edema. Older teeth with increased dentin, decreased pulp, and a near closed apex cannot accommodate as much swelling, which can result in pressure necrosis of moderate to severely traumatized pulp.[7] The time interval between fracture and evaluation is the next parameter to consider. A long interval between fracture and evaluation/repair negatively affects the prognosis because of increasing bacterial infiltration, irritation from feed and saliva, and worsening inflammation. Moderate to severe chronic dental fractures usually result in pulp necrosis and even death in the horse.

Fracture severity as determined on oral examination is the third critical parameter. When examining a fractured tooth, the fracture is evaluated for length, width, and pulp exposure. Fractures involving solely the clinical crown have a better prognosis, because the periodontal structures surrounding the tooth are uninvolved. Fractures involving the reserve crown and/or root require more consideration because of involvement of regional supporting structures. Fractures limited to cementum and enamel are minor and need little treatment, because the pulp remains intact. If a fracture extends deep into the dentin or involves the pulp, it is considered significant and treatment requires either intervention or close monitoring. The pulp is located on the labial aspect of the incisors and varies in shape from ribbon to oval depending on its position within the tooth (**Fig. 2**). The American Veterinary Dental College (AVDC) has established a classification system to describe dental fracture (**Table 1**).[18] As an adaptation for the hypsodont tooth, the classification system refers to the hypsodont reserve crown and root as the root because of the involvement of the periodontal system. Although this classification system is not ideal for hypsodont teeth because of the differing pulpal configurations within the hypsodont reserve crown and brachydont root, it does provide a basis for discussing and recording disorders.

In addition, radiographic appearance of the fracture is the last major parameter to consider. Radiographs determine the full extent of subgingival fracture, tooth vitality, periodontal involvement, and surrounding alveolar and adjacent bone damage. Tooth vitality is gauged by the width and appearance of the pulp horns, pulp chamber, and root canals. As a tooth ages, increasing dentinal thickness decreases the diameter of the pulp horn and root canal, and asymmetry between similar teeth in endodontic width and shape should be viewed with suspicion. A dead tooth ceases to create new dentin and thus has a larger endodontic space. The exuberant reparative response of the equid tooth also sometimes leads to the radiographic appearance of pulp stones, pulpal irregularities, or partial/complete sclerosis of the endodontic space. All of these are signs of past inflammation, and should be evaluated closely.

A   **B**

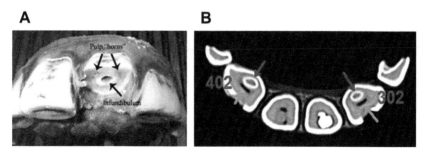

Fig. 2. (*A*) Normal pulp horn anatomy in a fully developed incisor. The two *upper black arrows* illustrate the pulp horns along the labial aspect of the incisor. The *lower black arrow* shows the infundibulum. (*B*) Computed tomography (CT) of the coronal aspect of young incisors with single oval pulp horns (*green arrows*) and infundibulum (*red arrows*). Root canal therapy has been performed on tooth 301. ([*A*] *Courtesy of* Robert Baratt, DVM, Salem, CT.)

Table 1
AVDC classification of dental fractures. Note that the AVDC system considers that the hypsodont reserve crown and root comprise the root in this system

Classification	Abbreviation	Description
Enamel infraction	EI	An incomplete fracture (crack) of the enamel without loss of deeper tooth substance
Enamel fracture	EF	A fracture with loss of crown substance confined to the enamel
Uncomplicated crown fracture	UCF	A fracture of the crown that does not expose the pulp
Complicated crown fracture	CCF	A fracture of the crown that exposes the pulp
Uncomplicated crown-root fracture	UCRF	A fracture of the crown and root that does not expose the pulp
Complicated crown-root fracture	CCRF	A fracture of the crown and root that exposes the pulp
Root fracture	RF	A fracture involving the root

From AVDC Nomenclature Committee. American Veterinary Dental College. Dental Fracture Classification. 2009. p. 6–16.

Signs of periapical disorders (apical lucency, apical osteosclerosis, root resorption or blunting, hypercementosis) coupled with endodontic irregularities signals a nonvital tooth. Signs of past endodontic inflammation and no periapical or periodontal disorders reveal an equine tooth that may be healing from injury and should be monitored closely radiographically (every 6 months) to determine a trend.

Reversible Versus Irreversible Pulpitis

Pulp exposure and near pulp exposure result in pulpitis (inflammation of the pulp). Pulpitis results from the tooth's initial response to injury and infection and is maintained until the inciting injury is repaired via medical intervention or natural pathways and the bacterial contamination ceases. Pulpitis can be reversible or irreversible.[19,20] Reversible pulpitis refers to a state of inflammation within the pulp that retains the potential to overcome infection and quiet inflammation. Irreversible pulpitis refers to pulp that is irreversibly damaged and cannot recover from injury and infection. The degree and extent of pulpitis and consideration of the reparative process of the equine tooth dictates the treatment plan. A vital partial pulpectomy procedure with restoration is indicated if the pulpitis is reversible. The goal of vital pulp therapy is to remove the irreversibly inflamed pulp so that the remaining pulp may heal and form new dentin. At present, there are no statistical data in horses to accurately determine the maximum time interval for treating reversible pulpitis, but 5 to 10 days between injury and treatment is suggested, with a potentially decreasing prognosis for longer time frames. If the pulpitis is irreversible, root canal therapy or extraction is recommended.

Examples of Common Dental Fractures

Uncomplicated crown fracture
An incisor fracture of tooth 102 without pulp exposure is shown in **Fig. 3**. This type of fracture is uncomplicated because there is no pulp involvement. The time interval is not as sensitive when there is no pulp involvement. The main concerns are possible regional decay and periodontal inflammation caused by abnormal feed, debris, and

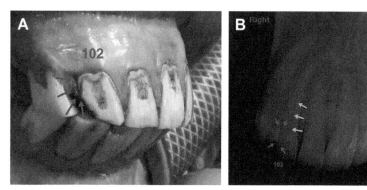

Fig. 3. (A) Uncomplicated crown fracture of tooth 102. Note the distal fragment (*red arrows*). (B) Uncomplicated crown fracture of 102 (*red arrows*). Normal pulp of 102 (*green arrows*).

plaque accumulation and continued fracture. Therefore treatment should involve regional debridement and restoration (if possible), and 2 to 3 mm of occlusal odontoplasty to reduce occlusal forces that might worsen the fracture.

Complicated crown fracture: acute

Acute incisor fractures roughly 36 hours after trauma in a 4-year-old quarter horse (QH) that involves teeth 301 and 401 are shown in **Fig. 4**A. These fractures are

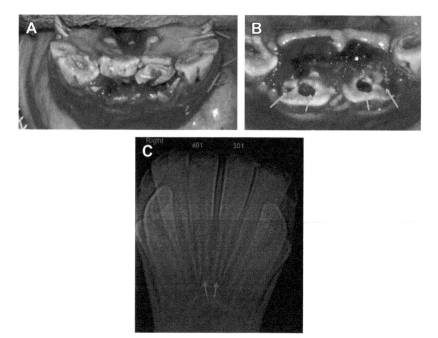

Fig. 4. (A) Complicated crown fracture of teeth 301 and 401. (B) Complicated crown fracture. Dental fragments removed. Note the pulp horns (*green arrows*). (C) Complicated crown fracture, acute. Both reserve crowns are intact with a good apical vascular supply (*red arrows*).

complicated crown fractures because there is pulp involvement. With the dental fragments removed, pulp horns are evident with each tooth (see **Fig. 4**B). Radiographic evaluation reveals that both reserve crowns are intact with good apical vascular supply (see **Fig. 4**C). A vital pulp therapy is indicated with an acute complicated crown fracture.

Complicated crown fracture: subacute

A subacute incisor fracture 10 days after trauma with pulp exposure involving tooth103 in a 6-year-old warmblood is shown in **Fig. 5**A. The significance of the extended time interval is reflected in the radiograph (see **Fig. 5**B). Radiographic evaluation suggests an open apical foramen appropriate for dental age, slight increased radiolucency in the region of the apex and apical periodontal ligament, and mild increased radiodensity of the apical alveolar bone. The dental age indicates improved ability to accommodate pulpal swelling and reparative qualities. The mild abnormal findings in the apical region suggest an active pulpitis extending past the apical aspect of the tooth. Vital pulp therapy may be considered, but owners should be made aware of the increased risk for treatment failure.

Complicated crown fracture: chronic

An incisor with a chronic complicated crown fracture involving tooth 201 in a 10-year-old QH is shown in **Fig. 6**A. The tooth has been fractured for 14 months. Exploration with an endodontic file reveals only a necrotic pulp. An intraoral radiograph shows an open blunt apex suggesting past tooth resorption caused by chronic inflammation (see **Fig. 6**B). Based on the history, examination, and radiograph, tooth 201 is considered not vital. Treatment options include root canal therapy or extraction.

Traumatic Injuries to the Rostral Maxilla and Mandible

Oral trauma to the incisive bone or mandible can lead to tooth avulsion, dental fracture, fracture of adjacent bony structures, and laceration of soft tissue structures. The most common jaw fracture sustained by horses is in the region of the rostral mandible.[21] Injury is more common in young horses and can be incurred during

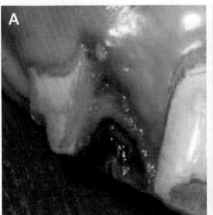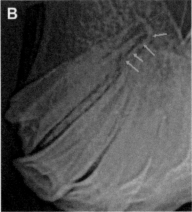

Fig. 5. (*A*) Subacute complicated crown fracture. A fracture of 103 evaluated 10 days after the trauma. (*B*) Subacute complicated crown fracture. Initial intraoral radiograph shows an open apical foramen and mild increased radiolucency (*red arrow*) and slight increased radiodensity of apical alveolar bone (*green arrows*).

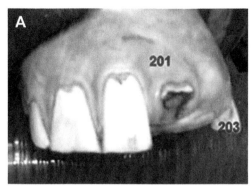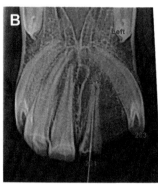

Fig. 6. (*A*) Chronic complicated crown fracture of tooth 201. Tooth 202 is missing. (*B*) Chronic complicated crown fracture with endodontic file in canal. The apex has undergone resorption leaving only an open blunted structure behind (*red arrows*). Tooth 202 is missing.

play behavior with other horses or interaction with barn and pasture inanimate objects.[22] Partial or complete tooth avulsion involving 1 or more teeth is common for these injuries. Avulsion typically involves fracture of a least 1 bony alveolar wall, tearing of the periodontal ligament, and damage to the apical pulp. Fractures involving the rostral mandible and incisive bone may affect the periodontal structure of peripherally involved teeth and/or the roots/apices of involved teeth. Because many of these injures occur in young animals, deciduous teeth, unerupted permanent teeth, and tooth buds may also be involved. Radiography is essential for complete evaluation of regional trauma and for long-term monitoring of dental health in the traumatized region.

Although periodontal structures and apical blood supply can be severely traumatized or even completely avulsed in some cases, the prognosis for healing and return to normal function is favorable.[23] Management of regional trauma involves gentle flushing and debridement of contaminated structures, possible suturing of soft tissue wounds, and stabilization of teeth and fracture with wires and/or a dental splint fashioned with dental composites or nonexothermic acrylic. Debridement should be vigorous enough to remove debris and potential sequestra but preserve periodontal and apical tissue to allow for dental healing. Tooth buds and unerupted teeth should be avoided if possible during debridement to prevent future damage and maleruption of permanent teeth. If tooth buds and developing adult teeth are involved in the fracture, owners need to be informed that teeth may be nonvital, malformed, or misplaced on eruption and reexamination and radiographs may be necessary. If a complicated crown or crown-root fracture is present, extraction of the tooth is usually recommended. Temporary replacement of fatally damaged teeth may be indicated if stabilization of the bone fracture is needed; however, a fractured tooth with pulp exposure left in place needs close monitoring because of increased risk for developing periodontal and apical disease. If necessary, it can be extracted or a root canal therapy performed at a later date.[24,25] Only 1 study to date has tracked the dental outcome following repair of a variety of rostral mandibular and incisive fractures with dental involvement, and it shows the equine's robust dental reparative and regenerative response to trauma.[1]

Typical Case of Incisive Bone Trauma

A 16-year-old warmblood gelding presented with trauma to the left incisive bone (**Fig. 7**A, B). The left incisor bone was fractured dorsally and ventrally in the apical

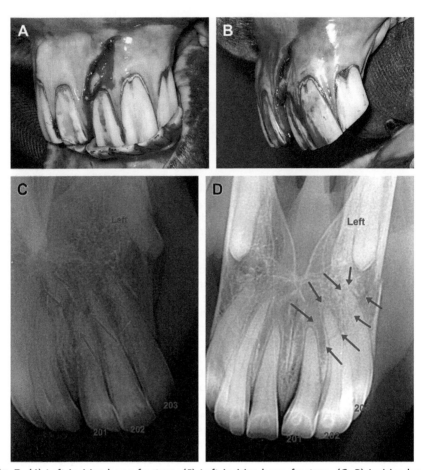

Fig. 7. (*A*) Left incisive bone fracture. (*B*) Left incisive bone fracture. (*C, D*) Incisive bone trauma, initial intraoral radiographs. Note the 2 incisive bone fracture lines (*red arrows*). (*E*) Incisor teeth avulsion. Acrylic splint pulled into place with the interdental wiring. (*F*) Incisive bone fracture, postrepair intraoral radiograph. (*G*) Incisive bone fracture, postrepair intraoral oblique radiograph. The *green arrows* illustrate the reduced fracture line immediately post surgical repair.

region of teeth 201 to 203 allowing the fracture fragment to flip ventrocaudal against the hard palate. The apices of teeth 201 to 203 were avulsed from the apical alveolar sockets, and the mesial periodontal ligament of tooth 201 was completely torn. Intraoral radiographs show the fracture lines extending through the apical region of all three incisors (see **Fig. 7**C, D). An acrylic splint was formed along the palatal aspect of the fracture, incorporating large wire loops. Interdental wires were tightened along the labial aspect of the teeth, which pulled the acrylic splint against the hard palate to give support to the incisive bone fracture (see **Fig. 7**E).[26] Intraoral radiographs were taken following the procedure to evaluate the reduction of the fracture (see **Fig. 7**F, G).

DIAGONAL INCISOR MALOCCLUSION

A diagonal incisor malocclusion (DIM) refers to an abnormal incisor occlusion in which diagonally opposite incisors are excessively long, creating a tilted or slanted incisor

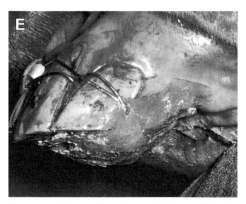

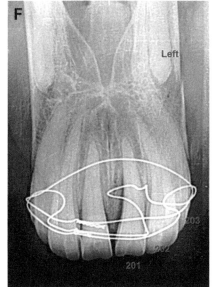
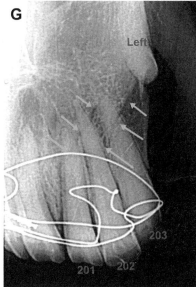

Fig. 7. (continued)

occlusal table.[27] In the past, treatment recommendations for this type of malocclusion in the horse have been to perform odontoplasty to the overlong incisors without considering the potential symmetry of the head and facial bone.[28–30]

Forty-two horses affected with DIM were recently evaluated for skeletal abnormalities of the skull, maxilla, mandibles, and dentition.[31] Oral and radiographic examinations were performed on all horses in the study. Oral examination of the hard palate and cheek teeth arcades revealed asymmetry in 41 of 42 horses. Radiographic examination showed skull asymmetry in all 42 horses. Only 2 of the 10 control horses with normal incisor occlusion showed asymmetry of the hard palate and cheek teeth arcades. Radiographic examination of the control group revealed no asymmetry of skulls.

The main conclusion of the study was that skull asymmetry is typically associated with DIM. This conclusion raises many questions as to the validity of performing incisor odontoplasty on DIM overlong incisors. Treatment of a DIM should be approached like any other malocclusion, with premolar and molar evaluation and treatment before incisor work remembering that the most important tenant of equine dentistry is maximizing a functional occlusion. Many DIM horses require only minor adjustments.[32,33] Equalizing the arcades so that they are of similar occlusal angle is not necessary and potentially destroys the normal occlusal bite of the patient. Once the premolars and molars have a functional occlusion, attention should be focused on the DIM to see whether any specific incisor is causing a problem. It is the author's experience that by removing the enamel points of the cheek teeth, most DIM cases are able to have a functional premolar/molar occlusion. Only occasionally is additional minor odontoplasty needed with the incisors.

Typical DIM Case

A 15-year-old QH cross gelding presented with a DIM resulting from right deviation of the maxillary incisor bone (**Fig. 8**A). **Fig. 8**B and C show the palatal asymmetry with the left hard palate rolling in (steeper arch) creating a greater than normal left occlusal angle and the right hard palate rolling out (flattened) with a resultant shallower than normal right occlusal angle. An extraoral radiograph shows deviation of the incisive and vomer bones (see **Fig. 8**D). The mandible is symmetric. An intraoral radiograph of the maxilla shows the asymmetrical incisive and vomer bones (see **Fig. 8**E). In

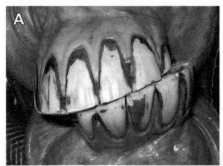

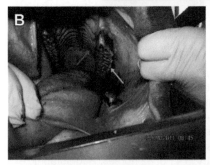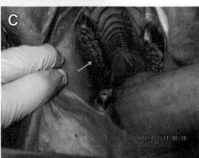

Fig. 8. (*A*) DIM. Right deviation of the maxilla and incisive bone. (*B*) DIM: left caudal mouth. Note the left hard palate rolling in (*red arrow*) causing the occlusal angle to steepen/increase (*green arrow*). (*C*) DIM: right caudal mouth. Note the right hard palate rolling out (*red arrow*) causing the occlusal angle to flatten (*green arrow*). (*D*) DIM. Red line, maxilla; green line, mandible; yellow line, incisive bone; blue line, vomer. (*E*) DIM. Right deviation of the incisive bone (*red arrows*) and vomer (*yellow arrows*). Rolling out of the right maxillary cheek teeth (*orange arrows*) and rolling in of the left maxillary cheek teeth (*blue arrows*). (*F*) Hard palate (*green arrows*) and cheek teeth (*red arrows*) asymmetry shown with a CT image.

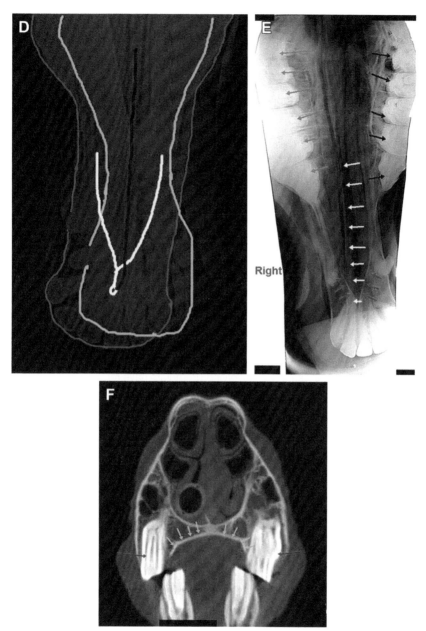

Fig. 8. (*continued*)

addition, the steep positioning of the left cheek teeth and the flattening of the right cheek teeth are evident. Only enamel point reduction and minor incisor odontoplasty were necessary to manage this case appropriately. Hard palate and cheek teeth asymmetry is shown in a similar case with a computed tomography (CT) image of the skull (see **Fig. 8**F).

TOOTH RESORPTION AND/OR HYPERCEMENTOSIS

In the last decade, an emerging disorder involving tooth resorption and hypercementosis has been recognized within the equine population. Tooth resorption is not new, and it is found in commonly studied species. A recent published study in dogs showed the presence of resorptive lesions at a rate of 53.6%.[34] These findings are similar to those of a study published approximately 30 years ago, in which a prevalence rate of tooth resorption was determined to be 43.5%.[35] A similar study in cats has shown the prevalence to be between 38.0% for mixed-breed cats and up to 70% in pure-breed cats.[36] Comparisons with canine and feline tooth resorption are tempting to draw, but the cause and pathophysiology of equine tooth resorption are still under investigation and showing some distinct differences, namely hypercementosis or invasive irregular cementum. The condition was first described in 2004 as a periopathogenic disease involving the incisor and canine teeth of the horse,[37] and, in 2006, a study formally recognized cemental hyperplasia and hypoplasia associated with the disease.[38] In 2007 and 2008, tooth resorption was described as a major component of this disorder, and the disease was termed equine odontoclastic tooth resorption and hypercementosis (EOTRH).[39,40] A detailed study was recently completed of 18 horses with advanced stages of the disease. The study evaluated radiographs, histopathology, nutrition, and hematology. Although not yet published, the initial results of the study suggest that many variables are associated with this disease and there may be more than one pathologic process occurring, suggesting that all cases might not fit cleanly under 1 diagnosis, EOTRH, in the future.[41]

Tooth resorption and hypercementosis affect both the incisors and canine teeth of horses typically greater than 15 years of age.[40] A small number of anecdotal reports of resorption and irregular cementum involving premolars have recently been confirmed by histopathology. The disease is characterized by internal and external resorption of dental structures sometimes associated with excessive production of irregular cementum on the exterior and interior of the tooth. The apical one-third to one-half of the tooth is commonly affected. The disease tends to start along the lingual/palatal aspect of the tooth with expansion in a mesial and distal direction (**Fig. 9**A). As the disease progresses, the pulp, dentin, periodontal ligament, and alveolar bone become inflamed and infected, leading to reduced structural support for the teeth, degradation of gingiva, increased incisor angle, fistula formation, tooth fracture, and pain. Periodontal inflammation is reported as a possible initiating trigger for tooth resorption, and it is suspected that chronic inflammatory mediators, particularly prostaglandin E2, an inflammatory factor that plays a primary role in the stimulation of osteoclasts, perpetuate the resorptive process.[42] Osteoclastic activity has been shown to be influenced by several hormones and cytokines as well.[43] A reparative reaction involves fibroblasts, odontoblasts, and cementoblasts invading spaces between the osteoclasts to produce a cementumlike tissue to fill the dental defects. Depending on individual animal and tooth reaction, the balance between resorption and cementum deposition can vary, resulting in the variety of stages seen sometimes in one mouth.[42]

Histopathology of resorptive lesions and proliferative cementum has shown abnormal location and activity of osteoclasts, odontoclasts, and cementoblasts. Osteoclasts in normal dentition typically reside against the bone surface occupying shallow hollowed-out depressions they have created called Howship lacunae.[44] Histopathologic examinations of resorptive lesions revealed osteoclasts and odontoclasts residing in large, atypical lacunae within bone, cementum, enamel, and dentin (see **Fig. 9**B).[40] Additional cellular components included mostly inflammatory cells, neutrophilic granulocytes, macrophages, plasma cells, and lymphocytes. In some of

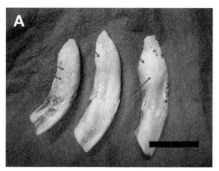
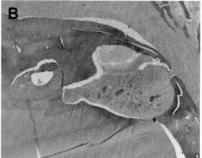
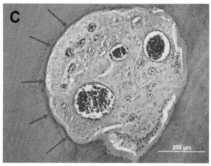

Fig. 9. (A) Tooth resorption and hypercementosis with mesial and distal advance of the disease (*red arrows*). (B) Tooth resorption: abnormally large Howship lacunae (*red arrows*) within the dental structures. The large scalloped lytic foci typically contain necrotic cellular debris either primarily neutrophilic or lymphocytic in nature with granulating fibrosis. (C) Infiltration of irregular cementum/fibrodentin (*red arrows*) on the inner surface of a pulp cavity. (*Courtesy of* [A] Laurelyn Keener, DVM, Duluth, MN, and Victor S. Cox, DVM, PhD, St Paul, MN; and [B, C] Rebecca Smedley, DVM, MS, Lansing, MI.)

the large lacunae, irregular cementum was invading the resorbed surfaces, and the irregular cementum was described as an abnormal cellular type of cementum with intrinsic collagen fibers. In addition to invading the lacunae, the irregular cementum was invading normal cementum, enamel, dentin, and even the inner walls of the pulp (see **Fig. 9**C).[40] The term hypercementosis has been used in pathology reports to describe hyperplasia of normal cemental tissue and proliferation of irregular cementum, and this nondescript use of the word has led to questions regarding the true nature of the cemental change reported in the past. Research into improved recognition and classification of the different forms of equine hypercementosis may help further reveal the nature of its association with tooth resorption and importance as a possible primary disorder.

Tooth resorption in general is a painful disease, and the level of pain seems to intensify with the severity of the lesions. A common initial sign of incisor pain reported by owners is a reduced ability/desire to grasp apples and carrots. Other signs of pain include sensitivity to bitting, head shaking, ptyalism, resistance to turning during work, shyness about the head, periodic inappetence, weight loss, and decreased use of incisors for grasping and grazing. Some horses become adept at grasping feed with the lips, sliding it past the incisors and moving it into the mouth through the bar region. Watching how a horse eats hay before an oral examination is a good way to gauge the animal's discomfort and stage of disease. Some horses that are in the early stages of disease, or with primarily hypercementosis, may have no apparent signs of discomfort; however, level of pain is a subjective assessment and difficult to evaluate in the horse. Oral examination can be challenging because patients are resistant to manipulation of the lips and pressure on affected teeth. Placement and opening of an oral speculum can elicit alert and possibly dangerous behavior even under heavy sedation because of pain. Oral examination findings can include enlarged mandibular lymph nodes, decreased incisor angle not appropriate for age, prominent juga, loss of dental papillae, gingival and mucogingival fistulas, severe regional inflammation, purulent drainage, calculus and feed accumulation, missing teeth, hyperplastic gingiva, gingival recession, bulbous enlargement of dental structures, tooth mobility, and supragingival regions of dental resorption. Resorptive lesions in older horses can be found under excessive calculus deposition on the mandibular (more common) and maxillary canine teeth. Exposing these lesions after removal of calculus causes discomfort for the horse and the practitioner should be prepared to address the problem.

Evaluating tooth resorption and hypercementosis necessitates intraoral radiographs of both the incisors and canines to properly formulate a treatment plan. Radiographic findings typically include varying levels of dental resorption and hypercementosis, loss of the periodontal ligament space, disruption of alveolar and regional cancellous bone, osteomyelitis, and tooth fracture. A radiographic classification system for tooth resorption based on location was found to be useful in categorizing the type of resorptive lesions present in dogs.[34,45] The system radiographically evaluated lesions for 7 types of resorption, which included external surface resorption, external replacement resorption, external inflammatory resorption, external cervical root surface resorption, internal surface resorption, internal replacement resorption, and internal inflammatory resorption. In this recent study, all types of resorption were evident in the dog except for internal replacement resorption.[34] In 2012, a new study was initiated to try to identify and categorize resorptive lesions radiographically and establish the incidence among the horse general population.[46]

Treatment planning depends heavily on clinical examination, radiographic findings, and the patient's level of pain. Horses with mild subgingival resorption and no regional osteitis or alveolitis can be monitored with oral examination and radiographs because the pace of disease progression varies between teeth and individuals. It is common to see radiographically a variety of disease stages ranging from normal to severe throughout the incisors and canines. Once supragingival lesions, alveolitis, osteomyelitis, tooth fractures, and extensive resorption of the reserve crown and root are detectable radiographically, extraction is recommended. Moderate to severe cases require staged or complete extraction of the affected incisor and canine teeth to alleviate infection and pain caused by this disease. Incisor extraction can be accomplished in 2 ways depending on the nature and severity of the disorders associated with the tooth/teeth. Singular incisor extraction can be accomplished simply in mild to moderately affected teeth by elevation and avulsion.[47] In cases of multiple incisor and canine tooth extraction with severe disease, a surgical approach is necessary to allow for complete removal of dental material, visualization of tooth and diseased structures, debridement, and closure. In addition, a surgical approach increases the surgeon's ability to deal with complicated extractions in which reserve crowns and roots have fractured because of initial trauma and resorption.

Three Distinct Presentations of EOTRH

Tooth resorption predominate

Primary tooth resorption is shown in an 18-year-old QH gelding (**Fig. 10**A). The owners noted that the horse was sensitive around the face. In addition, they had noticed that

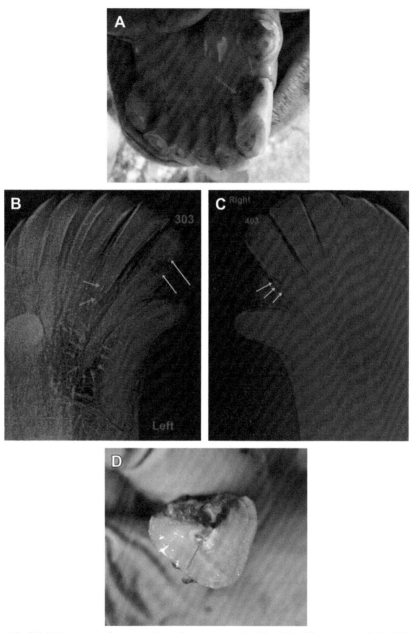

Fig. 10. (*A*) Primary tooth resorption demonstrated with 303. (*B*) Intraoral left oblique radiograph demonstrates primary tooth resorption (internal surface resorption) with 303 (*green arrows*), apical remodeling and resorption of 303 (*red arrows*) and primary resorption of 302 (*orange arrows*). (*C*) Intraoral right oblique radiograph demonstrates primary tooth resorption (external surface resorption) with 403 in the reserve crown (*green arrows*). (*D*) Cross section of 303 following extraction demonstrates the resorption process extending into the pulp (*orange arrow*).

he was rubbing his lower incisors back and forth against the wooden stall wall. An intraoral radiograph reveals a large resorptive lesion involving the crown of 303 (see **Fig. 10**B). A contralateral oblique intraoral radiograph shows a smaller resorptive lesion in the reserve crown of 404 (see **Fig. 10**C). The lesion associated with 303 appears to be an internal surface resorption, whereas the 404 could be classified as an external surface resorption. Following extraction of 303, a cross section of the tooth shows the resorption process extending into the pulp (see **Fig. 10**D). At the 2-week follow-up examination, the owners commented that the horse was no longer rubbing his teeth against the wall. It was decided to watch 403 and monitor the resorptive lesion in the reserve crown.

Hypercementosis predominate
Severe irregular cemental infiltration and layering is shown in an 18-year-old Arabian stallion. The stallion was presented for weight loss, head shyness, and depression. Note the large bulging juga caused by the layering of the invasive irregular cementum and the alveolar bone expansion (**Fig. 11**A, B). **Fig. 11**B shows the massive expansion of cementum as it pushes through the gingiva. An intraoral radiograph shows the large areas of cemental expansion involving 102, 103, 202, and 203, and the resorption process has blunted the reserve crowns/roots of 101 and 201(see **Fig. 11**C). This presentation is common for the central incisors. Cases that radiographically appear to be mostly cemental proliferation can still have extensive regions of resorption as seen on CT of a similar case indicating that the excessive radiodensity of severely thickened cementum can hide underlying resorption (see **Fig. 11**D). An intraoral radiograph of the mandibular incisors reveals a moderate level of irregular cementum infiltration with areas of resorption evident (see **Fig. 11**E). The treatment plan was to extract the maxillary incisors and monitor the mandibular incisors. During the 1-month follow-up examination, the owner commented that the stallion was eating better and was less depressed, but still not his normal happy personality. A recommendation of extracting the mandibular incisors was suggested; however, the owner wanted to wait and see how he progressed. In managing similar cases, the author has noticed a more dramatic improvement when all of the incisors are extracted.

Combined tooth resorption and hypercementosis
Combined resorption and irregular cementum infiltration is shown in a 24-year-old thoroughbred gelding. Note the bulging juga and alveolar bone expansion involving teeth 103 and 203 (**Fig. 12**A, B). There are also moderate irregular cementum and alveolar bone changes associated with 303 and 403 (see **Fig. 12**A, C). The gelding presented with weight loss, sensitivity around the face, and difficult eating. Intraoral radiographs reveal extensive cemental infiltration and layering associated with 103, and moderate cemental changes involving 203, 303, and 403. Resorptive lesions are also evident within the teeth and irregular cementum of 103, 203, 303, and 403 (see **Fig. 12**D, E). The extraction of the incisors was staged. Following extraction of teeth 103 and 203, the owner noted that there was some improvement with the face sensitivity and eating. This case shows radiographically the combination of resorptive and cemental lesions, with lysis/resorption occurring within the irregular cementum.

COMBINED PERIODONTAL-ENDODONTIC INFECTIONS

The interrelationship between endodontic and periodontal infection must be evaluated before determining treatment options. Endodontic and periodontal infections are classified into 5 categories: primary endodontic lesion, primary endodontic lesion with

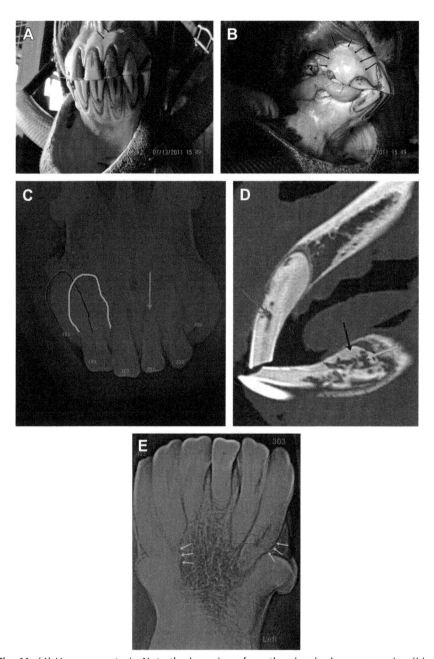

Fig. 11. (*A*) Hypercementosis. Note the large juga from the alveolar bone expansion (*blue arrows*). (*B*) Hypercementosis. Massive expansion of cementum as it pushes through the gingiva (*orange arrows*). (*C*) Hypercementosis of teeth 102 to 103 and 202 to 203 where the reserve crown/root is more severely affected than the crown, and the resorption process has blunted the reserve crowns/roots of 101 and 201 (*orange arrow*). The cementum of 103 (*blue line*) is superimposed over the cementum of 102 (*green line*) making it difficult to distinguish between the two teeth. (*D*) CT imaging of tooth resorption and hypercementosis. Irregular cementum (*blue arrow*), with lytic resorption (*green arrow*). Lytic resorption with possible internal inflammatory resorption (*red arrow*). (*E*) Intraoral radiograph of a case with hypercementosis predominate (*green arrows*) with some evidence of resorption (possible internal inflammatory resorption - *red arrows*). ([*D*] *Courtesy of* Laurelyn Keener, DVM, Duluth, MN, and Victor S. Cox, DVM, PhD, St Paul, MN.)

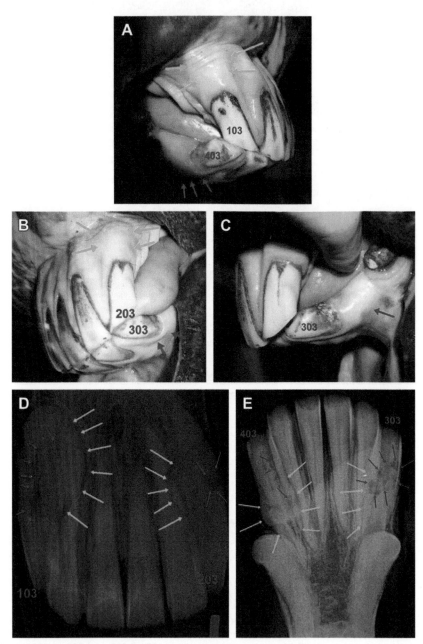

Fig. 12. (*A*) Combined irregular cementum and resorption. Alveolar bone expansion/remodeling with 103 (*green arrows*) and 403 (*red arrows*). (*B*) Combined irregular cementum and resorption. Alveolar bone expansion/remodeling with 203 (*green arrows*) and 303 (*red arrows*). (*C*) Combined irregular cementum and resorption. Moderate alveolar bone remodeling of 303 (*red arrows*). (*D*) Combined tooth resorption (*red arrows*) and infiltrative irregular cementum (*green arrows*). (*E*) Combined tooth resorption (*red arrows*) and infiltrative irregular cementum (*green arrows*). (*Courtesy of* Jeff Reiswig, DVM, PhD, Pataskala, OH.)

secondary periodontal involvement, primary periodontal lesion, primary periodontal lesion with secondary endodontic involvement, and true combined lesions.[48] With primary endodontic lesions, the extension of disease typically progresses from the crown through the apical opening of the root canal and extends into the surrounding periapical alveolar bone and soft tissue structures only. Primary endodontic lesions with secondary periodontal involvement are an extension or continuation of primary endodontic lesions in which the disorder extends into the surrounding periodontal structures either through the apex or lateral channels of the root canal. Inflammation of the periodontal ligament may be so extensive that drainage extends into the gingival sulcus and/or results in gingival recession. Primary periodontal lesions involve infection of the gingiva and periodontium extending apically along the periodontal ligament. Periodontal pocket formation, accumulation of plaque and calculus, and furcation involvement are common features of this disease. Primary periodontal lesions with secondary endodontic involvement occur when periodontal infection extends into the pulp via the apex of the tooth, dentinal tubules, or lateral channels, resulting in pulpal inflammation. True combined lesions are endodontic and periodontal infections that are independent. These disease processes can advance and merge, making it difficult to distinguish which lesion incited the initial disease process. When evaluating an endodontic periodontal infection, as the severity of the periodontal component increases, the prognosis for treatment of the tooth decreases.[48–50] Distinguishing between these categories may at first seem academic, but knowledge and recognition of endodontic and periodontal interrelationships is critical for appropriate treatment planning, especially if the practitioner is considering therapy other than extraction.

Examples of Periodontal-Endodontic Lesions

Primary endodontic lesion with secondary periodontal involvement

An example of a primary endodontic lesion with secondary periodontal involvement is shown in **Fig. 13**A. Chronic pulp exposure was created 15 years earlier with severe crown odontoplasty to tooth 304. An intraoral radiograph (see **Fig. 13**B) reveals that the chronic pulpal inflammation has led to severe decay and resorption of the coronal one-third of the tooth. Expansion of the pulpal disease into the periodontal structure through the apex, lateral channels, or dentinal tubules is evident with increased radiodensity of the apical alveolar bone and loss of supporting periodontal structures. External inflammatory resorption is evident along the apical third of the tooth (see **Fig. 13**B, C). The extension of the periodontal disease is also evident in **Fig. 13**A with the gingival inflammation and overgrowth.

During the last 20 years, it was common practice to file and/or amputate the canine teeth. These teeth are prominent in male horses. There is no apparent function of these teeth other than that they can be used for fighting. Without regard to the consequence of chronic pulp exposure, traditional dental practice has been to reduce these teeth for comfort and biting purposes. Chronic pulp exposure involving a canine tooth initiates a resorptive process that may show decay in 1 to 2 years or slowly progress over 15 to 20 years; therefore, it is recommended to discontinue this practice.

Primary periodontal lesion with secondary endodontic involvement

An example of a primary endodontic lesion with secondary periodontal involvement is shown in **Fig. 14**A, B. The oral examination of tooth 404 reveals heavy supragingival calculus and a deep periodontal pocket ($\sim$35 mm) along the mesial aspect. An intraoral radiograph discloses a large periodontal abscess associated with tooth 404 (see **Fig. 14**C). The periodontal infection has extended to the apical half of the tooth creating external inflammatory resorption and exposure of dentinal tubules

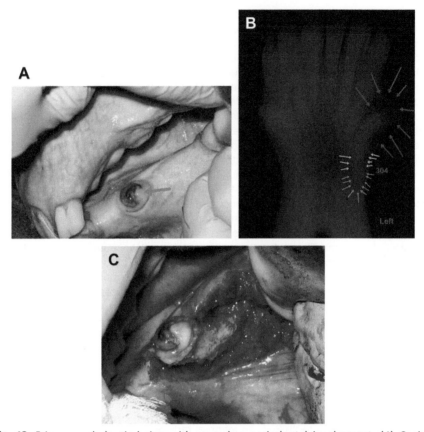

Fig. 13. Primary endodontic lesion with secondary periodontal involvement. (*A*) Canine decay and resorption of 304 (*orange arrow*). (*B*) Intraoral radiograph of 304 demonstrates expansion of the pulpal disease to the peridontium with severe decay and resorption of the coronal 1/3 (*red arrows*), loss of supporting periodontal structures (*green arrows*) and increased radiodensity of the apical alveolar bone with external inflammatory resorption of the apex (*orange arrows*). (*C*) Surgical extraction of 304.

leading to pulpal tissue inflammation and decay of the tooth. The decay of 404 is so severe that the apical half of the tooth crumbled and fractured during surgical extraction (see **Fig. 14**D, E). The remaining reserve crown and root remnants are surgically extracted. Large amounts of inspissated pus are debrided and flushed and the surgical site is closed following a postoperative intraoral radiograph (see **Fig. 14**F–H).

Occasionally the lower canines build up large deposits of calculus. It is suspected that the constant bathing of the lower canines with saliva from the sublingual salivary ducts allows an active biofilm and plaque production that may develop into a heavy calculus surrounding these teeth. Plaque is composed of bacteria in a matrix of glycoproteins and extracellular polysaccharides.[51] Calculus is a hard deposit that forms by mineralization of the dental plaque. Saliva has been shown to be the source of mineralization for supragingival calculus. The key ingredient in saliva that seems to promote calculus formation is phosphorus. If saliva is high in phosphorous the mineralization of plaque occurs by binding calcium ions to carbohydrate-protein complexes, creating a

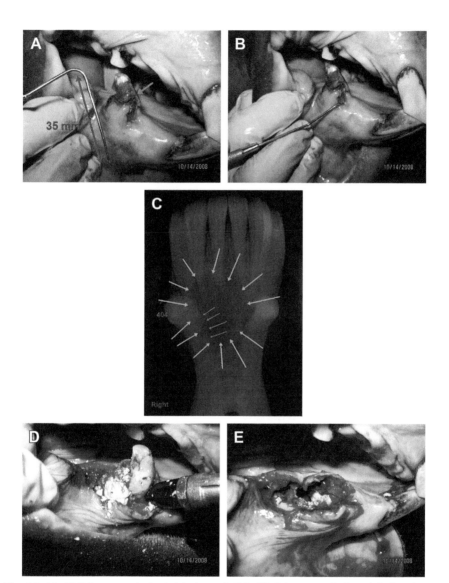

Fig. 14. (A, B) Primary periodontal lesion of 404. (C) Primary periodontal lesion (*green arrows*) with external inflammatory resorption leading to secondary endodontic disease (*orange arrows*). (D) Surgical extraction of 404. (E) Remaining periodontal abscess following extraction of 404.

precipitate of crystalline phosphate salts.[52] This heavy calculus may potentially lead to periodontal disease and pocketing that involves the lower canines.

GEMINATION

Developmental malformations of incisors are uncommon. Most permanent dental malformations are secondary to regional tooth bud damage during maturation, but

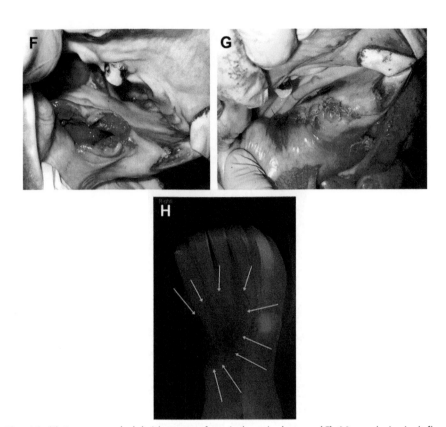

Fig. 14. (*F*) Lavage and debridement of periodontal abscess. (*G*) Mucosal-gingival flap closure. (*H*) Post surgical intraoral radiograph to evaluate extraction of 404 and periodontal abscess debridement.

periodically a malformation presents that seems to be truly developmental in origin. One type of developmental malformation is the appearance of a double crown on one tooth. A typical discussion regarding this condition involves the terms fusion, gemination, and concrescence. In the past, gemination was defined as a disorder in which a developing tooth bud attempts to divide with the resultant formation of a tooth with a double crown and usually a common root or root canal.[49] In contrast, fusion was defined as the union of 2 normally separated tooth buds with the resultant formation of a joined tooth with confluent dentin, and concrescence was the union of 2 teeth by cementum only.[53] Many clinicians have found these definitions unwieldy in a clinical setting, so more practical definitions have been created. Gemination is now defined as a single enlarged tooth or a joined tooth in which the tooth count is normal when the anomalous tooth is counted as 1, and fusion is defined as a single enlarged tooth in which the tooth count reveals a missing tooth when the anomalous tooth is counted as 1.[53] Concrescence remained the union of 2 adjacent teeth by cementum only with no change in the tooth count; moreover, concresence can occur during development or after inflammation, unlike gemination and fusion, which can solely occur during development.[53] However, these three conditions have favorable prognoses, and management usually involves only minor reduction of clinical crown overgrowth.

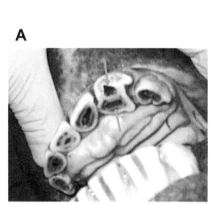
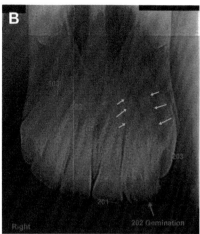

Fig. 15. (*A*) Incisor gemination of 202. (*B*) Intraoral radiograph reveals a 90 degree roatation of 202 with only one reserve crown and root (*green arrows*).

Case of Gemination

Oral examination of a 9-year-old paint gelding reveals a double crown involving tooth 202 (**Fig. 15A**). Because the tooth count including the anomalous tooth is normal, this is considered a case of gemination. An intraoral radiograph shows that the tooth is rotated ~90° and only 1 reserve crown and root is present (see **Fig. 15B**).

SUMMARY

This article presents the current knowledge and perspective of disease conditions that involve the incisor and canine teeth. Equine dentistry is rapidly advancing and it will be intriguing to review this article in 5 and 10 years. There will be new insight regarding diagnosis and treatment involving these conditions.

ACKNOWLEDGMENTS

The authors thank the following for their assistance: Rebecca M. Smedley, DVM, DACVP; Robert M. Baratt, DVM, FAVD/Eq, FAVD; Stephen M. Galloway, DVM, FAVD/Eq; Santiago Peralta, DVM, Diplomate AVDC; Laurelyn Keener, DVM; Vic Cox, DVM, VBMS; Jeff Reiswig, DVM, FAVD/Eq; Allison Dotzel, DVM.

REFERENCES

1. Dixon PM, Tremaine WH, Pickles K, et al. Equine dental disease Part 1: a long-term study of 400 cases: disorders of incisor, canine, and first premolar teeth. Equine Vet J 1999;31(5):369–77.
2. du Toit N, Burden FA, Dixon PM. Clinical dental examinations of 357 donkeys in the UK. Part 1: prevalence of dental disorders. Equine Vet J 2009;41(4):390–4.
3. Dixon PM, Dacre I. A review of equine dental disorders. Vet J 2005;169:165–87.
4. Dixon PM. Disorders of development an eruption of the teeth and developmental craniofacial abnormalities. In: Easley J, Dixon PM, Schumacher J, editors. Equine dentistry. 3rd edition. Philadelphia: WB Saunders; 2011. p. 99–114.

5. Dixon PM, du Toit N, Dacre I. Equine dental pathology. In: Easley J, Dixon PM, Schumacher J, editors. Equine dentistry. 3rd edition. Philadelphia: WB Saunders; 2011. p. 129–47.
6. Floyd MR. The modified Triadan system: nomenclature for veterinary dentistry. J Vet Dent 1991;8:18–9.
7. Dixon PM, du Toit N. Dental anatomy. In: Easley J, Dixon PM, Schumacher J, editors. Equine dentistry. 3rd edition. Philadelphia: WB Saunders; 2011. p. 51–76.
8. Lowder MQ, Mueller PO. Dental embryology, anatomy, development, and aging. Vet Clin North Am Equine Pract 1998;14(2):227–45.
9. Nanci A. Dentin-pulp complex. In: Nanci A, editor. Ten Cate's oral histology: development, structure, and function. 6th edition. St Louis (MO): Mosby; 2003. p. 192.
10. Trowbridge H, Syngeuk K, Suda H. Structure and functions of the dentin and pulp complex. Pathways of the pulp. 8th edition. St. Louis (MO): Mosby Inc; 2002. p. 411–26.
11. Towbridge H, Kim S, Suda H. Structure and functions of the dentin and pulp complex. In: Cohen S, Burns RC, editors. Pathways of the pulp. 8th edition. St Louis (MO): Mosby; 2002. p. 421, 423.
12. Shaw DJ, Dacre IT, Dixon PM. Pathological studies of cheek teeth apical infections in the horse: 2. Quantitative measurements in normal equine dentine. Vet J 2008;178:321–32.
13. Fitzgerald M, Chiego DJ, Heys DR. Autoradiographic analysis of odontoblast replacement following pulp exposure in primate teeth. Arch Oral Biol 1990;35: 707.
14. Marshall R, Shaw DJ, Dixon PM. A study of sub-occlusal secondary dentine thickness in overgrown equine cheek teeth. Vet J 2012;193:53–7.
15. Du Toit N, Kempson SA, Dixon PM. Donkey dental anatomy. Part 2: histological and scanning electron microscopic examinations. Vet J 2008;176: 345–53.
16. Dacre IT, Kempson S, Dixon PM. Pathological studies of cheek teeth apical infections in the horse: 1. Normal endodontic anatomy and dentinal structure of equine cheek teeth. Vet J 2008;178:311–20.
17. Staszyk C. Anatomy of the pulp of equine cheek teeth. Veterinary Dental Forum Proceedings. 2006. p. 115.
18. AVDC Nomenclature Committee. American Veterinary Dental College. Dental Fracture Classification. Haddonfield (NJ): AVDC; 2009. p. 6–16.
19. Cohen AS, Brown DC. Orofacial dental pain emergencies: endodontic diagnoses and management. Pathways of the pulp. 8th edition. St. Louis (MO): Mosby Inc; 2002. p. 32–53.
20. Wiggs RB, Lobprise HB. Basic endodontic therapy. Veterinary dentistry, principles and practice. Philadelphia (PA); 1997. p. 280–9, 646.
21. DeBowes RM. Fractures of the mandible and maxilla. In: Nixon AJ, editor. Equine fracture repair. Philadelphia: WB Saunders; 1996. p. 323–32.
22. Greet T, Ramzan PH. Head and dental trauma. In: Easley J, Dixon PM, Schumacher J, editors. Equine dentistry. 3rd edition. Philadelphia: WB Saunders; 2011. p. 115–27.
23. Henninger RW, Beard WL, Schneider RK, et al. Fractures of the rostral portion of the mandible and maxilla in horses: 89 cases (1979-1997). J Am Vet Med Assoc 1999;214(11):1648–52.
24. Manfra-Marretta S. Maxillofacial surgery. Vet Clin North Am Small Anim Pract Canine Dentistry 1998;28(5):1285–96.

25. Earley ET. Complications with extractions. AAEP Proceedings. 2012. p. 289–93.
26. Iacopetti I, De Benedictis GM, Faughnan M, et al. Treatment of incisive bone fracture in a horse using an acrylic splint. Equine Vet Educ 2009;346–51.
27. Delory MS. A retrospective evaluation of 204 diagonal incisor malocclusion corrections in the horse. J Vet Dent 2007;24(3):145–9.
28. Rucker BA. Incisor and molar occlusion: normal ranges and indications for incisor reduction. In: Proceedings of the 50th Annual Convention for the AAEP. Denver (CO): 2004. p. 7–12.
29. Stubbs CR. Dentistry of equine cheek teeth. In: Proceedings of the 50th Annual Convention for the AAEP. Denver (CO): 2004. p. 1–6.
30. Foster DL. Incisor corrections using a hand-held belt sander. In: Proceedings of the Focus on Dentistry, AAEP. Indianapolis (IN): 2006. p. 285–8.
31. Earley E. Skeletal abnormalities in the equine skull. In: Proceedings of the Focus on Dentistry, AAEP. Albuquerque (NM): 2011. p. 131–3.
32. Baratt RM. How to recognize and clinically manage class I malocclusions in the horse. In. Proceedings of the 56th Annual Convention for the AAEP. Baltimore (MD): 2010. p. 458–64.
33. Baratt RM. Perspectives on management of common malocclusions and the surrounding controversy. In: Proceedings of the 26th Annual Dental Forum. Seattle (WA): 2012. p. 143–50.
34. Peralta S, Verstraete FJ, Kass PH. Radiographic evaluation of the types of tooth resorption in dogs. Am J Vet Res 2010;71:784–93.
35. Hamp SE, Olsson SE, Farso-Madsen K, et al. A macroscopic and radiological investigation of dental diseases of the dog. Vet Radiol 1984;25:86–92.
36. Giard N, Servet E, Biourge V, et al. Feline tooth resorption in a colony of 109 cats. J Vet Dent 2008;25(3):166–74.
37. Klugh DO. Incisor and canine periodontal disease. In: Proceedings of the 18th Annual Dental Forum. 2004. p. 166–9.
38. Gregory RC, Fehr J, Bryant J. Chronic incisor periodontal disease with cemental hyperplasia and hypoplasia in horses. In: Proceedings of the Focus on Dentistry, AAEP. Indianapolis (IN): 2006. p. 312–6.
39. Baratt RM. Equine incisor resorptive lesions. In: Proceedings of the 21st Annual Dental Forum. Minneapolis (MN): 2007. p. 123–30.
40. Staszyk C, Bienert A, Simhofer H, et al. Equine odontoclastic tooth resorption and hypercementosis. Vet J 2008;178:372–9.
41. Earley ET, Smedley RM, Baratt RM, et al. AVD Research grant presentation: clinicopathologic and histopathologic findings in horses with EOTRH. In: Proceedings of the 26th Annual Dental Forum. Seattle (WA): 2012. p. 165.
42. Schatzle M, Tanner SD, Bosshardt DD, et al. Progressive, generalized, apical idiopathic root resorption and hypercementosis. J Periodontol 2005;76:2002–11.
43. Stepaniuk K. Biphosphate related osteonecrosis of the jaws: a review. J Vet Dent 2011;28(4):277–81.
44. Nanci A, Whitson SW, Bianco P. Bone. In: Nanci A, editor. Ten Cate's oral histology: development, structure, and function. 6th edition. St Louis (MO): Mosby; 2003. p. 111–43.
45. Andreasen FM, Andreasen JO. Luxation injuries of permanent teeth: general findings. In: Andreasen JO, Andreasen FM, Andersson L, editors. Textbook and color atlas of traumatic injuries to teeth. 4th edition. Copenhagen (Denmark): Blackwell Munksgaard; 2007. p. 372–403.
46. Rice M, Henry T. Prevalence of incisor and canine tooth resorption. In: Proceedings of the 26th Annual Dental Forum. Seattle (WA): 2012. p. 167–8.

47. Tremaine W, Schumacher J. Exodontia. In: Easley J, Dixon P, Schumacher J, editors. Equine dentistry. 3rd edition. London: Saunders-Elsevier; 2011. p. 321–2.

48. Wang HL, Glickman GN. Endodontic and periodontic interrelationships. In: Cohen S, Burns R, editors. Pathways of the pulp. 8th edition. St. Louis (MO): Mosby; 2002. p. 651–60.

49. Wiggs RB, Lobprise HB. Veterinary dentistry, principles and practice. Philadelphia (PA): Lippincott-Raven; 1997. p. 287–9, 646.

50. Kerns DG, Glickman GN. Endodontic and periodontic interrelationships. In: Hargreaves KM, Cohen S, editors. Pathways of the pulp. 10th edition. St. Louis (MO): Mosby; 2011. p. 655–67.

51. Quirynen M, Teughels W, Haake SK, et al. Microbiology of periodontal disease. Chapter 9. In: Carranza's clinical periodontology. 10th edition. St. Louis (MO): Saunders-Elsevier; 2006. p. 134–47.

52. Hinrichs JE. The role of dental calculus and other predisposing factors. Chapter 10. In: Carranza's clinical periodontology. 10th edition. St. Louis (MO): Saunders-Elsevier; 2006. p. 170–6.

53. Neville BW, Damm DD, Allen CM, et al. Oral and maxillofacial pathology. 3rd edition. Philadelphia: WB Saunders; 2009. p. 84–5.

A New Understanding of Oral and Dental Pathology of the Equine Cheek Teeth

Miriam Casey, MVB, MSc, MRCVS*

KEYWORDS

- Equine dental pathology • Equine periodontal disease • Equine cheek teeth
- Dental regeneration

KEY POINTS

- Equine periodontal disease is common and painful, but the periodontium has the regenerative capacity to respond well to treatment. This disorder is more common in older horses but is also important in younger horses.
- The spectrum of normal anatomy in relation to occlusal angles and infundibular cemental defects is much broader than is conventionally believed.
- Mild or moderate infundibular defects do not commonly advance to cause apical disease or dental fractures. The maxillary 09 teeth are relatively more prone to severe infundibular caries that progresses to clinically significant disease.
- Equine dental pulpitis commonly has no obvious portal of entry for bacteria to the pulp.
- When the odontoblasts lining the pulp chamber are compromised by pulpitis, they may cease to produce dentine, and a secondary dental defect (open pulp horn) will eventually become apparent with attrition on the occlusal surface.
- Equine oral and dental neoplasia is rare, but should be kept in mind as a differential for clinical signs of cranial, oral, and upper airway disease.

INTRODUCTION

Equine hypsodont cheek teeth have adapted for mastication of abrasive foodstuffs over prolonged periods. Lifelong eruption of the dental reserve crown, constant turnover of the periodontium, high rates of dentinogenesis, infundibula, peripheral cement, and dentine that can tolerate occlusal exposure all manifest as part of this adaptation. These specializations mean that only limited inference from human and small animal dentistry can be made to equine dental pathology.

Equine dental science is emerging from its nascence with increasing numbers of peer-reviewed publications every year. There are logistical challenges in examining

School of Veterinary Sciences, University of Bristol, Langford House, Langford, Bristol BS40 5DU, UK
* Corresponding address: Flat 2/3, 37 Kelvindale Court, Glasgow G12 0JG, Glasgow.
E-mail address: m.casey.2@research.gla.ac.uk

Vet Clin Equine 29 (2013) 301–324
http://dx.doi.org/10.1016/j.cveq.2013.04.010
0749-0739/13/$ – see front matter © 2013 Elsevier Inc. All rights reserved.

Key Abbreviations Box

The Triadan system of dental nomenclature[1] is used in this article and throughout this issue. Triadan positions 06, 07, and 08 correspond to the second, third, and fourth premolars. Triadan positions 09, 10, and 11 correspond to the first, second, and third molars.

---

oral abnormalities in the live animal. Processing equine dental tissues for pathologic investigation can also be challenging. The use of methods such as oral endoscopy and computed tomography has greatly facilitated meeting these challenges and improving our understanding of equine dental anatomy and pathology.[2–12]

Anatomic studies in horses with no history of dental disease and case-control studies have also questioned what is deemed to be pathologic (a structural or functional disorder) rather than normal anatomic variation. Conventional opinions about the normal occlusal angle, the etiology of mucosal ulceration, and the clinical relevance of maxillary infundibular changes have been challenged.[3,13–15] Much remains to be discovered about the etiology and pathogenesis of clinically important disorders such as pulpitis and periodontal disease. However, new insights on these topics are emerging.[5,16–18]

This review aims to summarize what is known about the more prevalent diseases of equine cheek teeth, highlighting recent developments and new ideas emerging from the literature.

GENERAL ESTIMATES OF PREVALENCE OF EQUINE DENTAL DISEASE

The prevalence of equine dental disease is estimated to be 36% to 85%.[19–23] One postmortem study of 355 skulls from an abattoir population in Ireland found a prevalence of 37%, 31%, 17%, and 13% for periodontal disease, caries, wear abnormalities, and maleruption, respectively. Further postmortem reviews in the United Kingdom and Belgium also revealed a high prevalence of these conditions.[20,23] Similarly, surveys of live horses in the United States and Europe have reported prevalences of 24% to 85% for oral disorders, mostly related to malocclusions, overgrowths, and periodontal disease.[21,24] The reported prevalence of idiopathic fractures of equine cheek teeth is 0.07% to 5.9%.[25] Apical disease is relatively less common in the general equine population, but is the most common reason for referral of horses for specialist dental investigation and treatment.[26]

PERIODONTAL DISEASE
Prevalence of Periodontal Disease

Periodontal disease is the most painful disease of the horse's mouth.[27] Abattoir surveys report prevalences of 52% to 60% in horses older than 15 years.[19,28] A recent clinical endoscopic survey of horses referred with dental problems noted that 75% of these horses had at least 1 diastema.[11,29] Prevalence in the general equine population is reported to be 49.9%.[30]

Overview of Periodontitis and Grading System

The periodontium is the supporting structure of the tooth and consists of the dental cement, the periodontal ligament, alveolar bone, and gingiva. Disease of these structures is characterized and graded clinically through the appearance of gingival ulceration and regression (**Fig. 1**), cemental discoloration, probing depth in the periodontal space (**Table 1**), loss of attachment and mobility of the tooth, radiographic evidence of

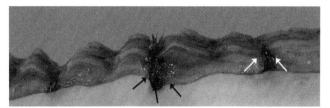

Fig. 1. Gingival recession associated with a diastema between 2 mandibular cheek teeth in a cadaver. There is also food pocketing and cemental discoloration (*black arrows*). The interproximal space to the right of the image has plaque lesions, possibly also due to food accumulation at this site (*white arrows*).

alveolar bone loss, and radiographic evidence that periodontal disease has reached the endodontic system and has caused apical disease.[31]

Periodontitis Associated with the Emerging Dentition

Transient periodontal disease may occur during the normal dental eruption process in the immature equine mouth. For example, if food gets trapped around a loose deciduous tooth or an irregular recently erupted tooth, gingival and periodontal lesions may ensue. This condition normally resolves as soon as the adult dentition comes into wear.

Periodontitis Associated with Diastemata

The majority of periodontal disease that produces clinical signs in the horse is associated with diastemata, or abnormal gaps between the cheek teeth.

Diastemata are most commonly observed between the caudal mandibular cheek teeth, at Triadan locations 09 to 10 and 10 to 11 in horses referred for periodontal disease treatment, and at position 07 to 08 in the population examined by first-opinion veterinarians.[11,30] However, they may occur at any location in the mandibular or maxillary cheek-tooth rows. The greatest forces are generated in the caudal mandibular area while chewing, which may be a reason for more severe food impaction and clinical signs arising from diastemata between the caudal mandibular teeth.[32]

Proposed etiology of diastemata
Diastemata may be congenital or acquired.

Developmental diastemata Misalignment of the tooth buds of the permanent dentition may result in reduced interproximal compression of cheek teeth at the alveolar crest in

Table 1		
One aspect of periodontal disease grading based on periodontal pocket depth		
Grade of Periodontal Disease	**Descriptive Grade**	**Sulcus/Periodontal Pocket Depth from Normal Gingival Margin (mm)**
0	No disease	0–4
1	Mild disease	5–9
2	Moderate disease	10–14
3	Severe disease	>15

Data from Klugh D. Equine periodontal disease. Clin Tech Equine Pract 2005;4:135–47; and Cox A, Dixon P, Smith S. Histopathological lesions associated with equine periodontal disease. Vet J 2012;194(3):386–91.

the adult horse, allowing food impaction and subsequent periodontal disease. Tooth buds may develop spatially too far apart, in misalignment or at abnormal angles to one another.[4,33] Misalignment may also result from overcrowding caused by teeth erupting too near to each other. Diastemata commonly occur between supernumerary or dysplastic cheek teeth and their neighbors.[33,34] Misalignment of single or multiple cheek teeth, especially in the mandible, is an important cause of valve diastemata and severe periodontal disease in young age groups as well as in older horses.[4,27,35]

Acquired diastemata A common reason for acquired diastemata is age-related reduction in coronal cross-sectional area and reduction in reserve crown length, with subsequent loss of rostrocaudal compressive forces on the row of cheek teeth.[35] It is these types of diastemata that cause such high reported prevalence of diastemata in older horses.[28] Diverted eruption as a result of large overgrowths is thought to be a cause of diastemata in some circumstances.[35] Dental extraction by repulsion is reported to cause multiple diastemata and periodontal disease in the affected row,[36] but per os extraction is not associated with diastemata remote from the extraction site or periodontal disease.[37]

How diastemata result in periodontitis
When food impacts in the interproximal space as a result of diastemata, it damages the gingiva and promotes bacterial growth. There is subsequent inflammation, gingival ulceration, and cemental destruction. This process provides more space for the impacted food to travel more deeply into the interproximal space, advancing the level of inflammation and tissue destruction in a vicious cycle. Valve diastemata are widest at or below the gingival margin and narrowest near the occlusal level (**Fig. 2**).[38] Valve diastemata are associated with more severe dental disease and are the most prevalent type of diastemata reported.[30] Open diastemata are the same width occlusally and gingivally, and are generally associated with less severe periodontal disease and clinical signs. The prevalence of open diastemata increases with age.[30]

Pathologic Findings with Periodontal Disease
Once pocketed food is removed, gross pathologic features of equine periodontitis range from gingivitis to gingival recession, bleeding, and purulent exudate.[11,31] Severe periodontitis may be associated with loss of periodontal attachment, bacteria reaching the apex and causing endodontic disease (**Fig. 3**). Between the caudal maxillary

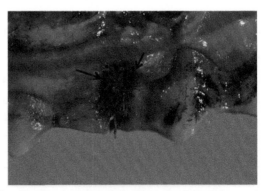

Fig. 2. A severe valve diastema between 2 maxillary cheek teeth in a cadaver. There is hardly any gap between the teeth at the occlusal end of the diastema, but there is much food impaction and a wider space at the gingival (upper) end of the diastema (*arrows*).

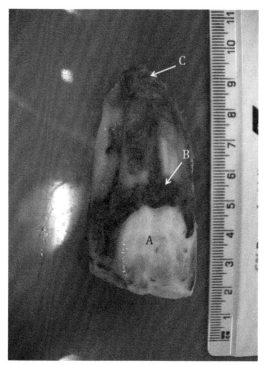

Fig. 3. A rotated maxillary tooth that was associated with severe periodontal disease. Loss of periodontal attachment is apparent (A). There is inflamed periodontium adherent to the middle section of the tooth (B). The tooth apex has lost any root structure and is covered by a granuloma (C).

cheek teeth, severe lesions may erode through the alveolar bone and cause oro-sinus fistulation, with subsequent sinusitis.[39] End-stage periodontitis is associated with tooth loosening and loss (**Fig. 4**). Alveolar bone destruction and osteomyelitis have been identified in some severe cases post mortem. One histopathologic study of periodontitis has been conducted on periodontal lesions from 21 randomly selected equine cadavers. Gingival erosion and ulceration, neutrophilic exudate, bacterial rods, cocci, and spirochetes were associated with periodontitis. Of note, there were few reported histopathologic changes in the equine periodontal ligament, and none

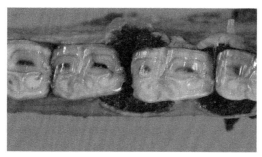

Fig. 4. End-stage diastemata in a cadaver mandible. There is extensive food impaction to the depth of the alveolar bone, and the teeth involved with the lesions are loose.

of the pathologic changes present were deemed irreversible.[18] The equine peridontium is constantly remodeling to enable hypsodont tooth eruption at 2 to 4 mm per year and has regenerative and stem cell cell populations within it.[40] Therefore, the equine periodontium may well have better facilities to recover form mild or moderate disease than its brachydont counterparts.[41]

EQUINE DENTAL PULPITIS (APICAL INFECTION)
Prevalence of Apical Infections of Cheek Teeth

Relative to equine dental disease in general, findings consistent with dental pulpitis (apical infection) are less common in the general equine population. Wafa[19] reported 9 cheek teeth with evidence of pulpitis from his survey of 355 skulls. Uhlinger[24] reported 6 (intact) cheek teeth with evidence of infection in her survey of 233 horses. By contrast, pulpitis features dominantly in the population of horses referred to specialist institutions because of challenging dental disorders. In a large case series, 162 of 400 horses were referred for specialist dental investigation because of signs of pulpitis.[26] This proportion was higher than for any other dental disorder.

Terminology

The disorder termed pulpitis here has also been called "tooth root abscess," "apical abscess,"[42] "apical infection,"[26,43] "peri-apical infection,"[19,44] "dental sepsis,"[45] and "dento-alveolar infection."[46] The clinical syndrome to which all of these terms refer includes external bony swellings and discharging tracts with unilateral nasal discharge that are due to apical disease of a tooth. Less common clinical signs are epiphora, bitting problems, head shaking, dysmastication, and weight loss.[26]

Etiology

Bacteriology

Anaerobic bacteria predominate among those cultured from periapical abscesses, necrotic pulp, and sinus contents in cases of dental sinusitis.[47,48] Bacteria have also been demonstrated histologically in the dentinal tubules of diseased teeth.[17] However, it is unknown whether the bacteria are primary etiologic agents or whether they gain access secondarily to the pulp and dentine of a tooth that is already compromised.

Portals of entry for bacteria to the pulp

Proposed portals of entry for bacteria into the pulp of equine cheek teeth are through caries extending to the dentine-pulp complex,[49] coronal fractures, periodontal transmission to the apex,[27] occlusal pulpar exposure,[19] pulp necrosis with secondary bacterial colonization through transient impaction during eruption,[44] and anachoresis (Fig. 5).[16,17] However, most horses showing clinical signs of pulpitis have no evidence of coronal fracture or periodontal disease (Fig. 6).[16,17,26]

Teeth with No Obvious Portal of Entry for Bacteria to the Pulp: Proposed Anachoresis (Blood- or Lymphatic-Borne Infection)

Extension of caries into the endodontium is an uncommon portal of entry of bacteria to the pulp, and dentinal defects are likely to be a result, rather than a cause, of pulpitis.[16,17] Anachoretic infections, progression of infundibular caries, coronal fractures, and periodontal disease may cause pulpitis. The absence of other precipitating lesions was cited as evidence (by exclusion) for anachoretic infection in 51% of maxillary and 59% of mandibular cheek teeth.[16,17] Anachoretic infection was considered to be responsible for 68% of teeth with pulpitis in a further study.[50] However, anachoretic infection is rare in brachydont teeth,[51,52] where exposure of the dental pulp to the

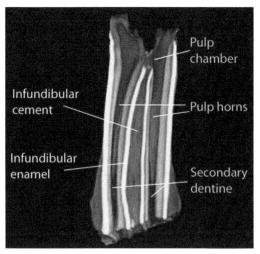

Fig. 5. A computed tomographic reconstruction of a maxillary cheek tooth representing a sagittal section through the tooth. Possible routes for bacteria to reach the pulp horse are from the apical vessels, via the periodontal space, via defects in the secondary dentine, via defects in the peripheral enamel and dentine, or via defects in the infundibular cement, enamel, and dentine.

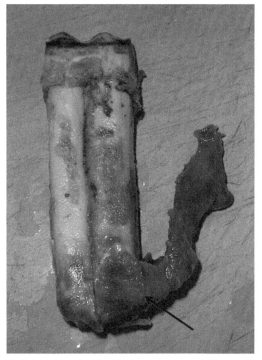

Fig. 6. An 08 mandibular tooth extracted from a 4-year-old horse. There was no obvious portal of entry for bacteria to the pulp. An apical granuloma is evident (*arrow*).

oral cavity is the most common portal of pulpal infection. Anachoretic pulpar infection could not be induced experimentally in vital canine teeth unless they were inflamed[53] and, in the monkey, teeth with experimentally devitalized pulp remained sterile for 6 months.[54]

The hypsodont nature of equine teeth may be a possible explanation for this difference between species. In contrast to brachydont teeth, equine odontoblasts continue to secrete dentine at high rates after emergence of the teeth. In the brachydont tooth germ, when the odontoblasts are engaged in high rates of dentinogenesis, the blood vessels supplying them are fenestrated to allow greater fluid and cell transfer, and do not seal until after the bulk of dentinogenesis is complete.[55] As rates of dentinogenesis remain high throughout the life of the equine tooth, it is possible that the blood vessels supplying the odontoblasts remain fenestrated, allowing greater transfer of blood contents to the pulp. Increased permeability of its blood vessels would make the equine pulp more vulnerable to infection with blood-borne bacteria.

Impaction of equine cheek teeth, anachoresis and pulpitis
Mandibular 08s and maxillary 07s and 09s predominate among the Triadan positions of equine cheek teeth afflicted by pulpitis.[26,56] The median ages of horses referred for treatment of mandibular and rostral maxillary (Triadan 06–08) pulpitis are 5 and 6 years, respectively.[26] Hence these teeth are causing signs of pulpitis within 3 years or less of their emergence times.[57] Clinical external signs of pulpitis that are recognized in horses (bony swellings, discharging tracts, and nasal discharge) reflect an advanced dental disease state.[58] Transient impaction during tooth emergence, pulpar insult and, possibly, increased vascular permeability is a possible explanation for how cheek teeth in young horses with no obvious coronal abnormality can develop pulpitis. Overt cheek-tooth impaction whereby there is complete failure of the tooth to emerge into the oral cavity (**Fig. 7**) has also been described in association with signs of pulpitis.[59,60]

Infundibular Caries and Pulpitis
The high percentage of maxillary 09s among the teeth causing signs of pulpitis[19,26,56] cannot be explained by transient impaction during emergence, as they are the first of the molars to emerge at approximately 1 year old.[61] Furthermore, the median age of horses with caudal maxillary cheek-tooth pulpitis ranges from 8 to 14 years, which is too old for temporal association with tooth emergence.[26,56] There is no significant

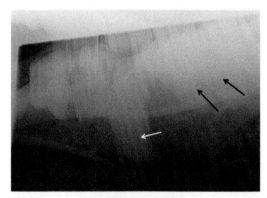

Fig. 7. A lateral-45° ventral to lateral oblique radiograph of the mandibular cheek teeth of a 5-year-old Connemara pony. The 08 tooth (*white arrow*) has not emerged above the gingival margin. The 09 and 10 teeth are angled forward (*black arrows*).

difference in the prevalence of infundibular caries in maxillary cheek teeth extracted from horses with pulpitis in comparison with matched controls. However, infundibular caries progressing to the infundibular enamel, or progressing beyond the enamel to involve dentine, is more common in teeth extracted from cases of pulpitis than in teeth from asymptomatic controls, and is also more common in maxillary cheek teeth from Triadan position 09.[62] In an etiopathologic study, infundibular caries was implicated as the cause of 16% of apical infections of maxillary cheek teeth.[17]

Other Causes of Pulpitis

Some coronal fractures, especially sagittal fractures through maxillary infundibula, may result in pulpitis (see later discussion on cheek-tooth fractures and caries).

Pathologic Changes Associated with Pulpitis

The earliest histologic signs of pulpitis reported are pulpar edema and hyperemia. More chronic cases have destruction of the pulp, neutrophilic inflammation, absence of predentine, and eventually caries extending from the pulpar area into the dentine (see **Figs. 8** and **9** for the histologic appearance of normal pulp and that from a tooth with pulpitis).[17,63] Inflammatory changes in the periodontium surrounding the apex of the tooth have been described.[63] In many cases, there is reduced dentinal thickness owing to destruction of the odontoblasts lining the pulp cavity and subsequent cessation of dentinogenesis.[64] In advanced cases, there may be complete pulpar exposure, food pocketing in the dentinal defect, and secondary caries.[16,56] Reactive and reparative dentinogenesis and extensive pulpar calcification, previously undescribed in horses, as well as reactive cemental deposition have also been recently identified.[63] The cheek teeth of horses appear vulnerable to pulpitis, especially that which is related to impaction and anachoresis. However, the equine dentine-pulp complex appears to be able to respond to insult in a dynamic fashion with deposition of reparative calcified tissue.

CARIES

Peripheral and infundibular cemental caries are the most common types of caries in equine teeth. The embryology, anatomy, and physiology of equine coronal and infundibular cement is unique to hypsodont teeth. Dental cement in brachydonts is limited

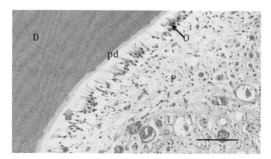

Fig. 8. A normal pulp horn and associated dentine from a 6-year-old horse. The pulp (P) has the appearance of loose connective tissue. There is a palisade of odontoblasts (O) lining the pulp horn producing predentine (pd) that mineralizes to become dentine (D). The slight shrinkage of the odontoblasts away from the dentine is a processing artifact, but it exposes part of the odontoblast processes (*thick blue arrow*) that normally run inside the dentinal tubules (decalcified section; hematoxylin and eosin [H&E] stain, bar = 100 μm).

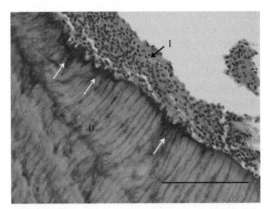

Fig. 9. Histologic section of the dentine and pulp of an 07 mandibular tooth from a 5-year-old horse. This tooth was extracted because of clinical signs of pulpitis. It had no obvious portal for bacteria to the pulp. The pulp in this section is filled with polymorphonuclear leukocytes (inflammatory cells) (I). The normal structure of odontoblasts and predentine is not visible. The dentine (D) adjacent to the pulp has an irregular border with the pulp horn (*white arrows*). (H&E, bar = 100 μm).

to that which is below the gingival margin. Hence, limited inference can be made from studies on caries in humans, primates, and carnivores. Caries may also progress from cement to include enamel and dentine, and dentinal caries may also be a consequence of the development of defects in the secondary occlusal dentine.

Peripheral Cemental Caries

There are high levels of peripheral caries in domesticated horses.[11,65] It is most prevalent in the caudal 3 maxillary and mandibular cheek teeth. Gray, plaque-like material and partially masticated food have been observed endoscopically over many peripheral carious lesions. However, there is no association between food pocketed within interproximal diastemata between cheek teeth and peripheral caries.[11] A histopathologic study corroborates this, reporting plaque overlying areas of cemental destruction, but no significant association between the periodontal disease score and the level of plaque and cemental destruction present.[18]

Dentinal Caries

Caries may extend from cement and enamel lesions to reach dentine. In the case of pulpitis or another insult to the odontoblasts, dentine production may halt, after which a secondary dentinal defect develops; food and bacteria from the oral cavity then enter the dentinal defect, and a carious lesion of the dentine ensues (**Fig. 10**).[17,66]

Maxillary Infundibular Lesions

Terminology
Terms used to describe infundibular lesions include hypoplasia,[2,3,15,43,67] necrosis,[28,49] and caries.[12,15,19,43,68]

Infundibular cemental hypoplasia
Absence of cement in areas within the infundibulum, with underlying enamel exposed but without dark staining of the tissues, is referred to as infundibular hypoplasia.[15,43,67] These areas sometimes contain folds of soft tissue and are associated with the

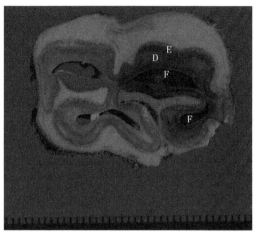

Fig. 10. Transverse section from a mandibular 07 tooth from a 9-year-old horse that was causing clinical signs of pulpitis. There is food impacted into the caudal buccal and caudal lingual pulp areas (F). The dentine (D) and enamel (E) adjacent to where the food is pocketed has a dark color consistent with caries.

remnant of the central vascular channel, and are more common in the apical portion of the infundibulum.[2,15] Recent anatomic studies concluded that only 10% to 11.7% of infundibula from horses with no history of dental disease were completely filled with cement.[2,15] Hence infundibular hypoplasia may be viewed as an anatomic variation rather than a pathologic condition (**Fig. 11**).

Infundibular caries
Caries is a bacterial disease of the calcified tissues of the teeth characterized by demineralization of the inorganic substance and destruction of the organic substance of the tooth.[69] Grossly, infundibular cemental caries is recognized as dark-colored destruction of cementum that may extend through the full length of the infundibulum (**Fig. 12**).[15] A grading system for caries adapted from one used in man based on the number of calcified tissues (cement, enamel, and dentine) involved in the carious lesion and the effect of the lesion on the structural integrity of the tooth has been applied to equine peripheral and infundibular caries (see **Fig. 12**, **Table 2**).[68,70]

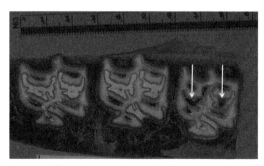

Fig. 11. Transverse sections of 07, 08, and 09 maxillary cheek teeth from a 6-year-old horse with no history of dental disease, 40 mm below the occlusal surface. The 09 tooth on the right of the image has defects in the cementum of both its infundibula (*white arrows*).

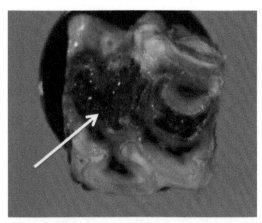

Fig. 12. A maxillary cheek tooth with infundibular caries. The rostral infundibulum (*white arrow*) has advanced caries of the cement, enamel, and dentine that has caused the fracturing away of part of the tooth; this corresponds to Honma grade 4 caries. The caudal infundibulum on the right of the image also has caries of its cement and of parts of the infundibular enamel.

Histologic and pathologic findings in infundibula

The presence of viable cementocytes and blood vessels in the apical portion of the infundibulum of an 09 tooth 2 years after emergence contradicts the conventional belief that infundibular cement is an inert substance and that the apical infundibular enamel cup is always fully intact.[15] Other investigators have also supported the possibility of an apical blood supply to the infundibula.[2,70,71] Carious destruction of infundibular cement and enamel has been demonstrated histologically.[17]

Etiology of infundibular lesions

Proposed developmental etiology In the developing equine tooth, enamel needs to be laid down fully and then partially resorbed, before cementogenesis can commence.[67,72,73] Amelogenesis spreads from the top of the future occlusal surface in

Table 2
Modified Honma system for grading infundibular caries

Caries Grade	Description
0	No evidence of caries on a macroscopic level. May include hypoplastic tissue
1	Caries of infundibular cementum only
1 (i)	Small darkly pitting superficial spot
1 (ii)	Extensive destruction and loss of cementum
2	Carious infundibular cementum and infundibular enamel
3	Carious infundibular cementum, infundibular enamel and dentine
4	Integrity of the whole tooth is affected, ie, it has fractured

Adapted from Honma K, Yamakawa M, Yamauchi S, et al. Statistical study on the occurrence of dental caries of domestic animals. Jpn J Vet Res 1962;10:31–6; and Dacre IT. Equine dental pathology. In: Baker GJ, Easley J, editors. Equine dentistry. 2nd edition. Philadelphia: Elsevier Saunders; 2005. p. 102–4.

an apical direction, hence the initial cementogenic stimulus will be near the future occlusal surface. The area in the central apical portion of infundibular cement will be the last area in the infundibulum to encounter the cementogenic stimulus traveling in the occlusal to apical direction. This fact may explain the high prevalence of hypoplasia in the apical region of maxillary infundibula. Although the 09 tooth germ is partially mineralized at 275 days of gestation,[74] it is possible, as it emerges in advance of the other permanent teeth, that it has not had time to fully deposit cement in the apical region of its infundibulum. The 09 tooth may subsequently be prone to more extensive infundibular hypoplasia, leaving it more vulnerable to carious damage when this hypoplastic area is eventually exposed through attrition. This hypothesis may explain the dramatic overrepresentation of more severe caries in maxillary 09 teeth of older dental ages that has been repeatedly found in many different studies.[15,19,23,28] Further anatomic or tomographic studies of the 09 maxillary teeth of very young horses are necessary to confirm this.

Managemental etiology If there are foodstuffs trapped within or around the tooth that contain simple carbohydrates, favorable conditions for cariogenic bacteria exist. Caries is reported to be rare in wild equids and in horses fed exclusively on hay-based diets.[46,75] Feeding high levels of silage with added acid, as well as processed maize feedstuffs, has been associated with outbreaks of severe generalized equine caries.[76] High levels of caries found in a population of Swedish horses were also believed to be associated with feeding of haylage.[65] The feeding of mollassed feed grains and grasses with high levels of fructans may also explain the higher levels of caries in domestic equids.

Fibrous foodstuffs rather than pellets also provide the horse with more opportunity to clear food from around their teeth. Mandibular excursion during chewing is greater with hay than with pellets.[77] With a normal dentition, chewing hay to create an appropriate bolus to swallow takes longer than for pellets, allowing greater production of saliva and movement to clear entrapped food from around the teeth, thus reducing the chances for caries to form. However, contrary to this, if a horse has diastemata, hay may become entrapped and make the problem worse, calling for alternative considerations. Painful lesions in the horse's mouth, such as periodontal disease or mucosal trauma from points on the teeth, may also predispose to reduced chewing movement, food pocketing, and caries.

Clinical significance

Extension and coalescence of rostral and caudal infundibular caries is suspected to cause midline fractures of the maxillary cheek teeth of horses.[78] This fracture configuration makes up 16% to 17% of all idiopathic fractures of equine cheek teeth.[25,79] It is also the fracture configuration most commonly associated with clinical signs of pulpitis.[79] In a study of 57 maxillary cheek teeth with pulpitis, infundibular caries was the proposed route of infection of the pulp in 16% of the teeth.[17] However, prevalences of up to 79% of infundibular caries in older horses were found in an abattoir study of skulls.[28] Furthermore, no direct relationship between infundibular lesions and apical pathologic changes could be ascertained from a study of computed tomographs from 17 horses, with the prevalence of infundibular lesions being high in both normal and apically diseased teeth.[7] The investigators did note higher prevalences of both infundibular and apical lesions in maxillary 09s, however. A question mark remains over the clinical significance of many infundibular lesions; however, those in the maxillary 09 teeth are often more severe than those in other teeth, and appear to be more frequently clinically significant.

DENTAL FRACTURES
Prevalence of Dental Fractures

Trauma, especially in the case of kicks near the more rostral mandibular cheek teeth, can result in dental fractures above or below the gingival margin. The American Veterinary Dental College classification of dental fractures is shown in **Table 1** of the article by Earley and Rawlinson elsewhere in this issue. Idiopathic fractures of the cheek teeth can also occur without any history of trauma.

The estimated prevalence of idiopathic fractures of equine cheek teeth observed by first-opinion veterinarians and technicians ranges from 0.07% to 5.9%. As many of these fractures are not associated with overt clinical signs and their observation requires careful oral examination, this estimate is likely to be lower than the true prevalence.[25] The most common fracture configurations are buccal slab fractures through both buccal pulp horns in maxillary cheek teeth, followed by sagittal fractures through both maxillary infundibula (**Figs. 13** and **14**). Mandibular cheek teeth may also have buccal slab fractures or fracture patterns going through various combinations of the mandibular pulp horns (**Fig. 15**). The maxillary 09 is the one most commonly afflicted by fractures.[25,50,78,79]

Clinical Relevance of Idiopathic Fractures of the Cheek Teeth

The most common clinical problem caused by cheek-tooth fractures is oral pain caused by mucosal trauma or food pocketing, and periodontitis around the fractured tooth (see **Fig. 14**).[79] It is remarkable that many fractures that traverse through pulp horns do not result in signs of pulpitis or apical disease.[25,79] Generalized pulpar exposure indicating pulp insult and signs of apical disease occur more commonly with maxillary sagittal fractures.[79]

Pathology of Cheek-Tooth Fractures

Buccal slab fractures
Only 25% of teeth with fractures had evidence of long-term cessation of dentine production, and these were thought to be the result of, rather than the cause of, the

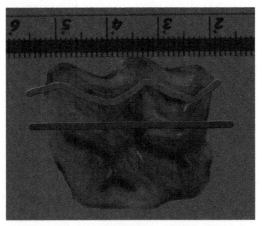

Fig. 13. Occlusal surface of a maxillary cheek tooth, with representations of the most common maxillary cheek-tooth fracture configurations using data from Dacre and colleagues.[78] The pink line represents buccal slab fractures through the buccal pulp horns, the most common configuration. The blue line represents sagittal fractures through both infundibula.

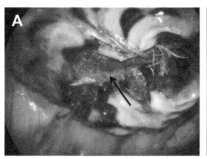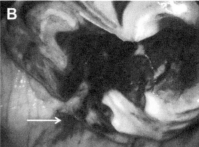

Fig. 14. (A) An oral endoscopic image of a maxillary 11 tooth with a buccal slab fracture. Food is impacted within the fracture (*black arrow*). (B) When the food has been cleared away, trauma to the soft tissue caudal to the fracture is evident (*white arrow*). (*Courtesy of* Dr Jack Easley, DVM, MS, DABVP, Shelbyville, KY.)

fracture.[78] Buccal slab fractures are also less likely than other fracture types to be associated with pulpar exposure,[50] although this discounts weakened or defective dentine as a possible cause of for these slab fractures. No conclusive cause for fractures through the pulp chambers has been ascertained. However, it is postulated that they may be sites of anatomic weakness that are more vulnerable to fracturing under masticatory forces.[78] Ultrastructural examination clarified that caries did not play a major role in these fractures.[78] While some of these fractures result in apical disease[79] many do not, reflecting a remarkable performance of the equine dentine-pulp complex in walling off the oral environment subsequent to the fracture.

Maxillary sagittal fractures
Severely carious infundibula coalesce to form sagittal fractures of maxillary cheek teeth,[78] linking the etiology of this disease to that proposed for severe infundibular

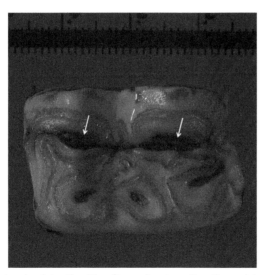

Fig. 15. A mandibular cheek tooth with a fissure line traveling through both buccal dentinal areas (*white arrows*). It is unknown why these fissures occur; they may progress to a buccal slab fracture.

caries discussed earlier. The maxillary 09 teeth are especially prone to this fracture configuration. Sagittally fractured teeth are more likely to be associated with apical disease than other fracture configurations.[79]

NEOPLASIA OF THE DENTAL AND ORAL TISSUES

Neoplasia is rare in the equine oral cavity, but must be borne in mind as a possible differential for loose or displaced teeth, mandibular, maxillary, or other cranial swellings, facial distortion, noise while breathing, or nasal discharge.

Classification of Neoplasms of Dental Origin

In the embryo, the equine dentition is formed from an initial dental lamina lining the developing oral cavity. The dental lamina is folds of ectoderm filled with underlying tissue that has undergone ectomesenchymal transformation. As the tooth germs develop, the dental lamina breaks up. Remnants of the fragmented dental lamina may sometimes persist to cause dental cysts, supernumerary teeth, or tumors of dental tissue.[55]

Tumors of equine dental tissues are classified based on the embryonic germ layer from which they are derived: ectoderm (ameloblasts) or mesoderm (odontoblasts), or both. Tumors are also classified based on the ability of the neoplastic tissues to induce changes in the tissues around them, and whether the tumor is benign, locally aggressive, or malignant.

Examples of Tumors of Dental Origin

An ameloblastoma is the most commonly reported tumor of the dental tissues in the mandible.[80] It is benign but locally invasive, and is characterized histologically by palisades of epithelial cells. It has no inductive effect on surrounding tissues, but commonly distorts the mandible and can result in multiple loose teeth. Other tumors of dental origin, such as complex odontomas (benign) or ameloblastic odontomas (locally invasive), have inductive effects on the surrounding tissues and may be associated with enamel or dentine production. Cementomas are benign, and commonly occur in association with the cheek-tooth apices. It is difficult to differentiate them from the proliferative reaction of the cementoblasts to insult, which also manifests as extra cement deposited around the apex or reserve crown (**Fig. 16**).

Tumors of Nondental Tissues in the Oral Cavity

Although ossifying fibromas are more regularly encountered than other tumors in the rostral mandible of young horses, osteomas, osteofibromas, and osteosarcomas have all been reported.[80]

Soft-tissue carcinomas and adenomas or pharyngeal lymphomas can occur in the mouth and sinuses (**Fig. 17**).[81,82] Many of tumors that have been reported are locally aggressive. Except for some benign fibrous and osseous tumors, they carry a poor prognosis.[81]

Nonneoplastic Growths

Nonneoplastic growths in the head unassociated with dental tissue

Epithelial-lined cysts in the head may be classified by their type of lining into dermoid cysts, dental residue cysts, or cysts lined by respiratory epithelium.[81] The latter occur more commonly than the other types, and mostly in the paranasal sinuses.[81,83,84] These cysts may expand and cause facial deformity and sinusitis resulting from impaired drainage, but respond well to excision.[83,85] Progressive ethmoid hematomas

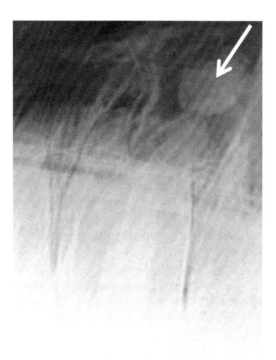

Fig. 16. A lateral-30° dorsal to lateral radiograph of the apex of a maxillary cheek tooth. This tooth had no clinically evident abnormality, but there is extracemental deposition near the caudal aspect of its apex (*white arrow*), sometimes termed a cementoma or cementosis.

are understood to be a discrete entity from respiratory lined cysts, and are most commonly associated with the ethmoid turbinates within the nasal cavity or the paranasal sinuses. These hematomas are encapsulated, are associated with progressive hemorrhage and chronic inflammatory changes, and may cause serosanguinous nasal discharge.[83,84]

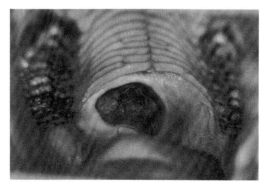

Fig. 17. A squamous cell carcinoma of the soft palate. This horse presented with halitosis and a malodorous nasal discharge. Though much rarer than dental pathologic conditions, neoplasia must be borne in mind as a possible differential for clinical signs relating to the oral cavity, head, and upper respiratory tract.

Nonneoplastic growths associated with dental tissue

The term "dental cyst" is sometimes used to refer to the physiologic mandibular and maxillary remodeling around the developing apices and lengthening reserve crowns of the cheek teeth in young horses. Abnormal cysts derived from dental tissue, or dentigerous cysts, may rarely occur. These cysts are commonly located in the temporal region, are associated with discharging tracts, and may be unilateral or bilateral. Partially or fully developed cheek teeth may be present within the cyst, and salivary tissue has also been reported.[86,87] These cysts are likely to be derived from aberrant fragments of the embryonic dental lamina (ectoderm and ectomesenchyme).[55] It is unknown why the temporal region is a site of predisposition for these cysts, although it may be associated with the dynamics of the developing stomatodeum and head structure at the time of dental laminar fragmentation.

DENTAL OVERGROWTHS AND ORAL MUCOSAL ULCERATION
Overview of Dental Overgrowths

Areas of reduced dental attrition commonly occur on opposing missing teeth, worn teeth in aged horses, dysplastic teeth, broken teeth, and diastemata, or as a consequence of cheek-tooth malocclusion (eg, the maxillary cheek-tooth rows lying further rostrally than the mandibular rows). An overgrowth opposing a diastema may confound periodontal disease by further impacting food into the interproximal area (**Fig. 18**).

Proposed Etiology for Oral Mucosal Ulceration and Recent Research on This Topic

It is believed that horses with painful oral lesions or those on a diet low in forage[77] have less lateral excursion of their mandibles during the masticatory cycle, and subsequently have less attrition on the lingual corners of their mandibular teeth and the buccal corners of their maxillary teeth. Conventionally, these sharp corners were thought to cause buccal mucosal and lingual ulcers (**Fig. 19**). However, free-living horses are reported to have as many enamel points as those that are stabled,[88] and an anatomic survey has reported the range of the normal occlusal angle for the cheek teeth to be much more variable than was originally thought.[13] A recent case-control study has shown that horses that were ridden in bridles had more ulcers opposite their 06 teeth and lips than those that were not bridled.[14] It is likely that the bit, noseband, and cheek-pieces of the bridle are important in the etiology of some cases of oral ulceration.

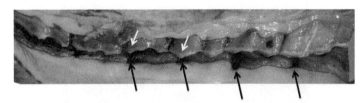

Fig. 18. Opposing mandibular and maxillary cheek-teeth rows (in the masticatory "power stroke" position) in a cadaver. There are multiple diastemata between the mandibular cheek teeth (*black arrows*). The teeth opposing the diastemata have areas of reduced attrition (*white arrows*), which are taller than the surrounding dentition and increase the impaction of food into the diastemata.

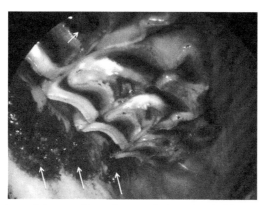

Fig. 19. An oral endoscopic image of buccal mucosal ulceration (*white arrows*) adjacent to the caudal maxillary cheek teeth. (*Courtesy of* Dr Jack Easley, DVM, MS, DABVP, Shelbyville, KY.)

SUMMARY

Recent anatomic and pathologic work in equine dentistry has broadened the spectrum of what is considered anatomic variation rather than abnormality. Periodontal disease is increasingly being recognized as an important dental disorder in the horse. However, new insights into the regenerative capacity of the equine periodontium are being gained. Caries, pulpitis, and idiopathic dental fractures are also important. There have been new insights into the etiology and pathogenesis of these disorders.

ACKNOWLEDGMENTS

The processing and photography of pathologic material for many of the images in this review were greatly facilitated by the support of Bob Brafield, Donna Harraway, Andy Phillips, Sheila Jones, and Andy Skuse of the University of Bristol's Department of Veterinary Pathology, and Tracey Dewey and John Conibear from the photography department. Professor Geoff Pearson gave much guidance on the interpretation of histopathologic sections. Miriam Casey's clinical training scholarship in equine dentistry was generously funded by the Horse Trust. Mr Henry Tremaine supervised Miriam Casey's Clinical Training Scholarship and gave valuable advice on many aspects of equine dental pathology and clinical treatment.

REFERENCES

1. Floyd MR. The modified Triadan system: nomenclature for veterinary dentistry. J Vet Dent 1991;8:18–9.
2. Windley Z, Weller R, Tremaine WH, et al. Two-dimensional and three-dimensional computer tomographic anatomy of the enamel, infundibulae and pulp of 126 equine cheek teeth. Part 1: findings in teeth without macroscopic occlusal or computer tomographic lesions. Equine Vet J 2009;41:433–40.
3. Windley Z, Weller R, Tremaine WH, et al. Two-dimensional and three-dimensional computer tomographic anatomy of the enamel, infundibulae and pulp of 126 equine cheek teeth. Part 2: findings in teeth with macroscopic occlusal or computer tomographic lesions. Equine Vet J 2009;41:433–40, 441–7.
4. Ramzan P. Cheek tooth malocclusions and periodontal disease. Equine Vet Educ 2010;22:445–50.

5. Lupke M, Gardemin M, Kopke S, et al. - Finite element analysis of the equine periodontal ligament under masticatory loading. (special issue: motion analysis in animals). Wien Tierarztl Monatsschr 2010;97:101–6.

6. Henninger W, Frame EM, Willmann M, et al. CT features of alveolitis and sinusitis in horses. Vet Radiol Ultrasound 2003;44:269–76.

7. Veraa S, Voorhout G, Klein WR. Computed tomography of the upper cheek teeth in horses with infundibular changes and apical infection. Equine Vet J 2009;41: 872–6.

8. Tremaine WH. Dental endoscopy in the horse. Clin Tech Equine Pract 2005;4: 181–7.

9. Simhofer H, Griss R, Zetner K. The use of oral endoscopy for detection of cheek teeth abnormalities in 300 horses. Vet J 2008;178:396–404.

10. Ramzan PH, Palmer L. Occlusal fissures of the equine cheek tooth: prevalence, location and association with disease in 91 horses referred for dental investigation. Equine Vet J 2010;42:124–8.

11. Ramzan PH, Palmer L. The incidence and distribution of peripheral caries in the cheek teeth of horses and its association with diastemata and gingival recession. Vet J 2011;190:90–3.

12. DuToit N, Burden FA, Kempson SA, et al. Pathological investigation of caries and occlusal pulpar exposure in donkey cheek teeth using computerised axial tomography with histological and ultrastructural examinations. Vet J 2008; 178(3):387–95.

13. Brown SL, Arkins S, Shaw DJ, et al. Occlusal angles of cheek teeth in normal horses and horses with dental disease. Vet Rec 2008;162:807–10.

14. Tell A, Egenvall A, Lundström T, et al. The prevalence of oral ulceration in Swedish horses when ridden with bit and bridle and when unridden. Vet J 2008;178: 405–10.

15. Fitzgibbon CM, Du Toit N, Dixon PM. Anatomical studies of maxillary cheek teeth infundibula in clinically normal horses. Equine Vet J 2010;42:37–43.

16. Dacre IT, Kempson S, Dixon PM. Pathological studies of cheek teeth apical infections in the horse: 4. Aetiopathological findings in 41 apically infected mandibular cheek teeth. Vet J 2008;178:341–51.

17. Dacre I, Kempson S, Dixon PM. Pathological studies of cheek teeth apical infections in the horse: 5. Aetiopathological findings in 57 apically infected maxillary cheek teeth and histological and ultrastructural findings. Vet J 2008; 178:352–63.

18. Cox A, Dixon P, Smith S. Histopathological lesions associated with equine periodontal disease. Vet J 2012;194(3):386–91.

19. Wafa NS. A study of dental disease in the horse [MVM thesis, University College Dublin. MVM]. Ireland: University College Dublin; 1988.

20. Brigham EJ, Duncanson GR. An equine post-mortem dental study: 50 cases. Equine Vet Educ 2000;12:59–62.

21. Peters JE, de Boer B, Broezeten-Voorde GB, et al. Survey of common dental abnormalities in 483 horses in the Netherlands. Proceedings, American Association of Equine Practitioners, AAEP Focus Meeting, 2006, Indianapolis, IN, USA. Indianapolis (IN): 2006. Available at: www.ivis.org. Accessed July 15th, 2013.

22. Baker GJ. A study of dental disease in the horse. PhD. University of Glasgow; 1979.

23. Vlaminck L, Desmet P, Steenhaut M, et al. Dental disease in the horse: a survey on 283 equine skulls. Proceedings, Tenth Annual Scientific Meeting of the European College of Veterinary Surgeons. Velbert (Germany): 2001:213–5.

24. Uhlinger C. Survey of selected dental abnormalities in 233 horses. Proceedings, 33rd Annual Convention of the American Association of Equine Practitioners. 1987. Available at: www.ivis.org.
25. Taylor L, Dixon PM. Equine idiopathic cheek teeth fractures: Part 2: a practice-based survey of 147 affected horses in Britain and Ireland. Equine Vet J 2007; 39:322–6.
26. Dixon PM, Tremaine WH, Pickles K, et al. Equine dental disease part 4: a long-term study of 400 cases: apical infections of cheek teeth. Equine Vet J 2000;32: 182–94.
27. Dixon PM, Tremaime WH, Pickles K, et al. Equine dental disease part 2: a long term study of 400 cases: disorders of development and eruption and variations of position of the cheek teeth. Equine Vet J 1999;31:519–28.
28. Baker GJ. Some aspects of equine dental disease. Equine Vet J 1970;2:105–10.
29. Dixon PM, Barakzai S, Collins N, et al. Treatment of equine cheek teeth by mechanical widening of diastemata in 60 horses (2000-2006). Equine Vet J 2008;40:22–8.
30. Walker H, Chinn E, Holmes S, et al. Prevalence and some clinical characteristics of equine cheek teeth diastemata in 471 horses examined in a UK first-opinion equine practice (2008 to 2009). Vet Rec 2012;171:44.
31. Klugh D. Equine periodontal disease. Clin Tech Equine Pract 2005;4:135–47.
32. Huthmann S, Staszyk C, Jacob HG, et al. Biomechanical evaluation of the equine masticatory action: calculation of the masticatory forces occurring on the cheek tooth battery. J Biomech 2009;42:67–70.
33. Casey MB, Tremaine WH. Dental diastemata and periodontal disease second-ary to axially rotated maxillary cheek teeth in three horses. Equine Vet Educ 2010;22:439–44.
34. Quinn GC, Tremaine WH, Lane JG. Supernumerary cheek teeth (n = 24): clinical features, diagnosis, treatment and outcome in 15 horses. Equine Vet J 2005;37: 505–9.
35. Collins NM, Dixon PM. Diagnosis and management of equine diastemata [Special issue: Equine dentistry]. Clin Tech Equine Pract 2005;4:148–54.
36. Vlaminck L. Post-extraction molariform tooth drift and alveolar grafting in horses. PhD. Universiteit Gent; 2007.
37. Townsend NB, Dixon PM, Barakzai SZ. Evaluation of the long-term oral conse-quences of equine exodontia in 50 horses. Vet J 2008;178:419–24.
38. Carmalt JL. Understanding the equine diastema. Equine Vet Educ 2003;15: 34–5.
39. Hawkes CS, Easley J, Barakzai SZ, et al. Treatment of oromaxillary fistulae in nine standing horses (2002-2006). Equine Vet J 2008;40:546–51.
40. Mensing N, Gasse H, Hambruch N, et al. Isolation and characterization of multi-potent mesenchymal stromal cells from the gingiva and the periodontal ligament of the horse. BMC Vet Res 2011;7:42.
41. Staszyk C, Bienert-Zeit A. The equine periodontium: the (re)model tissue. Vet J 2012;194(3):280–1.
42. Dixon PM, Dacre I. A review of equine dental disorders. Vet J 2005;169:165–87.
43. Dacre IT. A pathological, histological and ultrastructural study of diseased equine cheek teeth. PhD. The University of Edinburgh; 2004.
44. Crabill MR, Schumacher J. Pathophysiology of acquired dental diseases of the horse. Vet Clin North Am Equine Pract 1998;14:291–307.
45. Mueller PO, Lowder MQ. Dental sepsis. Vet Clin North Am Equine Pract 1998; 14:349–63.

46. Miles AE, Grigson C. Colyer's variation and diseases of the teeth of animals. Revised edition. Cambridge (United Kingdom): Cambridge University Press; 1990.

47. Mackintosh ME, Colles CM. Anaerobic bacteria associated with dental abscesses in the horse and donkey. Equine Vet J 1987;19:360–2.

48. Bienert A, Bartmann CP, Verspohl J, et al. Bacteriological findings for endodontical and apical molar dental diseases in the horse. Dtsch Tierarztl Wochenschr 2003;110:358–61 [in German].

49. Baker GJ. Dental disease in horses. Practice 1979;1:19–26.

50. van den Enden MS, Dixon PM. Prevalence of occlusal pulpar exposure in 110 equine cheek teeth with apical infections and idiopathic fractures. Vet J 2008; 178:364–71.

51. Nair PN. Pathobiology of primary apical periodontitis. In: Cohen S, Hargreaves KM, editors. Pathways of the pulp, vol. Philadelphia: Mosby Elsevier; 2006. p. 541–79.

52. Orstavic D, Pitt Ford TR. Apical periodontitis: microbial infection and host responses. In: Orstavic D, Pitt Ford TR, editors. Essential endodontology: prevention and treatment of apical periodontitis. London: Blackwell; 2007. Chapter 1. p. 1–9.

53. Gier RE, Mitchell DF. Anachoretic effect of pulpitis. J Dent Res 1968;47:564–70.

54. Moller AJ, Fabricus L, Dahlen G, et al. Influence on periapical tissues of indigenous oral bacteria and necrotic pulp tissue in monkeys. Eur J Oral Sci 1981;89: 475–84.

55. Nanci A. Ten Cate's oral histology. 7th edition. Philadelphia: Mosby Elsevier; 2008.

56. Casey MB, Tremaine WH. The prevalence of secondary dentinal lesions in cheek teeth from horses with clinical signs of pulpitis compared to controls. Equine Vet J 2010;42:32–6.

57. Ramzan PL, Palmer L, Barquero N, et al. Chronology and sequence of emergence of permanent premolar teeth in the horse: study of deciduous premolar 'cap' removal in Thoroughbred racehorses. Equine Vet J 2009;41:107–11.

58. Berman LH, Hartwell GR. Diagnosis. In: Cohen S, Hargreaves KM, editors. Pathways of the pulp, vol., 9th edition. Philadelphia: Mosby Elsevier; 2006. p. 21–3.

59. Edwards GB. Retention of permanent cheek teeth in 3 horses. Equine Vet Educ 1993;5:299–302.

60. Tremaine WH, McCluskie LK. Removal of 11 incompletely erupted, impacted cheek teeth in 10 horses using a dental alveolar transcortical osteotomy and buccotomy approach. Vet Surg 2010;39:884–90.

61. Martin TM. American Association of Equine Practitioners guide for determining the age of the horse. Lexington (KY): 2002.

62. Casey MB. Occlusal findings in 44 cheek-teeth extracted from horses with clinical signs of pulpitis. MSc. University of Bristol; 2011.

63. Casey MB, Pearson GR, Perkins JD, et al. Pathological and CT findings in mandibular cheek-teeth extracted from horses with pulpitis. Proceedings, British Equine Veterinary Association Annual Congress. Liverpool (United Kingdom): p. 179.

64. Dacre IT, Shaw DJ, Dixon PM. Pathological studies of cheek teeth apical infections in the horse: 3. Quantitative measurements of dentine in apically infected cheek teeth. Vet J 2008;178:333–40.

65. Gere I, Dixon PM. Post mortem survey of peripheral dental caries in 510 Swedish horses. Equine Vet J 2010;42:310–5.

66. Casey MB, Tremaine WH. The prevalence of secondary dentinal lesions in cheek teeth from horses with clinical signs of pulpitis compared to controls. Equine Vet J 2009;41:30–6.

67. Kilic S, Dixon PM, Kempson SA. A light microscopic and ultrastructural examination of calcified dental tissues of horses. 4. Cement and the amelocemental junction. Equine Vet J 1997;29:213–9.
68. Honma K, Yamakawa M, Yamauchi S, et al. Statistical study on the occurrence of dental caries of domestic animals. Jpn J Vet Res 1962;10:31–6.
69. Soames JV, Southam JC. Dental caries. In: Soames JV, Southam JC, editors. Oral pathology, vol., 3rd edition. Oxford (United Kingdom): Oxford University Press; 1998. p. 21–35.
70. Dacre IT. Equine dental pathology. In: Baker GJ, Easley J, editors. Equine dentistry. 2nd edition. Elsevier Saunders; 2005. p. 102–4.
71. Johnson TJ, Porter CM. Infundibular caries. Proceedings, 52nd Annual Convention of the American Association of Equine Practitioners, Indianapolis, USA, 2006. Available at: www.ivis.org.
72. Jones SJ, Boyde A. Coronal cementogenesis in the horse. Arch Oral Biol 1974; 19:605–10.
73. Sahara N, Moriyama K, Ozawa H. Coronal cementogenesis in the teeth of the horse. Proceedings, 81st General Session of the International Association for Dental Research, Goteborg. Sweden. June 25–28, 2003. Available at: http://iadr.confex.com/iadr/2003Goteborg/techprogram/abstract_28489.htm.
74. Soana S, Gnudi G, Bertoni G. The teeth of the horse: evolution and anatomo-morphological and radiographic study of their development in the foetus. Anat Histol Embryol 1999;28:273–80.
75. Maslauskas K, Tulamo RM, McGowan T, et al. Dental examination findings in two groups of Lithuanian horses with no history of dental prophylaxis or treatment. Veterinarija Ir Zootechnika 2009;47:60–5.
76. Dixon PM, du Toit N, Dacre IT. Equine dental pathology. In: Easley KJ, Dixon PM, Schumacher J, editors. Equine dentistry, vol., 3rd edition. Edinburgh (United Kingdom): Elsevier Saunders; 2010.
77. Bonin SJ, Clayton HM, Lanovaz JL, et al. Comparison of mandibular motion in horses chewing hay and pellets. Equine Vet J 2007;39:258–62.
78. Dacre IT, Kempson S, Dixon PM. Equine idiopathic cheek teeth fractures. Part 1: pathological studies on 35 fractured cheek teeth. Equine Vet J 2007;39:310–8.
79. Dixon PM, Barakzai SZ, Collins NM, et al. Equine idiopathic cheek teeth fractures: part 3: a hospital-based survey of 68 referred horses (1999-2005). Equine Vet J 2007;39:327–32.
80. Pirie RS, Dixon PM. Mandibular tumours in the horse: a review of the literature and 7 case reports. Equine Vet Educ 1993;5:287–94.
81. Head KW, Dixon PM. Equine nasal and paranasal sinus tumours. Part 1: review of the literature and tumour classification. Vet J 1999;157:261–78.
82. Dixon PM, Head KW. Equine nasal and paranasal sinus tumours: part 2: a contribution of 28 case reports. Vet J 1999;157:279–94.
83. Tremaine WH, Dixon PM. A long-term study of 277 cases of equine sinonasal disease. Part 1: details of horses, historical, clinical and ancillary diagnostic findings. Equine Vet J 2001;33:274–82.
84. Tremaine WH, Clarke CJ, Dixon PM. Histopathological findings in equine sinonasal disorders. Equine Vet J 1999;31:296–303.
85. Dixon PM, Parkin TD, Collins N, et al. Equine paranasal sinus disease: a long-term study of 200 cases (1997-2009): treatments and long-term results of treatments. Equine Vet J 2012;44:272–6.
86. Easley JT, Franklin RP, Adams A. Surgical excision of a dentigerous cyst containing two dental structures. Equine Vet Educ 2010;22:275–8.

87. Smith LC, Zedler ST, Gestier S, et al. Bilateral dentigerous cysts (heterotopic polyodontia) in a yearling Standardbred colt. Equine Vet Educ 2012;24: 573–8.
88. Masey O'Neill HV, Keen J, Dumbell L. A comparison of the occurrence of common dental abnormalities in stabled and free-grazing horses. Animal 2010;4: 1697–701.

Oral Examination and Charting
Setting the Basis for Evidence-Based Medicine in the Oral Examination of Equids

Robert Menzies, BVSc

KEYWORDS

- Equine • Dentistry • Oral examination • Dental charting • Evidence-based medicine
- Veterinary • Scientific method • Horse

KEY POINTS

- The tool most in need of improving is the clinician himself/herself.
- Oral examination findings need to be considered in light of the history, health of the whole horse, and results from further diagnostic tests when performed.
- Is a finding normal or abnormal for a particular horse?
- Each case is its own scientific experiment, which therefore requires:
  - A standardized set of material
  - A maneuver
  - An appraisal
- It is important to develop standardized clinimetrics and criteria for recording the oral examination findings and evaluating response to therapy.

INTRODUCTION

Oral examination of the equid is an integral component of assessing oral health. It is essential in the assessment of the equid's overall health, diagnosis of oral problems and conditions, monitoring of oral conditions and oral health, and evaluation of therapeutic effectiveness of any treatments performed (**Fig. 1**). By itself, the findings from the oral examination are relatively meaningless without being interpreted in light of the horse's history, overall health, and results of ancillary tests when indicated. Findings from the oral examination require appropriate documentation and interpretation. Oral care is complex, and should be administered by knowledgable and appropriately trained clinicians in a scientific manner.

Dentistry & Oral Surgery Service, Veterinary Teaching Hospital, University of Helsinki, PO Box 57, Koetilantie 4, FI-00014, Finland
E-mail address: menziesrobert@hotmail.com

Vet Clin Equine 29 (2013) 325–343
http://dx.doi.org/10.1016/j.cveq.2013.04.008
0749-0739/13/$ – see front matter © 2013 Elsevier Inc. All rights reserved.

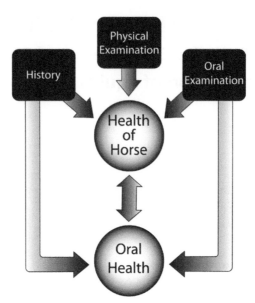

Fig. 1. Oral health cannot be considered without appreciation of the overall health of the animal.

EVIDENCE-BASED MEDICINE

The currently accepted standard of care for patients in human medicine is described under the banner of evidence-based medicine (EBM), a term established in 1992.[1] Proponents of developing similar standards in veterinary medicine adapted the term evidence-based veterinary medicine (EBVM) in 2003.[2] While few would question the benefits of EBVM, implementing it in a fashion similar to that of EBM has been problematic.[3] Five steps have been identified in performing EBM (**Box 1**).[3] EBM has been described as "… the conscientious, explicit, and judicious use of current best evidence in making decisions about the care of individual patients."[4] The best external evidence refers to (though certainly not limited to) systematic research, ideally randomized clinical trials, and meta-analyses, and depends on the type of question being posed (**Table 1**).[3,4] However, this presents a major problem in veterinary medicine: there is insufficient scientific information of adequate quality available to answer

---

Box 1
The 5 steps of evidence-based medicine

1. Form an answerable question
2. Perform a literature search
3. Assess the sources of information for internal validity
4. Integrate the best scientific evidence with clinical expertise and information specific to the patient
5. Critically review decision-making process and outcomes for efficacy and efficiency

Data from Vandeweerd JM, Kirschvink N, Clegg P, et al. Is evidence-based medicine so evident in veterinary research and practice? History, obstacles and perspectives. Vet J 2012;191:28–34.

Table 1
Study design is an important consideration depending on the type of evidence-based medicine question being asked

Question	Study Design
Treatment	Randomized controlled trial
Risk	Retrospective cohort study, case-control study
Frequency	Transversal study (prevalence study)
Diagnosis	Transversal study
Prognosis	Prospective cohort study

From Vandeweerd JM, Kirschvink N, Clegg P, et al. Is evidence-based medicine so evident in veterinary research and practice? History, obstacles and perspectives. Vet J 2012;191:29.

questions for the vast majority of veterinary fields.[3] In equine medicine, well-controlled clinical trials are uncommon[5]; in the subspecialty equine dentistry, they are a rarity.

The concepts of EBM are relevant to veterinary medicine for scientific, medicolegal, economic, and ethical reasons.[6] The practice of equine dentistry, while being one of the oldest fields of veterinary medicine, is one of the least developed and therefore one of the most challenged when it comes to implementing EBVM principles.[7] Despite so little research, clinicians and other people have not tempered their enthusiasm for "doing."[8] This perspective reflects the lack of proper attention that the field has generally received from people with appropriate knowledge and training. Medical convention sees "knowing" as the first step in a long journey toward "doing"; however, equine dentistry has more often reflected an inversion of the concepts reflected in Miller's pyramid (**Fig. 2**).[9,10] In the absence of sufficient information for EBVM in equine dentistry, an ethical and scientific approach is still possible, and indeed should be considered mandatory.

THE ART AND SCIENCE

In common with any branch of clinical medicine, the performance of equine dentistry comprises both art and science. The art refers to how the data are obtained in the clinical setting, such as the history taking, physical examination, and oral examination,

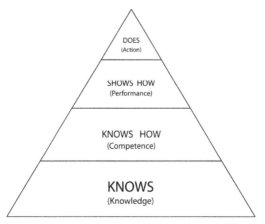

Fig. 2. Miller's framework for clinical assessment. (*From* Miller GE. The assessment of clinical skills/competence/performance. Acad Med 1990;65:S63; with permission.)

and the science for the information gleaned from the laboratory, such as clinical pathology, histopathology, and radiology.[11] Interpreting the data in light of clinical experience has been referred to as "clinical judgment."[12] The science tells the clinician what to examine, and the art provides the method for examination.[13] The art provides the data for the science, and the science provides the reason for the art.[13] To care for the patient and client requires art; to provide therapy in an ethical and scientific manner requires science.[11]

ESTABLISHING A SCIENTIFIC BASIS

The development of a scientific field has been described using the four "Phases of Knowledge": the Age of Experts; the Age of Professionalism; the Age of Science; and the Age of Evidence.[14] The progression of equine dentistry has been recognized to be entering the third phase, the Age of Science, meaning that much of the knowledge in the field is merely the opinion of "experts."[7] It is important that scientific validity and proof be central to the techniques used by those practicing clinical medicine.[11] Good knowledge in the basic sciences such as physiology, microbiology, pharmacology, and biochemistry, and of the data that express these functions in health and in disease, is essential for all clinicians.[11] For those practicing equine dentistry, a good understanding is also necessary in areas such as embryology and development, anatomy, periodontics, endodontics, orthodontics, orthopedics, radiology, and dental materials. As researchers continue to investigate the etiology and pathogenesis of equine oral conditions, clinicians are required to advance the knowledge of prognosis and therapy.[13]

Prognosis and therapy are in the domains of the clinician because they are aspects of oral care that are best studied in the naturally diseased animal.[13] The clinician's skills make him or her the most appropriate tool for gathering data. Meaningful and measurable data need to be collected and disseminated to the profession from clinical cases.[7] Clinical observation has been key in indicating what sort of laboratory investigations may be worthwhile. Conversely, knowledge gained from bench-top research has helped direct what sort of clinical observations may be useful.[15]

ORAL HEALTH AS A SCIENCE

Medical care may be viewed as the endeavor to repeat or surpass the most successful experiments of the past.[16] The thought processes used in both laboratory work and clinical care may be the same; however, the execution of the experiment differs considerably (**Table 2**).[11] Common to both are the principles of scientific method. The "experiment" may be divided into three distinct and essential phases or components (**Table 3**):

1. Preexperimental design
2. Experimental maneuver
3. Appraisal of response[11,16]

1. THE PREEXPERIMENTAL DESIGN

The premaneuver step is necessary to ensure the repeatability of the experiment. It comprises of preparing the subjects, calibrating the apparatus used for measurement (the clinician), and dividing the subjects into treatment and control groups.[13]

In clinical medicine preparation of the subjects (patients) is an intellectual process of classification and the establishment of homogeneous groups.[11] It involves identifying, classifying, and organizing a patient into a group of patients with similar individual

Table 2
Comparisons between the 2 types of "experiments": laboratory-based and clinical care

Component	Laboratory	Clinical Practice
Purpose	To gain new knowledge	To reproduce the best results of previously successful therapeutic experiments To prevent or alter any or all of the entities of disease
Responsible for advances in:	Etiology, pathogenesis, diagnosis, pharmacology, surgery	Prognosis, therapy
Materials	Samples from patient	Patient
Material preparation	Scientist prepares "diseased" material from "healthy" material. Is able to reproduce process	No physical preparation: patient comes with naturally occurring disease. Preparation of material is an intellectual one of classification and ordering
Tools	Various laboratory equipment	Clinician, clinical skills
Calibration of tools/apparatus	Data accurately measured using apparatus precisely calibrated and standardized Apparatus and techniques used for preparation of material usually differ from those used to observe the result Essential	Same degree of precision and accuracy not possible Same "tool" used to determine the material as to assess its outcome, ie, the clinician Much more challenging
Division of material	Inanimate material can be physically divided into identical parts	Naturally diseased patients are divided into similar, comparable groups
Method of observation	Particular to the experiment	Clinical examination
Period of observation	Usually short	Usually extended
Environment	Laboratory	Clinic
Methodology of acquiring and arranging numbers	Measure and equate	Classify and count
Data	Describes the disease Based on measurement	Describes the diseased patient Based on descriptions: signs, symptoms, and individual data
Maneuver	Uncompromising	May have to be modified or countermanded by many patient factors
Identification of cause	Looks at the maneuvers	Considers both: 1. The effect of the maneuvers 2. Original cause of the disease

Data from Feinstein AR. Scientific methodology in clinical medicine. III. The evaluation of therapeutic response. Ann Intern Med 1964;61:944–65.

Table 3
Clinical care portrayed in the 3 essential components of an experiment

The Experimental Design	The Experimental Maneuver	The Appraisal of Response
Pretreatment	Treatment	Posttreatment
The arrangement of material (patients)	Best to treat one problem at a time if possible	Successful treatment of the primary cause usually results in resolve of secondary problems
Purely intellectual techniques of identification and classification	Treatment to be as specific as possible	
To group patients of similar individual characteristics, with the same disease, and similar clinical symptoms and signs	Initial treatment may target both symptomatic and causal components	Successful treatment/ resolution of primary problem does not require ongoing treatment
Allows for reproducibility of the experiment		Treatment of only secondary effects and not the primary cause requires ongoing treatment
Allows for the determination of prognosis		
Allows establishment of criteria used in the appraisal for success/ failure		
Propose what abnormalities are primary (causal) and what are secondary		

Data from Feinstein AR. Scientific methodology in clinical medicine. I. Introduction, principles, and concepts. Ann Intern Med 1964;61:564–79; and Feinstein AR. Scientific methodology in clinical medicine. III. The evaluation of therapeutic response. Ann Intern Med 1964;61:944–65.

data, disease, and illness (**Fig. 3**).[11] Once done it allows for therapy that has been performed on similar cases in the past to be provided, and enables a prognosis to be made based on the outcomes of the previous "experiments". The disease is defined by data from laboratory analysis (eg, histopathology, clinical pathology); the illness is the effect of the disease on the host and is described in terms of clinical findings.[11,17] To identify the subject and ensure that it is placed in the right group, the patient, the disease, and the illness all need to be identified. In patients with similar individual data and laboratory information, and the same disease, it is the clinical features that differentiate the groups further, and help determine prognosis and aid selection of appropriate therapy. Examples of clinical features that may differentiate patients include:

- Patterns of symptoms
- Severity of illness
- Effects of comorbid conditions
- Timing of phenomena
- Rate of progression of illness
- Functional capacity
- Other clinical distinctions[18]

The maneuver is the intervention applied to the homogeneous group of subjects. In clinical medicine, it is the treatment used by the clinician to intervene in the natural course of the disease and resulting illness.[16] Ideally this should be a single intervention

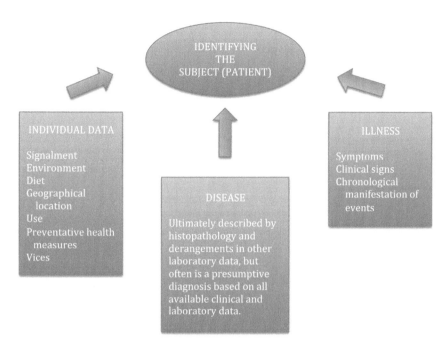

Fig. 3. Types of data necessary to appropriately categorize the patient. (*Data from* Feinstein AR. Scientific methodology in clinical medicine. III. The evaluation of therapeutic response. Ann Intern Med 1964;61:944–65.)

that is as specific as possible to allow for more effective appraisal. Often in clinical medicine the initial treatments will involve a component to treat the disease and a component to treat the symptoms. Concomitant disease may also require treatment. Before instigating a maneuver it is essential that the clinician understands the natural course of the disease, and therefore knows what he or she are trying to achieve by intervening.[11] Criteria for success, indifference, and failure, and an appropriate time frame for reappraisal, should be clearly established before treatment. In many instances where the natural course is not understood, ongoing monitoring without immediate intervention may be more prudent and in the animal's best interests.

The postmaneuver appraisal determines the effect of the maneuver on the subjects and is assessed using predetermined criteria. The dynamic and complex nature of the equid oral cavity, while posing significant challenges in identifying the primary cause, often displays many secondary changes that may resolve on successful treatment of the primary cause. An overview of the process of clinical care is given in **Fig. 4.**

A SCIENTIFIC APPROACH TO THE DATA

The first step in collecting the data is to appreciate how the data may be used at the end. The data need to be collected and used in a scientific manner that allows for its reproduction and critique. For this to occur the data need to be objective, precise, consistent, uniform, and reliable.[13] Different types of clinical data are displayed in **Tables 4** and **5.**

Objectivity

Objectivity is primarily a function of the mind-set of the clinician.[13] It is important that the facts from the history-taking process and evidence from the clinical examination

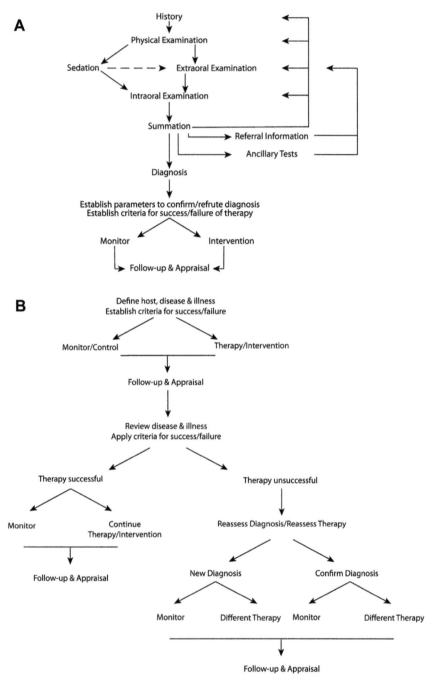

Fig. 4. The process of clinical care for equine dentistry. (*A*) The process for an individual visit of a case. (*B*) The process for the overall management of an individual case.

Table 4
Different types of data recorded in the practice of clinical care

Types of data	Variables expressed as numbers	Direct	Age
			Height
			Weight
			Length
			Body temperature
			Volume
		Indirect measurement	Noninvasive blood pressure
			Size of palpable mass
		Visual approximation	Angulation
		Counting	Pulse
			Respiration
		Semiqualitative gradings	Grade of heart murmur
			Grade of mast cell tumor
		Semiqualitative stages	Periodontal disease
			Tooth mobility
			Staging of tumors
		Semiqualitative indices	Gingival index
			Plaque index
	Major clinical variables not easily translated into numerical form		Color
			Shape
			Tenderness
			Texture
			Pulsation
			Movement
			Alertness
			Cooperation
	Functional clusters		Ability to walk
			Ability to feed
			Ability to perform

Data from Feinstein AR. Scientific methodology in clinical medicine. III. The evaluation of therapeutic response. Ann Intern Med 1964;61:944–65.

are obtained with an open mind, and not in light of how a clinician may expect a condition to present. The clinical findings should be recorded in terms of the raw evidence, in the most descriptive manner possible, and without interpretation. When receiving referral information, the initial examination should be made without knowing the

Table 5
Grading of infundibular caries as adapted by Dacre from Honma and colleagues[31,32]

Grade	Description
Grade 0	No visible caries
Grade 1	Caries of the infundibular cementum
Grade 2	Caries of infundibular cementum and surrounding enamel
Grade 3	Caries of infundibular cementum, enamel, and dentin
Grade 4	Splitting of the tooth as a result of caries
Grade 5	Loss of tooth due to caries

Data from Dacre IT. Equine dental pathology. In: Baker GJ, Easley J, editors. Equine dentistry. 2nd edition. Edinburgh (United Kingdom): WB Saunders; 2005. p. 103.

previous clinician's findings or conclusions, rather just an indication of which area to examine. Once a preliminary impression is formed and a summary made, all information available to the case should be considered before making a final diagnosis.

Precision

The data should be precise- that is, complete and accurate.[11] Clinical features not present but expected should be sought and confirmed as absent. It is imperative that the language used in recording observations is interpreted in the same way by all who may use it. Thus the language used should be consistent across scientific fields and species where possible. Anatomic terms should be consistent with those recorded in the *Nomina Anatomica Veterinaria*.[19] Leading bodies should ensure that there is appropriate and specific nomenclature for the field. The three steps in diagnostic reasoning—description, interpretation, and diagnosis—should be kept separate with notes made to illustrate the process of reasoning.

Consistency

For data to be interpreted in a consistent and, thus, reproducible manner, it must be done so in relation to explicit and specific criteria.[11] Criteria are important for determining abnormal from normal, making a diagnosis, and evaluating the clinical significance of post-therapeutic findings. Examples of criteria established in equine dentistry are given in articles elsewhere in this issue.

Uniformity

The uniformity of quality and of data are important features of the medical record.[11] Some information can be recorded using techniques such as photography or impression models; however, most information is written. Dental charts have been an integral part of the oral examination, ensuring certain information is complete and ordered. Abbreviations for use on dental records have been standardized by the American Veterinary Dental College (AVDC) and should be considered by those performing veterinary dentistry. The equine dental chart, while good at recording aspects of client and animal information, oral findings, and noting treatments performed, has often had insufficient room to record a complete and accurate history, clinimetrics, and measurements associated with each tooth, or to add progress notes that detail subsequent clinical observations, changes in therapy, and reasoning behind changes in therapy. Electronic medical records meet the demands of recording extensive detailed information per patient and facilitate appraisal of data with relative ease. Electronic records are not limited by the number of fields that may be incorporated within them or the amount of information recorded in each field. Advantages in keeping electronic records include: a patient's entire medical history can be readily available, which may include the results of many ancillary tests; data can be readily shared with other clinicians and visit summaries produced for the client; and the data from the various fields can readily be extracted and used in statistical analysis. The benefit of the statistical analysis is always limited by the scientific quality of the data originally entered. Much thought and care is required in the development of such electronic records and the type and quality of data entered.

Reliability

The reproducibility of the acquired data is an important scientific feature.[11] In clinical practice, this facet is challenging. Both the clinician and source of historical information need to be checked for reliability. The clinician needs to be checked against himself or herself and also against other clinicians. To do the latter, the clinician needs to meet with other clinicians and examine the same material to ensure standardization of data. In checking the reliability of the historical information, the clinician needs to carefully check and clarify the information throughout the examination process. The clinician needs to be aware of the bias that each of the sources of historical information brings; for example, the owner versus the trainer versus the rider. Establishing reliable historical information can require great care and tact, and is done throughout the management of the case. Absolute accuracy is rarely obtainable in the data used by the clinician for description, interpretation, and diagnosis; however, the reproducibility of the evidence (ie, the data and reasoning) is the more important feature.[13]

ACQUISITION OF HISTORICAL DATA

The art of acquiring a history that allows appropriate classification of the patient has been defined in two simultaneous processes by the Calgary-Cambridge guides (**Fig. 5**).[20,21] Data obtained through history taking is an essential part of defining the patient, the disease, and the illness. To be useful in diagnosis, prognosis, and therapy, it should include[11]:

1. The precise reason why the patient has presented for examination: the iatrotropic stimulus. In many cases this may be the chief complaint, but in cases where the client perceives no problems, or the problems are of a chronic nature, the stimulus

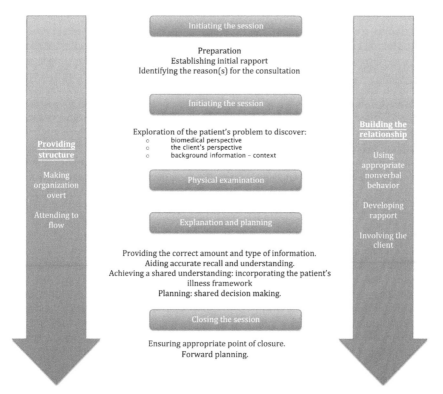

Fig. 5. Marrying content and process in the Calgary-Cambridge guides. (*Adapted from* Kurtz S, Silverman J, Benson J, et al. Marrying content and process in clinical method teaching: enhancing the Calgary-Cambridge guides. Acad Med 2003;78:802–9; with permission.)

for making the appointment should be sought. Use the client's own words to define the iatrotropic stimulus to avoid errors in interpretation.
2. Characterization of the symptoms in a detailed and descriptive manner. Symptoms not spontaneously offered need to be extracted, and symptoms that are expected but missing need clarification that they are indeed absent.
3. The order and timing in which symptoms were noted to occur.
4. The date when the area of concern was last examined and found to be normal. This date is essential for the establishment of "time equal to zero." Without the last known time that the area of interest was normal, the data are incomplete. The performance of examinations and ancillary tests as a matter of routine is to establish a baseline for normal findings, as much as to detect unexpected abnormal findings.

DETERMINATION OF GENERAL HEALTH STATUS OF PATIENT

The general health of the patient is important in defining the host for classification purposes, diagnostic purposes, and the establishment of an appropriate sedative or anesthetic regime to facilitate a thorough oral examination. In addition to the historical data, a general physical examination and possibly ancillary tests are necessary. The problem list needs to be complete and described in the most descriptive terms possible.[22]

FACILITATION OF ORAL EXAMINATION

It is important for the oral examination to be performed in a controlled environment-[23] avoid potential distractions that could stimulate the equid. A dedicated indoor facility is optimal. Reduction of auditory stimuli to the equid may be achieved using ear covers or earplugs.[24] Appropriate ambient lighting is necessary, and good-quality intraoral illumination is essential to enable a thorough oral examination without causing clinician eye strain and fatigue. A task–ambient lighting ratio not exceeding 10 to 1 is recommended[25,26]; for example, good fluorescent ambient lighting and bright fiber-optic halogen task lighting. Flooring needs to have a nonslip surface and be conducive to hospital cleaning standards. Drainage systems need to be well designed to cope with large volumes of urine, fluids and solids from oral and sinus lavage procedures, and oral ingesta. Good head support should be provided to help stabilize the sedated equid and to provide ergonomic positioning of both the patient and the clinician. The head support should be adjustable for the different-sized equids seen by the clinician.

A thorough oral examination requires a compliant patient with relaxed muscles of mastication and of the tongue, so that all aspects may be examined and recorded in a complete and accurate manner. To achieve such a state almost invariably requires appropriate sedation. It may also require local or regional anesthesia, and analgesia. Where severe pain does not allow for a thorough oral examination, instigation of appropriate treatment (which may only be palliative) may be required for a period before being able to perform a thorough oral examination. For instance, a case of very painful periodontal disease may require removal of impacted ingested feed, a dietary change, and a course of anti-inflammatory and antimicrobial medications. A thorough oral examination should be performed as soon as the painful area is more comfortable.

A thorough oral examination should be performed during an interval that allows for detection and possible treatment of abnormalities while they are still of a minor nature. The appropriate interval will vary between individual equids and be dependent on factors such as their stage of development, their anatomy, their use, previous treatments performed, oral conditions present, other historical information, and the clinician's expertise. The first oral examination should be performed at birth for the presence of congenital problems. In an equid without abnormalities, timely examinations following periods of significant development, such as eruption and succession of dentition, are recommended.

EQUIPMENT USED IN PERFORMING THE ORAL EXAMINATION

To perform a thorough oral examination, the equipment must facilitate:

- Easy and safe access to the oral cavity
- Removal of all oral ingesta including any impacted feed between teeth or within periodontal pockets
- Removal of dental calculus that may prevent proper assessment of the underlying tooth and associated periodontal structures
- Good visualization of all oral tooth surfaces and oral mucosal surfaces
- Accurate measurement of periodontal pockets and other defects
- Tactile investigation of periodontal and dental features
- Assessment of tooth mobility
- Specific provocation

Equipment that satisfies the aforementioned criteria and assists in the performance of a thorough oral examination includes:

- Full-mouth oral speculums
- Light source for intraoral illumination
- Oral and periodontal irrigators
- Forceps
- Dental mirrors
- Dental explorers
- Periodontal probes
- Scalers and curettes
- Air syringe

The equipment is commercially available or can be adapted from other areas of dentistry to meet the requirements of the equid oral cavity.

Intraoral cameras and endoscopes are able to provide improved visualization of many dental and oral features. The benefits of rigid endoscopy in aiding the diagnostic process of the oral examination procedure have been demonstrated, and should be considered basic equipment for the oral examination.[27,28]

PROCESS OF ORAL EXAMINATION

Following a general physical examination of the equid to assess its general health, temperament, and determination of an appropriate sedation regime, a closer examination of the structures of the head is performed (**Tables 6** and **7**). The extraoral examination involves: a visual appraisal of soft and hard tissue; palpation of masticatory muscles, salivary glands, lymph nodes, guttural pouches, and bony structures; percussion of sinuses; assessment of nasal odor (in areas where zoonoses, such as Hendravirus, are not suspected to occur); detection of ocular discharge, nasal discharge, or draining tracts; evaluation of vision; and assessment of incisor bite.

Once sedated, reevaluate any areas of concern or areas that were difficult to examine properly in the unsedated animal. Examine visually and by palpation the lips, mucosa of the rostral oral cavity, the rostral bite, incisor and canine teeth, and

Table 6		
Summary of features examined as part of the extraoral examination		
Bony Structures	**Soft-Tissue Structures**	**Sensory Organs**
Contour of skull	Muscles of mastication	Vision
Symmetry of skull	Lymph nodes	Hearing
Conformation of skull	Salivary glands	Response to palpation
Percussion of sinuses	Lips	
	Skin	

anatomic diastemata of the mandible and maxilla. Count the teeth and discern which belong to the deciduous dentition and which to the permanent dentition. Remove any foreign material present. Assess the periodontal characteristics using a periodontal probe, explore the occlusal surfaces with an explorer, and note pertinent anatomic features. Many clinimetric scales and indices routinely used in human and small animal dentistry are yet to be validated and standardized in equids. Although this does not mean that similar measurements and grading should not be performed, it should be written down precisely as to how each set of variables are obtained and later interpreted.

Use a full-mouth oral speculum to safely and thoroughly examine the more caudal areas of the oral cavity. Remove all ingesta and foreign material from the oral cavity using a combination of lavage, oral picks, and forceps. Examine the oral mucosa, hard and soft palates, and tongue. Assess tooth number, dentition, morphology, orientation, alignment, relation to adjacent and opposing teeth, mobility, and patterns of attrition and abrasion. Assess in detail the different dental hard tissues, first by careful visualization and then in a tactile manner using a dental explorer, paying particular attention to the occlusal dentin associated with each pulp horn.[29] Perform periodontal measurements and assess periodontal health surrounding each tooth. Describe diastemata using measurements. Dental mirrors, intraoral cameras, and endoscopes are all helpful in performing an oral examination.

Components of the extraoral and intraoral examination may need to be repeated to clarify a point of interest. The stimulus for doing this may be the discovery of an abnormal or equivocal finding on examination, new information gained from the client during the process of the examination, or the findings from an ancillary test such as a radiographic series. If a diagnosis of oral/dental origin is made, the effect of the condition on the body in general should be evaluated. Aspects of the general physical examination may need to be repeated along with further history taking from the client.

ANCILLARY TESTS

Ancillary tests are often performed to provide data for classification of the patient, disease, and illness, determination of diagnoses, evaluation of therapies, and

Table 7		
Summary of features examined as part of the intraoral examination		
Bony Structures	**Soft-Tissue Structures**	**Dental Hard Tissues**
Symmetry of oral cavity	Oral mucosa	Morphology
Conformation of oral cavity	Gingiva	Arrangement
Mandibular diastema	Tongue	Occlusion
	Lips	Mobility
	Salivary ducts	Defects

monitoring when no therapy is performed (**Table 8**). Certain ancillary tests, such as radiography, are so commonly indicated and provide invaluable information when investigating problems of dental origin that an oral examination whereby such tests are indicated should be considered incomplete until performed. Diagnostic radiographic studies of the skull and teeth using intraoral and extraoral techniques should be possible by all clinicians performing dentistry when indicated (see article written by Baratt and his colleagues elsewhere in this issue). It is important that the data obtained and interpreted from the ancillary tests also be objective, precise, consistent, uniform, and reliable. The findings from any ancillary test are incomplete until considered in light of the history and examination findings, and may indicate repeat examination of the area of interest and/or more ancillary tests.

DOCUMENTATION

The evidence of the clinical examination is the medical record, and clinical findings should be written in terms of the evidence.[11] Sections of interpretation and diagnosis should be clearly defined. Rationale for the diagnostic and therapeutic process should be evident. The medical record should portray the level of diagnostic resolution achieved and what remains to be resolved.[22] By explicitly stating what is known, the clinician is forced to acknowledge what is not known and to provide a plan for further diagnostic workup.

With the science of equine dentistry still in its infancy, interpretation of oral and extraoral findings can be challenging. The development of suitable and valid criteria for interpretation of clinical findings is an ongoing process. When considering whether a finding is abnormal or normal, not only is comparison with the wider horse population relevant, but most importantly the finding needs to be considered in the context of the

Table 8	
Additional tests useful in diagnosing and monitoring oral conditions	
Ancillary Tests	
Imaging	Upper respiratory endoscopy
	Radiography
	Computed tomography
	Scintigraphy
	Magnetic resonance imaging
	Ultrasonography
Provocation	Percussion
	Manipulation
	Hot/cold
	Desiccation (air syringe)
Microbiological tests	Anaerobic cultures
	Aerobic cultures
	Polymerase chain reaction
Clinical pathology	Blood tests
Cytology	Fine-needle aspirates
Parasitology	Egg identification
	Larval identification
Histopathology	Biopsy specimen
Exploratory surgery	Sinusotomy

individual patient. For example, skeletal asymmetry may result in variation in the dental occlusion that is outside the normal range for the general population; however, for the individual the occlusion cannot be improved upon, and any attempt to do so may only be to the detriment of the animal.

2. THE "EXPERIMENTAL" MANEUVER

The maneuver (treatment) should be as specific as possible and ideally directed toward the primary cause. Restricting therapy to one intervention at a time allows for easier evaluation of the therapy's effectiveness. By seeking to treat only the primary cause, the resolve of secondary problems may be used as indicators that the primary cause has been correctly identified and successfully treated.

Therapy may be directed at:

- The primary disease
- Abnormal findings in ancillary tests
- The symptoms and clinical signs of the illness or concomitant illnesses[11]

The aim of therapy may be to prevent or alter any or all of the aspects. Disease may be treated or prevented by removing factors conducive to its development; by eliminating the pathogen; or by increasing the host immunity.

3. THE APPRAISAL OF RESPONSE

Case follow-up should occur in a biologically appropriate time frame and be performed to predetermined criteria. Terms used to describe clinical progression, such as "unchanged," "worse," "markedly improved," or "resolved," should be well defined before the examination; this would be analogous to some of the information contained in the "Methods" section of a laboratory experiment.[11] In reviewing data, sufficient numbers of subjects should be included to ensure that results are not due to just chance alone. When correlations are made, data on both sides of the correlation should be robust. If significant correlations are found they should be evaluated as to whether the relationship is direct, indirect, causal, or coexistent.[16] Do the results and conclusions make sense? Are the subjects representative of the greater population to which the new knowledge may be applied? Finally, it is important to remember that despite the sophistication of current statistical programs, no amount of genius will make up for input data of poor scientific quality.[13]

GOING FORWARD

So how should the clinician operate in an environment where standards of care in human medicine, dentistry, and other veterinary fields are much more developed?

1. By caring for the patient[30]:
   a. Being knowledgable in dentistry and medicine
   b. Performing a detailed and complete oral examination when making an assessment relating to oral health
   c. Treating only after diagnosing
   d. Using efficacious treatments
   e. Appreciating that being able to change something is no guarantee that the change is for the better for the horse (for every action there is a consequence—we hope too much that it is positive)
   f. Being conservative with interventions in the absence of EBVM

g. Knowing as much as possible and doing as little as possible for the desired effect
h. Taking meticulous records
i. Reviewing collected data
j. Ensuring that data collected are as free from bias as possible
2. By realizing that each case in itself is an experiment, thus ensuring that it contains all of the components to satisfy basic scientific methodology
3. By ensuring the data obtained is precise, accurate, objective, uniform, complete, and preserved
4. By performing a thorough oral examination during an interval that allows for detection and possible treatment of abnormalities while they are still of a minor nature

SUMMARY

The oral examination is by no means a stand-alone feature of oral care. It is an integral part of a much bigger process that has the health and well-being of the patient as its goal. The process of oral care is complex and demanding. Evidence-based decision making is core to the integrity of the modern clinician. It is particularly challenging because of the lack of scientific evidence available in equine dentistry. It is every clinician's responsibility to obtain the evidence and improve the way in which they administer oral care, to generate, interpret, and reflect on clinical data in a manner that is scientific. Despite the limitations and imperfections in clinical work, much scientific validity can be achieved by adhering to the timeless principles of scientific method on an everyday basis. While the science takes time to develop, clinicians can be guided by caring for their patients and clients.[30]

ACKNOWLEDGMENTS

The author would like to acknowledge Dr Torbjörn Lundström for his contributions in preparing the article.

REFERENCES

1. Evidence-Based Medicine Working Group. Evidence-based medicine. A new approach to teaching the practice of medicine. JAMA 1992;268:2420–5.
2. Cockcroft PD, Holmes MA. Handbook of evidence-based veterinary medicine. Oxford (United Kingdom): Blackwell Publishing; 2003.
3. Vandeweerd JM, Kirschvink N, Clegg P, et al. Is evidence-based medicine so evident in veterinary research and practice? History, obstacles and perspectives. Vet J 2012;191:28–34.
4. Sackett DL, Rosenberg WM, Gray JA, et al. Evidence based medicine: what it is and what it isn't. BMJ 1996;312:71–2.
5. Cohen ND. The John Hickman memorial lecture: colic by numbers. Equine Vet J 2003;35:343–9.
6. Muir W. Is evidence-based medicine our only choice? Equine Vet J 2003;35:337–8.
7. Galloway SS, Easley J. Establishing a scientific basis for equine clinical dentistry. Vet J 2008;178:307–10.
8. Carmalt JL. Evidence-based equine dentistry: preventive medicine. Vet Clin North Am Equine Pract 2007;23:519–24.
9. Miller GE. The assessment of clinical skills/competence/performance. Acad Med 1990;65:S63–7.

10. Lurie SJ. History and practice of competency-based assessment. Med Educ 2012;46:49–57.
11. Feinstein AR. Scientific methodology in clinical medicine. III. The evaluation of therapeutic response. Ann Intern Med 1964;61:944–65.
12. Feinstein AR. Scientific methodology in clinical medicine. II. Classification of human disease by clinical behavior. Ann Intern Med 1964;61:757–81.
13. Feinstein AR. Scientific methodology in clinical medicine. IV. Acquisition of clinical data. Ann Intern Med 1964;61:1162–93.
14. Bader JD. Stumbling into the age of evidence. Dent Clin North Am 2009;53:15–22, vii.
15. Engel GL. Clinical observation: the neglected basic method of medicine. JAMA 1965;192:849–52.
16. Feinstein AR. Scientific methodology in clinical medicine. I. Introduction, principles, and concepts. Ann Intern Med 1964;61:564–79.
17. Feinstein AR. Clinical judgment in the era of automation. Ann Otol Rhinol Laryngol 1970;79:728–37.
18. Feinstein AR. "Clinical judgment" revisited: the distraction of quantitative models. Ann Intern Med 1994;120:799–805.
19. International Committee on Veterinary Gross Anatomical Nomenclature. Nomina anatomica veterinaria. 5th edition. Hannover (Germany), Columbia (MO), Gent (Belgium), Sapporo (Japan): Editorial Committee; 2005.
20. Kurtz S, Silverman J, Benson J, et al. Marrying content and process in clinical method teaching: enhancing the Calgary-Cambridge guides. Acad Med 2003;78:802–9.
21. Kurtz SM, Silverman JD. The Calgary-Cambridge referenced observation guides: an aid to defining the curriculum and organizing the teaching in communication training programmes. Med Educ 1996;30:83–9.
22. Kaplan DM. Perspective: whither the problem list? Organ-based documentation and deficient synthesis by medical trainees. Acad Med 2010;85:1578–82.
23. Menzies RA, Lewis JR, Reiter AM, et al. Essential considerations for equine oral examination, diagnosis, and treatment. J Vet Dent 2011;28:204–9.
24. MacFarlane PD, Mosing M, Burford J. Preliminary investigation into the effects of earplugs on sound transmission in the equine ear. Pferdeheilkunde 2010;26:199–203.
25. Young JM, Satrom KD, Berrong JM. Intraoral dental lights: test and evaluation. J Prosthet Dent 1987;57:99–107.
26. Preston JD, Ward LC, Bobrick M. Light and lighting in the dental office. Dent Clin North Am 1978;22:431–51.
27. Simhofer H, Griss R, Zetner K. The use of oral endoscopy for detection of cheek teeth abnormalities in 300 horses. Vet J 2008;178:396–404.
28. Ramzan PH. Oral endoscopy as an aid to diagnosis of equine cheek tooth infections in the absence of gross oral pathological changes: 17 cases. Equine Vet J 2009;41:101–6.
29. Casey MB, Tremaine WH. The prevalence of secondary dentinal lesions in cheek teeth from horses with clinical signs of pulpitis compared to controls. Equine Vet J 2010;42:30–6.
30. Peabody FW. The care of the patient. JAMA 1927;88:877–82.
31. Honma K, Yamakawa M, Yamauchi S, et al. Statistical study on the occurrence of dental caries of domestic animals: 1. Horse. Jpn J Vet Res 1962;10:31–6.
32. Dacre IT. Equine dental pathology. In: Baker GJ, Easley J, editors. Equine dentistry. 2nd edition. Edinburgh (United Kingdom): WB Saunders; 2005. p. 91–107.

FURTHER READINGS

Carranza's clinical periodontology. 11th edition. St Louis (MO): Saunders; 2011.

Cohen's pathways of the pulp. 10th edition. St. Louis (MO): Mosby Elsevier; 2011.

Easley J, Tremaine WH. Dental and oral examination. In: Easley J, Dixon P, Schumacher J, editors. Equine dentistry. Oxford (United Kingdom): Elsevier; 2011. p. 185–98.

Easley J. Oral and dental examination, in Proceedings. AAEP Focus on Dentistry. 2011. p. 28–34.

Galloway SS. How to document a dental examination and procedure using a dental chart, in Proceedings. AAEP 56th Annual Convention. 2010. p. 429–40.

Menzies RA, Lewis JR, Reiter AM, et al. Essential considerations for equine oral examination, diagnosis, and treatment. J Vet Dent 2011;28(3):204–9.

Tremaine WH, Casey MB. A modern approach to equine dentistry. 1. Oral examination. In Pract 2012;34(1):2–10.

Vandeweerd JM, Kirschvink N, Clegg P, et al. Is evidence-based medicine so evident in veterinary research and practice? History, obstacles and perspectives. Vet J 2012;191:28–34.

Incorporating Oral Photography and Endoscopy into the Equine Dental Examination

Stephen S. Galloway, DVM, FAVD/Eq[a],*, Jack Easley, DVM, MS[b]

KEYWORDS

- Dental examination • Oral photography • Oral endoscopy • Equine dentistry

KEY POINTS

- Dental photography provides visual documentation to supplement the dental record and to improve communication with colleagues and clients.
- Oral endoscopy supplements the conventional oral examination by facilitating visualization of areas in the horse mouth that are not within the dentist's line of sight.
- Oral endoscopy allows for detailed oral examination of subtle dental/oral conditions, promotes early recognition of oral pathology, and can be used to guide intraoral procedures.

INTRODUCTION

Improvements in digital photographic and video technologies and the associated decreasing cost of this electronic equipment have made the use of these visual imaging technologies in clinical practice more affordable. Dental photography has primarily been used by veterinary dentists as a means of documentation to enhance the patient's written dental record.[1,2] However, dental photographs also provide a visual platform to facilitate communication with colleagues and clients, optimize recording of lesion characterization, support treatment planning, improve accounting of treatment or lesion location, and aid client education. Many lesions and oral conditions are difficult to describe accurately without a photograph. Photographic presentations are a proven format of practice marketing, providing visual descriptions necessary for understanding and training. Additionally, photographic case presentations improve consultation with other veterinarians and facilitate the education of veterinary professionals through case-based learning. There is a digital camera system that will meet the clinical needs and practice budget for every equine practitioner.

Funding Sources: None.
Conflict of Interest: None.
[a] Animal Care Hospital, 8565 Hwy 64, Somerville, TN 38068, USA; [b] Easley Equine Dentistry, PO Box 1075, Shelbyville, KY 40066, USA
* Corresponding author.
E-mail address: achvet@yahoo.com

Because the conformation of the horse's oral cavity limits a dentist's unaided visual examination, some equine veterinarians are supplementing their conventional oral examination with oral endoscopy. Endoscopic examination facilitates a complete, detailed visual examination of the oral cavity with increased identification of subtle pathologic conditions. This early recognition of dental conditions promotes the prevention and the early treatment of oral diseases. This is the goal of dentistry! Although every equine veterinarian cannot justify the investment of an oral endoscope, practices with a significant dental caseload or those performing advanced procedures could improve their standard of care by offering oral endoscopy.

This article will discuss the significant features and use of digital cameras, intraoral cameras, and oral endoscopes in equine dental practice. Although the authors have listed system features believed to be important, specific system recommendations are purposely omitted, since each veterinarian must individually determine the best system to meet practice clinical needs and budget. This equipment can be a significant investment; therefore, veterinarians are encouraged to thoroughly research not only the camera/endoscope purchase but also the capabilities of the entire system, the compatibility of the system with different computer software programs, the reputation and service policies of the manufacturers, and references from other colleagues (**Box 1**).

DENTAL PHOTOGRAPHY

Producing a digital picture takes 3 steps:

1. Capturing the image with a camera
2. Storing the image file
3. Editing the image for presentation or printing

Most veterinarians own computers capable of storing digital files, and many software packages are readily available for editing digital pictures. The most time-consuming decision when instituting dental photography is typically which camera should be purchased. As with other electronic devices, there is usually a direct relationship between the expense and the quality, capability, and operational flexibility of a camera system. A 5 megapixel camera produces a quality image and has enough features for recreational photography. Therefore, the primary factor increasing camera

---

Box 1
Using photography as a marketing tool

Client education is a professional's marketing platform, and sight is the dominant sense for people. Therefore, photography provides a visual platform to facilitate communication. Visual communication enhances a client's understanding of dental conditions and treatments while reducing client stress and reinforcing the doctor–client relationship. Many owners have never looked inside their horse's mouth! Dental photography peaks an owner's interest in this area of health care. Most people remember stories and pictures, so, PowerPoint case presentations are an excellent way to educate clients about treatment plans and advanced procedures. Incorporating photographs into the patient's discharge instructions not only presents the examination findings and treatment results, but also increases the client's understanding of and perceived value for the services provided.

Social media has become the primary marketing resource for society, and experts advise that one should never post information without a picture! Dental photographs and videos can easily be edited to remove any case-sensitive material and posted onto Internet Web sites, Facebook, or YouTube as an information service to the public as well as veterinary clients.

expense should be the optics (lens) (**Box 2**). A private practitioner is faced with an overwhelming number of choices when purchasing digital equipment and must weigh the clinical applications for the equipment against the expected return on investment. Although the gold standard in human dental photography is the digital single lens

---

Box 2
Resolution confusion

Computer monitors

Poor image resolution? The monitor is probably not the problem! Most computer monitors are designed to view Internet images and have adequate resolution for most clinical applications. For improved resolution, most gaming computers/monitors usually produce high-definition, TrueColor resolution. For photography professionals, extremely high definition monitors are available. If one has poor image resolution, the camera optics are poor, or the image file size is too small!

Megapixels

1 megapixel (MP) = 1 million pixels. A pixel is a single point, or color component, in a graphic image. An "8 MP" camera set on the largest image file size (3456×2304) will produce pictures consisting 8 million pixels (ie, 3456×2304 pixels = 7,962,264 pixels). Assuming that all cameras are constructed equally, increased MP produces sharper images. However, once one gets above 5 MP, the optical qualities of the camera (primarily the lens) become more important than the file size, and some photography critics caution that increased MP is a market tactic to get consumers to purchase inferior cameras.

Pixels per inch

PPI (pixels per inch) is used to indicate the resolution (color accuracy, detail, and sharpness) of an image when viewed at a given distance. When viewed at arm's length, most printed pictures with 240 PPI are considered to be photographic quality. High-resolution images for most scholarly publications require 300 PPI. However, PPI also depends upon the physical size of the image. An image taken with a 5 MP camera (file size 2592×1944 pixels) printed at 240 PPI equals 10.8×8.1 in. If printed larger, the resolution will decrease proportionally to the size increase (eg, 150 PPI for a 17.3×13 in print). Similarly, decreasing the size of the picture will increase the resolution of the image (eg, 432 PPI for a 6×4.5 in print); however, image resolution above 500 PPI is visually indiscernible. As a practical point of reference, Microsoft Power-Point uses 3 image compression sizes: Print (220 PPI), Screen (150 PPI), and E-mail (96 PPI); therefore, image resolution less than 240 PPI does not necessarily make the image quality unacceptable. This discussion demonstrates why a 5 MP image will meet the resolution requirements for recreation photographers; however, because cropping an image during editing removes pixel dimensions, a 10 to 12 MP camera is recommended for equine dental applications. The demonstration of specific cheek tooth lesions often requires significant image cropping followed by image enlargement or resizing, and all editing processes have an additive effect on decreasing the final image resolution.

Dots per inch

This term (DPI), which is commonly misused for PPI, refers specifically to printers. Printers have a finite number of colored inks; therefore, to produce the correct color at each pixel of the image, the finite colors must be blended using smaller ink dots. Printers with larger DPI produce pictures with greater resolution and color accuracy; however, this increased resolution is associated with increased ink at an increased expense and slower production time. To optimize a printer's efficiency, the DPI should be adjusted to the lowest setting required to produce an acceptable picture.

reflex system (DSLR), some equine practitioners may find that the digital point and shoot camera system (P&S) or the basic subcompact camera (SCC) meets their clinical needs and budget. *Consumer Reports* recently tested 277 DSLR, P&S, and SCC digital cameras and DSLR lenses and reported findings and recommendations.[3] Digital Photography Review is also a good source for digital camera comparisons (see **Box 2**, **Table 1**).

Digital Single Lens Reflex System

The DSLR System, with the emphasis on system, produces the highest resolution images possible with complete color accuracy. This system is comprised of 3 required components:

1. Camera
2. Macro lens
3. Flash system

A marco lens, typically used for close-up wildlife photography, is required for dental photography. Macro lenses are not focused; the camera is moved toward or away from the target until the target comes into focus at the focal length for the specific lens. These lenses are manufactured for focal lengths of 60, 100, or 105 mm, and the longer focal lengths are preferred to increase the distance between the camera and the patient. Most dentists prefer a 100 or 105 mm lens, which allows approximately 4 in and 4.5 in standoff, respectively. However, increased focal length is associated with increased size, weight, and expense.

Although the DSLR camera houses a pop-up flash, the optical angle of this internal flash produces unacceptable shadowing of the target tissues during macrophotography. Therefore, a ring flash, which is designed specifically for macrophotography, is mounted on the front of the lens to provide a diffuse 360° illumination. The ring flash produces images with even lighting, color accuracy, and no shadows, but sometimes overillumination can flash-out slight texture and anatomy of the teeth. Two technologies have been produced to eliminate this overillumination. Through-the-lens metering (TTL) is available in many DSLRs to control flash exposure. Alternatively, the twin ring flash only flashes in 2 opposite quadrants on the ring, which can be rotated to optimize target illumination. When using a DSLR system, operators are cautioned that a shiny oral speculum will create an unacceptable flash-back even when using a ring flash.

Table 1
Digital image resolution chart

Megapixel	File Size	Monitor Resolution	Photo Quality 240 PPI	Publication Quality 300 PPI
0.3	640 × 480	Good	2.7 × 2 in	2.1 × 1.6 in
0.48	800 × 600	Excellent	3.3 × 2.5 in	2.7 × 2 in
1	1280 × 960	Excellent	5.3 × 4 in	4.2 × 3.2 in
2	1600 × 1200	Excellent	6.6 × 5 in	5.3 × 4 in
3	2048 × 1536	Excellent	8.5 × 6.4 in	6.8 × 5.1 in
5	2592 × 1944	Excellent	10.8 × 8.1 in	8.6 × 6.5 in
6	3032 × 2008	Excellent	12.6 × 8.4 in	10.1 × 6.7 in
8	3264 × 2448	Excellent	13.6 × 10.2 in	10.9 × 8.2 in
10	3872 × 2592	Excellent	16.1 × 10.8 in	12.9 × 8.6 in

The most popular DSLR systems are produced by Canon and Nikon. Most dentists recommend that a novice begin with a system produced by 1 of these manufactures instead of buying individual components and building a system.

Digital P&S System

Due to the high expense of the DSLR Systems, a flash diffuser (Promed International, Van Nuys, California) has been developed to diffuse the light emitted from the fixed flash on P&S cameras in a similar fashion to a ring flash. Although discerning cosmetic dentists prefer the superior resolution and operational flexibility provided by DSLR systems, most equine veterinarians will find that the Images produced by the P&S system are acceptable for clinical practice.

Subcompact Cameras

Due to the affordability and continuing improvements in camera design, SCCs are currently preferred by most equine veterinary dentists. Equine patients can damage equipment, and equine dentistry is often practiced in wet conditions, making quick and inexpensive replacement valuable. Waterproof models are also available.

Although image resolution may be inferior to that produced by the DSLR, the number of SCC images that have been published demonstrates the clinical acceptability of these cameras. Keep in mind, with the SCC there is a delay between the time the button is pushed and the picture is shot. All images in this article were taken with an SCC. The small lens of the SCC fits easily between the incisor plates of the full-mouth speculum, and the close proximity between the lens and flash produces acceptable shadowing. Because every camera model functions differently, each SCC must be tested to determine which combination of features produces the best quality image. The authors recommend starting with the following setting on

1. Set the camera in the portrait mode instead of the macro mode or the auto mode.
2. Turn the flash on, not to auto.
3. Use the widest view setting. Do not zoom on the target tissue.
4. Turn the automatic focus illuminator on, and do not shine a headlamp into the mouth.
5. Hold the camera 4 to 6 in outside of the horse's mouth, not between the speculum plates (**Fig. 1**).
6. Center the automatic focus illuminator on the target tissue.
7. Take 2 to 3 pictures and save the best one.

These steps will produce an image with a greater depth of focus, and the picture will be more versatile during editing. Macro mode and zooming increase the likelihood that the image will be out of focus. Use photoediting software to create an image of a specific tissue (**Fig. 2**).

Other Camera Features

Regardless of the camera system used, the image resolution on the camera should be set to the highest file dimension size available. Because dental photographs augment the patient record, the date stamp feature should be used to verify when photographs were taken. The image stabilizer feature available on most digital cameras minimizes image blurring caused by camera motion during exposure. Virtually all SCCs have video capabilities that produce acceptable videos for client education and teaching purposes. Most DSLRs and some SCCs can produce high-definition video (**Boxes 3** and **4**).

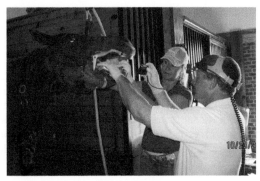

Fig. 1. Taking a photograph with a subcompact camera.

Dental Photography Technique

Patient positioning, sedation, and preparation

Most dental examinations and procedures can be performed in the standing, sedated patient restrained in stocks or a small stall. Restraint, sedation, and regional anesthesia techniques are elsewhere in this issue by Schilling and colleagues. To facilitate oral imaging and prevent equipment damage, the level of patient sedation and muscle relaxation must be sufficient to ensure that chewing, tongue movement, and head jerking are minimized. The patient's mandibles should rest on a headstand or suspended halter. Focus and motion are the most important considerations, because most other factors can be corrected or improved with software manipulation.

Oral examination photography

Oral photography is used to supplement the written dental chart by visually documenting the state of oral health during the oral examination and after treatments. Examination and charting techniques are discussed elsewhere in this issue by Menzies and colleagues. The following outlines the authors' oral examination photographic series:

1. The first photograph in the series should be a picture of the horse. This picture serves as the case divider for the numerous oral pictures on the memory card.
2. Any external abnormalities of the head (ie, enlargements, draining tracts, etc) should be noted and documented with photographs.
3. The incisors and canine teeth are rinsed to remove grass, feed, and debris.

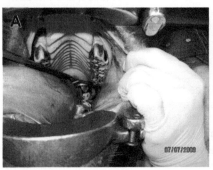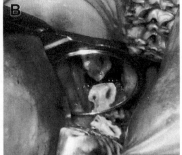

Fig. 2. (A) Original image taken with a subcompact camera. (B) Cropped image demonstrating periodontal disease in the interproximal space between 310 and 311.

Box 3
Image file formats

JPEG is a universal "lossy" file type designed for storing photographs, and most digital cameras save in JPEG format by default. The primary advantage of JPEG is its small file size, which is achieved through file compression of information that the eye is least likely to see. The primary disadvantage of this format is also file compression! JPEG images undergo resolution degradation, "loss," during file creation and each time a JPEG file is edited and saved. The original image should never be altered! Instead, a new file should be saved for each edited image produced. Overall, a JPEG is sufficient for most clinical and personal images. JPEG is the file type of choice for picture storage (small file size) on Secure Digital memory cards, the practice hard drive, and for Internet and PowerPoint applications. Some cameras can be switched to capture images in TIFF or RAW for improved image resolution, but this improvement may not be noticeable.

TIFF is a universal "lossless" file type. Although TIFF produces the best quality photographs, the file sizes are huge compared to JPEG. Few digital cameras use TIFF as a capture file type because fewer photos can be stored on the memory card; additionally, a longer wait between photographs is required as the image transfers to the card. Because TIFF is a "lossless" file, and file editing and compression does not result in image degradation, its primary use is as a working storage format for editing images in graphics programs. TIFF produces the highest quality photographs, but is only clinically applicable when detailed image analysis is required.

A RAW file is a nonuniversal, "lossless," read-only image capture format available on some cameras. RAW file size is similar to TIFF. The captured information must be transferred to a computer for image creation using the manufacturer's proprietary software, and finally saved as another file type (JPEG, TIFF, PNG). Although some photography critics argue that this format allows complete control of image quality and graphics software programs are being coded to read the more popular RAW files, other critics argue that the proprietary nature of this format make image archiving very risky and recommend conversion to a universal "lossless" file for long-term storage (eg, TIFF).

PNG is a "lossless" storage format with complete compression reversibility and superior color accuracy. Some discerning photography experts use this format.

GIF is a "lossless" storage format that has lost popularity to PNG due to limited colors.

BMP is Microsoft's proprietary format with limited popular use.

---

4. The photographer rolls the maxillary lips dorsally to expose the maxillary incisors, and an assistant rolls the mandibular lips ventrally to expose the mandibular incisors. Two to three pictures are taken of the facial aspect of the incisors (**Fig. 3**).
5. Next, the photographer and the assistant move to the left side of the head. The lips are rolled back as previously described, and the vestibular aspect of the left third incisors and canine teeth are photographed. The vestibular aspect of the right third incisors and canine teeth are photographed in the same fashion (**Fig. 4**).

Box 4
Price range of extraoral imaging equipment

Subcompact camera: $130–$430 (*Consumer Reports* recommended models)

P&S with flash diverter: $1500

DSLR systems (complete): $2500–5000

    Camera: $650–2000, macro lens: $750–1000

    Ring flash: $200–500, twin flash: $700–1000

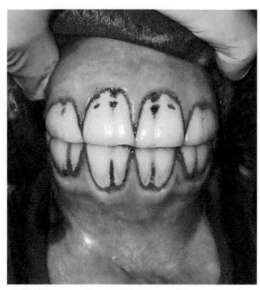

Fig. 3. Photograph of the facial aspect of the incisors of a 4-year-old pony.

6. If examination of the rostral teeth reveals pathologic or interesting conditions on other tooth aspects or associated soft tissues (eg, pulp exposure, tooth resorption, bar injuries) specific photographs can be taken to document these conditions (**Fig. 5**).
7. A full-mouth speculum is placed, the mouth opened, and the oral cavity rinsed to remove grass, feed, and debris.
8. A right-handed photographer retracts the right cheek of the horse with the left hand in a rostrolateral direction, and the assistant retracts the left cheek in a

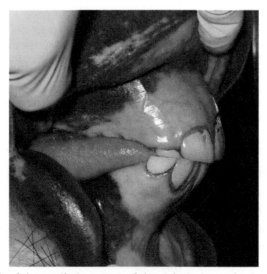

Fig. 4. Photograph of the vestibular aspect of the right incisors of a 4-year-old pony.

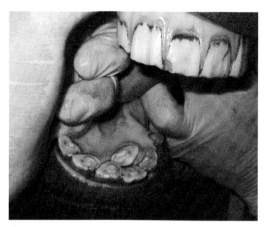

Fig. 5. Photograph demonstrating a mandibular incisor class 1 malocclusion in a teenage horse.

similar fashion to fully open the mouth. The palate, dorsal aspect on the tongue, and occlusal aspects of the maxillary cheek teeth can be photographed (**Fig. 6**).

9. Next, the right cheek is retracted rostrolaterally, and the tongue retracted to the left to expose the right cheek teeth for photography. The left cheek teeth are photographed in a similar fashion (**Fig. 7**).

10. If examination of the cheek teeth reveals pathologic or interesting conditions on other tooth aspects or associated soft tissues (eg, cheek, palate, and tongue trauma), specific photographs can be taken to document these conditions (**Fig. 8**).

11. Lesions on the occlusal aspects of the cheek teeth can be photographed by taking a picture of a dental mirror's reflection of the lesion. When a mirror is used, the camera should be focused on the surface of the mirror (see **Figs. 2** and **8B**).

12. The lingual aspects of the mandibular premolars can be photographed by retracting the tongue, taking the picture across the bars or with a mirror (**Fig. 9**).

13. The vestibular aspect of the premolars can be photographed by closing the horse's mouth and retracting the cheek with a cheek retractor (**Fig. 10**).

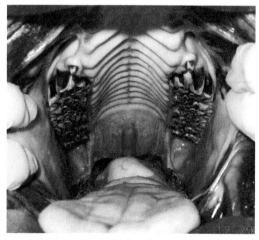

Fig. 6. Photograph imaging the oral cavity of a 4-year-old pony.

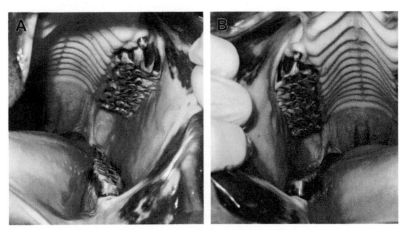

Fig. 7. Photograph imaging the right and left cheek teeth of a 4-year-old pony. Note color variations produced by subcompact camera.

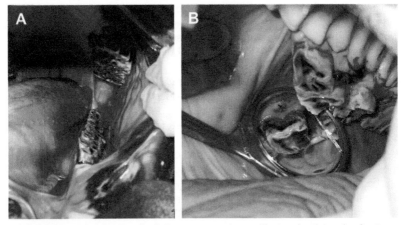

Fig. 8. (A) Photograph imaging the left tongue and mandibular cheek teeth of a 4-year-old pony. Note the sublingual inflammation caused by grass awns. (B) Photograph imaging the vestibular aspect of 107 to demonstrate a gingival tract.

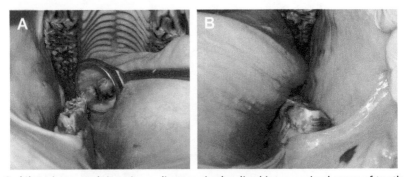

Fig. 9. (A) A photograph imaging a diastema in the distal interproximal space of tooth 408 in a teenage horse. (B) A photograph imaging a cementoma on lingual aspect of tooth 306 in a teenage horse.

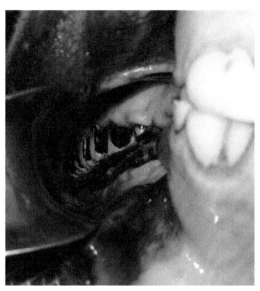

Fig. 10. Photograph imaging the vestibular aspect of the right cheek teeth of a 4-year-old pony used to demonstrate normal centric occlusion.

Examination photographs can be reviewed during treatment planning. Procedural photographs should be taken during and after treatments to document the procedures performed, as well as for comparison with the examination photographs (**Fig. 11**). Archiving the patient's photographs provides a visual case history that can be reviewed to determine the progress of pathologic conditions or the efficacy of treatments. Although the images produced by dental photography can document most oral conditions, these systems are limited to the dentist's line of sight and aspects of the mouth that can viewed using a mirror. Imaging of the vestibular and lingual aspects of caudal cheek teeth is difficult even in the most compliant horse (**Boxes 5** and **6**).

INTRAORAL IMAGING SYSTEMS

Research over the past two decades has improved the understanding of equine dental and oral pathologic conditions. In an effort to prevent or diagnose and treat these pathologic conditions as early as possible, dental diagnostic imaging techniques have also advanced in the modalities of radiography, computed tomography, magnetic resonance imaging, scintigraphy, and sinuscopy. Although advancements in equine dental sedation and anesthesia, restraint, and examination instrumentation have improved significantly over the past 2 decades, a detailed visual evaluation of all aspects of the oral cavity remains challenging because of the long and narrow anatomic configuration of the equine mouth and the limited spaces between dentition, cheeks, and tongue.[4] Most dental conditions can be diagnosed during a thorough visual and tactile oral examination using good illumination and a dental mirror, explorer, and probe[5]; however, under-recognition of subtle dental pathology and misdiagnosis is still commonly associated with traditional dental examination techniques. Therefore, some equine dentists advocate supplementing the traditional oral examination with an intraoral camera or endoscopic examination to provide a more detailed visual inspection of the dentition.[4,6–8]

Recent research has demonstrated that oral endoscopic evaluation allows for the detection of a higher number of cheek teeth dental conditions and abnormalities of

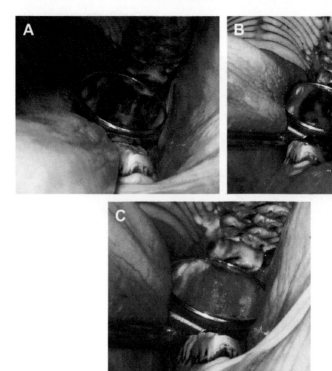

Fig. 11. Procedural photographs used to document: (*A*) instrument placement during surgical extraction of a 209 with a complicated crown fracture, (*B*) complete tooth root removal, and (*C*) alveolar healing at 2 months postoperatively.

Box 5
Storing image files

SD memory card storage capacity

Every 2 GB of memory holds about 770 × 10 megapixel images or 20 minutes of video in fine recording mode

Hard drive storage

Storage capacity is the same as the memory card

Consider an external hard drive to save space on computer hard drive

Store images in the original file format and large file size

Never alter the original image file; save edited images to a new file

Tips generated after ±50,000 images

Images can be stored by many veterinary management software programs, which will usually compress the images!

When downloading the images rename the original files (eg, IMG_0013) with the patient name and date, in YYMMDD (e.g. Aristotle 121031); this will help later when searching for or sorting images.

Store images in a master folder (eg, Dental Cases) with client subfolders (eg, Addams G) containing individual patient folders (eg, Aristotle, Bernice, and Cleopatra), each containing dated service folders (eg, Aristotle 121031), containing the original dated images for that service (eg, Aristotle 121031_001 through Aristotle 121031_033, Aristotle 121031 Video 001, and Aristotle 121031 RAD 001)

Rename edited images descriptively (eg, Aristotle 121031 INC EOTRH)

> **Box 6**
> **Photo editing/graphics programs**
>
> Images files should be edited before presentation based on their intended use, and the edited images should be saved to a new file. Basic programs come with most computer software packages, and graphics programs can be purchased for advanced editing applications. Most modern computers come with enough memory (4 GB RAM) to efficiently run graphics programs. MS Office Picture Manager is standard software on PCs and has basic image editing functions such as cropping, sizing, and basic color and contrast adjustment. Text can be added to images with MS Paint. Similarly, basic editing functions can be performed on MACs with iPhoto and Preview PDF and Image Viewer. Better graphics programs, such as Photoshop, Photo Suite, and Paint Shop Pro, allow more detailed editing of images, as well as layered editing, and allow JPEG image quality and file size to be viewed as a function of compression level, so that the editor can choose the balance between image quality and file size.
>
> Computer speed is inversely proportional to file size. Images should be sized based upon their intended use to improve computer efficiency. When sharing an image for general viewing over the Internet, resizing to around 0.5 MPs provides excellent monitor resolution. If sending an image to a colleague for detailed (magnified) analysis, resizing the image to 1 to 2 MPs is usually sufficient. High-speed Internet is capable of rapidly sending larger file sizes. PowerPoint has a compression function that can be used to simultaneously compress all images within the presentation.

eruption, especially in the caudal mouth, excluding gross dental malocclusions.[9] Endoscopic evaluation facilitates the detailed evaluation of subtle dental conditions such as pulp exposure from dental fractures, fissures in the enamel and secondary dentin, infundibular conditions, peripheral cemental caries, gingival recession and ulceration, diastemata and periodontal pocketing, and small occlusal malocclusions (**Fig. 12**).[8,10]

In addition to improving visualization during the oral examination, oral endoscopy is used by some veterinarians for visual guidance during intraoral dental and surgical procedures. In one human study, it was concluded that the use of an intraoral camera improved treatment decisions of the occlusal surface on posterior teeth.[11] During cheek tooth extraction and periodontal surgery, endoscopy helps minimizes proximal tissue trauma by ensuring correct instrument placement and precise wound inspection, debridement, and packing (**Figs. 13** and **14**). Oral endoscopy can also provide

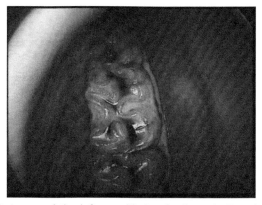

Fig. 12. Endoscopic image of the left mandibular cheek teeth. Noted the fissures in the secondary dentin and enamel of pulp horns 1 and 2 of the central tooth and in pulp horn 1 of the caudal tooth. (*Courtesy of* Jennifer Rawlinson, DVM, Ithaca, NY.)

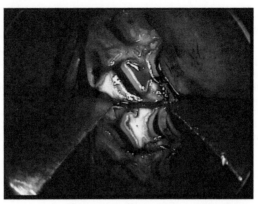

Fig. 13. Molar spreader placement is confirmed with an oral endoscope during a simple extraction of a maxillary cheek tooth. (*Courtesy of* Jennifer Rawlinson, DVM, Ithaca, NY.)

visualization for restorative procedures on cheek teeth, which have traditionally been performed in a blinded fashion (**Fig. 15**).

Most endoscopy systems have digital recording capabilities that can be used to save both photographic and video files. These files can be archived in the permanent patient record as discussed previously. The combination of detailed evaluation and recording capabilities makes intraoral imaging systems invaluable tools for research and education as well as clinical practice. For example, several studies about cheek tooth apical infection have been published. However, during oral endoscopic examination of horses with apical infections that lacked gross oral pathologic lesions, Ramzan discovered the previously unreported finding that 59% of horses had gingival recession of the apically infected tooth (**Fig. 16**).[7]

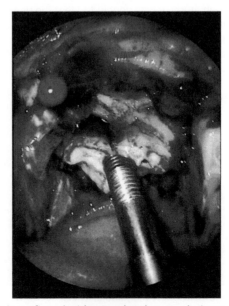

Fig. 14. Pin placement is confirmed with an oral endoscope during a surgical extraction of a maxillary cheek tooth. (*Courtesy of* Dr Manfred Stoll, Hohenstein, Germany.)

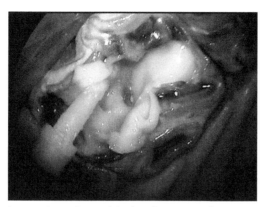

Fig. 15. An oral endoscope is used to guide the placement of a composite material during infundibular cavity repair. (*Courtesy of* Dr Manfred Stoll, Hohenstein, Germany.)

Equine veterinarians are currently using 3 types of intraoral imaging systems: oral endoscopes, human intraoral cameras, and industrial borescopes. Oral endoscopy and intraoral camera systems will be described. Borescopes are not discussed, because their nonmedical uses generate numerous product designs beyond the scope of this article. Because most intraoral camera systems produce 0.3 MP image files, photographic image quality is primarily determined by differences in optics (lens quality) and camera design. Images presented in this article represent several different systems with 0.3 MP file sizes.

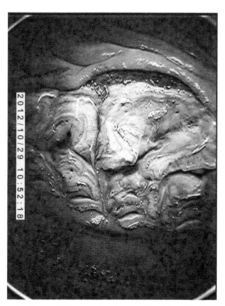

Fig. 16. Endoscopic examination of the palatal aspect of tooth 109 in a teenaged horse revealed a complicated crown fracture of pulp horn 5, which is closed by a dentin bridge. Also note the gingival recession associated with teeth 108 and 109. The combination of these findings warrants radiography.

Oral Endoscopic Systems

The limited product diversity and expense of the currently available equine oral endoscopic systems have relegated the placement of this visual technology into universities and referral centers. In an effort to incorporate this technology into private practice, some veterinarians are purchasing the system components separately and building their own systems. Since these systems consist of several equally important components, novices are advised to investigate system packages from established manufacturers and solicit references from colleagues before shopping for individual components that may not be compatible.

Most systems in clinical practice consist of a waterproof 40 to 60 mm rigid endoscope with a wide-angle lens at a viewing direction of 30° to 90°. For procedural applications, a viewing angle of 90° is probably most appropriate, because endoscopic task performance is optimized when the target plane (cheek tooth) is perpendicular to the optical axis of the endoscope.[12–14] Oral endoscopes have a short focal length. Therefore, the lens can be moved closer to the target to increase magnification or farther away to increase the field of view. Endoscopes require a strong light source (150 W is the industry standard.), and some manufacturers are offering LED options.

Most endoscopes are connected to a monitor or computer for real-time viewing and/or can be coupled with a camera capable of capturing either digital photographs or video, usually in a RAW file format. Some manufacturers now offer wireless feed to the video receiver/monitor. Because endoscope systems are designed for real-time viewing and video recording, pixel dimension capacity of most endoscopic cameras (industry standard is approximately 0.3 MP, 680 × 480 p) provides good resolution for digitally recorded video and acceptable photographs when viewed on a monitor in a small dimensional size but produces poor resolution when the image is enlarged for detailed evaluation. Some manufacturers have modified digital cameras with endoscope adapters that can produce photographic quality images and high-definition video. Also, because of the video-oriented design, some systems acquire photographic images very slowly and/or lack an image acquisition button on the endoscope. Such systems typically produce poor quality, blurry photographs and often require an assistant to capture the images.

Intraoral Dental Cameras Systems

Some equine dentists are using these systems as a less expensive, easy-to-use alternative to the oral endoscope (**Fig. 17**). These cameras, designed specifically for human dentistry, have a 90° to 105° lens and LED light system, usually in a ring configuration, mounted on the end of a 20 mm hand piece. Most are water resistant, not waterproof, and require some modification for use in the equine mouth (**Fig. 18**). The camera is USB linked into a docking station or directly into a computer. The short length of the camera hand piece often necessitates that the operating hand must be inserted into the horse's mouth to examine or image caudal structures (**Fig. 19**). The after-market equine application of these systems also brings the durability of the camera into question. An image acquisition button is sometimes positioned on the linkage cord, which makes image capture convenient. However, on most models, the image acquisition button is placed on the wand, which can make image acquisition of the caudal tissues difficult. Like oral endoscopes, the pixel dimension capacity (0.3 MP, 680 × 480 p) of most cameras provides adequate resolution for monitor viewing, but poor image resolution when the image is enlarged for detailed evaluation (**Box 7, Fig. 20**).

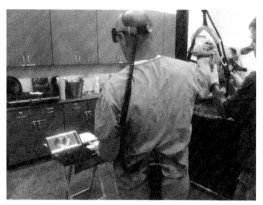

Fig. 17. An intraoral camera is being used to examine the cheek teeth of a horse. (*Courtesy of* Matt Evans, DVM, Driftwood, Texas.)

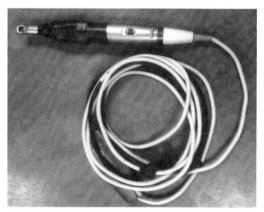

Fig. 18. An intraoral camera modified for use in the equine mouth. (*Courtesy of* Matt Evans, DVM, Driftwood, Texas.)

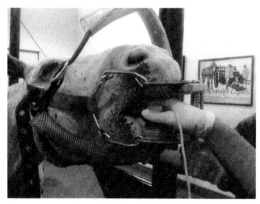

Fig. 19. The intraoral camera must be inserted into the horse's mouth to image the caudal cheek teeth. (*Courtesy of* Matt Evans, DVM, Driftwood, Texas.)

> **Box 7**
> **Price range of intraoral imaging systems**
>
> Human intraoral cameras: $200–$3500
>
> Equine intraoral endoscopes: $5000+, most $8000–10,000+

Intraoral Examination Technique

Patient positioning, sedation, preparation, and traditional examination techniques have previously been discussed. Due to the expense of most intraoral imaging systems, it is re-emphasized that to prevent equipment damage, the level of patient sedation and muscle relaxation must be sufficient to ensure that chewing and tongue movement are minimized and that the patient's mandibles rest on a headstand or suspended halter without head jerking (**Fig. 21**).

The following outlines the authors' oral endoscopic examination procedure:

1. The incisors and canine teeth are examined and imaged as previously described with a digital camera. Short video clips can also be taken with most cameras.
2. A full-mouth speculum is placed, the mouth opened, and the oral cavity rinsed to remove grass, feed, and debris.
3. The endoscopic examination is preceded by a complete oral examination.
4. The first image or video shot acquired should serve as case divider. The author usually images the patient identification section of the dental chart. If video recording the procedure, the recorder is left running, and the examination begins. If taking photographs, pathologic or interesting conditions are documented as they present during the examination.
5. Oral examination is facilitated by an assistant controlling the cheeks and tongue as described in the section on oral examination photography.
6. Dipping the lens plate in warm water or spraying it with an antifog solution may prevent fogging in cool climates.
7. The endoscopic examination begins by examining the vestibular aspect of the 100 cheek tooth arcade. The endoscope is advanced to the caudal buccal fold, and

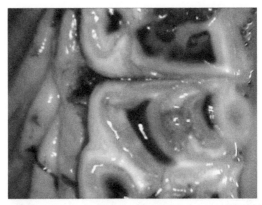

Fig. 20. An image taken with an intraoral camera of the maxillary cheek taken during evaluation of a palatal interproximal periodontal pocket. Also note the fissures in the secondary dentin of the fourth pulp horn of the rostral tooth. (*Courtesy of* Matt Evans, DVM, Driftwood, Texas.)

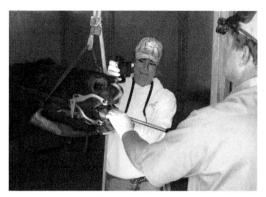

Fig. 21. A wireless oral endoscope is being used to image the left maxillary cheek tooth arcade. The assistant is holding the video monitor.

the distal aspect of the 111 is examined. The endoscope is retracted rostrally to view the vestibular aspects of the cheek teeth 111 to 106.

8. The endoscope is rotated 90°, inserted between the 100 and 400 cheek teeth arcades, and advanced caudally to examine the occlusal surfaces of the 106 through 111 cheek teeth arcades.

9. The endoscope is rotated 70° to 90° toward the palate and advanced rostrally to examine the palatal aspect of teeth 111 through 106.

10. Next, the 200 cheek tooth arcade is examined in a similar fashion, followed by the 300 and 400 arcades (see attached Video Endoscopic Tour of the Horse's Mouth).

Interpretation of Intraoral Findings

Although some recent articles imply that oral endoscopic findings are more valuable than those discovered during a traditional oral examination, it cannot be overemphasized that oral endoscopy supplements, and does not replace, a traditional oral examination. Oral endoscopy provides superior identification and visual evaluation of subtle dental lesions, but, periodontal disease is defined by attachment loss, which is determined by periodontal probing depth and radiographic bone loss, not visual gingival lesions (**Fig. 22**). Similarly, cavities and pulp exposures are suspected on visual examination, confirmed with a dental explorer, and graded with radiographs (**Fig. 23**). The successful diagnosis and treatment planning of dental diseases require the combination of oral examination and diagnostic findings.

The inexperienced equine practitioner can find the interpretation of oral endoscopic findings to be challenging. Magnified anatomic structures and normal age-related dental changes are easily confused with pathologic conditions. Therefore, a more detailed oral examination must be accompanied by a detailed understanding of dental anatomy, physiology, and pathology. This confusion can be compounded by the increased incidence of subtle dental conditions of unknown significance that are being identified by endoscope examination. For example, in a study of 300 consecutively examined horses, Simhofer et al found occlusal surface fissures and dental fractures in 54.3% and 22% of the all patients, respectively (see **Fig. 12**).[10] While most would agree that these findings are abnormal, the clinical relevance of such findings is undetermined.

Because minimal research has been performed to evaluate the clinical applicability and efficacy of oral endoscopy in horses, some veterinary authors have referenced

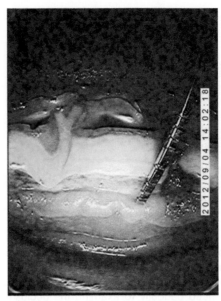

Fig. 22. This image demonstrates endoscopic assisted periodontal probing of the vestibular aspect of a mandibular cheek tooth that could not be visualized using a mirror. Note that the periodontal pocket in the proximal interproximal space does not extend across the vestibular aspect of the cheek tooth, which has a healthy gingival sulcular depth of less than 1 mm.

human studies reporting increased caries detection using intraoral imaging systems compared with conventional visual examination. Interestingly, one commonly cited study in people emphasizes the benefit of increased caries detection in the article's abstract, while minimizing the relevance of the data demonstrating that the use of intraoral imaging equipment also resulted in a significant number of false-positive diagnoses, which in clinical practice would result in the treatment of healthy teeth.[15] This conclusion was confirmed by another comparative study in people.[16] These human

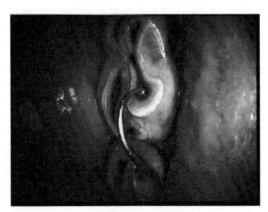

Fig. 23. This image demonstrates endoscopic assisted exploration of the third pulp horn of a mandibular cheek tooth. Also note the pulp exposure in the first pulp horn. (*Courtesy of* Jennifer Rawlinson, DVM, Ithaca, NY.)

studies caution dentists against overinterpretation of magnified findings and reinforce the need for thorough multimodal diagnostic evaluations.

SUMMARY

Documentation of dental procedures is required by both legal and ethical professional standards, and dental photography provides an accurate method of supplementing the written dental record. Additionally, dental photography provides a visual platform to improve communication with colleagues and clients. Due to advances in imaging technology, a digital camera is available that meets every practices' clinical needs and budget.

Additionally, oral endoscopy has proven to be beneficial in both documenting oral conditions as well as improving the detail and accuracy of the oral examination and intraoral dental procedures. The popularity of the currently available systems is limited by expense and operational capabilities. Market pressure for oral endoscopes purchased by private practitioners should encourage manufactures to design more affordable systems that better address the clinical needs of veterinary dentists.

ACKNOWLEDGMENTS

The authors would like to thank the following veterinarians for their clinical experiences and pictures from different imaging systems: Dr Lynn Caldwell, Dr Ed Early, Dr Matt Evans, Dr Rob Pascoe, Dr Jennifer Rawlinson, Dr Hubert Simhofer, and Dr Manfred Stoll.

REFERENCES

1. Earley ET. Computorized dental charting. In: Proceedings of American Association of Equine Practitioners. Focus on Dentistry. Indianapolis; 2006. p. 246–61.
2. Blazejewski SW. Photgraphic documentation for veterinary dentistry and oral surgery. J Vet Dent 2012;29(4):270–4.
3. Cameras. Consum Rep Dec 2012;40–3.
4. Collier MA, Balch KO, Alberts MK, et al. Use of an intraoral camera for identifying and documenting equine oral disease. In: Proceeding of the 44th American Association of Equine Practitioners Convention. Baltimore; 1998. p. 304–5.
5. Gieche JM. How to assess oral health. In: Proceedings of the 53rd Annual American Association of Equine Practitioners Convention. Orlando; 2007. p. 498–503.
6. Easley J. How to properly perform and interpret an endoscopic examination of the equine oral cavity. In: Proceedings. 54th Annual American Association of Equine Practitioners Convention. 2008. p. 383–5.
7. Ramzan PH. Oral endoscopy as an aid to diagnosis of equine cheek tooth infections in the absence of gross oral pathological changes: 17 cases. Equine Vet J 2009;41(2):101–6.
8. Tremaine WH. Dental endoscopy in the horse. Clin Tech Equine Pract 2005;4(2):181–7.
9. Goff C. A study to determine the advantages of oral endoscopy for the detection of dental pathology in the standing horse. In: Proceedings of the American Association Equine Practitioners Focus Dentistry Meeting. Indianapolis; 2006. p. 266–8.
10. Simhofer H, Griss R, Zetner K. The use of oral endoscopy for detection of cheek teeth abnormalities in 300 horses. Vet J 2008;178:396–404.

11. Erten H, Uctasli MN, Akarslan ZZ, et al. Restorative treatment decision making with unaided visual examination, intraoral camera, and operating microscope. Oper Dent 2006;31(1):55–9.
12. Hanna GB, Shimi S, Cuschieri A. Influence of direction of view, target-to-endoscope distance and manipulation angle on endoscopic knot tying. Br J Surg 1997;84:1460–4.
13. Hanna GB, Cuschieri A. Influence of axis-to-target angle on endoscopic task performance. Surg Endosc 1999;13(4):371–5.
14. Patil PV, Hanna GB, Cuschieri A. Effect of the angle between the optical axis of the endoscope and the intrument's plane on the monitor image and surgical performance. Surg Endosc 2004;18:111–4.
15. Erten H, Uctasli MB, Akarslan ZZ, et al. The assessment of unaided visual examination, intraoral camera and operating microscope for the detection of occlusal caries lesions. Oper Dent 2005;30(2):190–4.
16. Forgie AH, Pine CM, Pitts NB. The assessment of an oral intra-oral video camera as an aid to occlusal caries detection. Int Dent J 2003;53(1):3–6.

Advances in Equine Dental Radiology

Robert Baratt, DVM, MS

KEYWORDS

- Equine • Dental • Radiography • Imaging

KEY POINTS

- Digital radiography has enhanced the ability of the general practitioner to obtain diagnostic radiographs of the equine head. However, diagnostic images can be obtained with traditional rare-earth film-screen combinations.
- Diagnostic radiographic imaging depends on knowledge of the radiographic projections that are necessary for a complete study of the dentition and paradental structures.
- The radiographic signs of dental disease are most readily apparent when the disease is unilateral and the radiographs of the normal and abnormal (contralateral) side can be compared.

INTRODUCTION

The gross anatomy of the equine head is complex, therefore the normal radiographic anatomy can be challenging for the average equine practitioner. However, with adequate anatomic references, the practitioner can become comfortable with obtaining diagnostic images of the equine head and recognizing dental and paradental radiographic signs of pathologic conditions. With the widespread availability of digital radiography (DR) in equine practices, the practitioner can more readily learn the correct positioning for the various projections of the equine head that are used to evaluate the dentition and sinuses. Digital systems provide rapid processing of the image, enabling the practitioner to correct positioning errors and retake the image without significant delay.

The two digital systems in general use as of this writing are computed radiography (CR) and DR. Both systems can be used with the same portable x-ray generators that are commonly found in equine practice. The CR phosphor plate is physically transferred to a processor connected to a computer with software that generates a digital image, whereas the DR sensor is directly attached to the computer with software, which generates the digital image. Although the DR system is faster and facilitates learning the correct positioning for each radiographic projection, the DR equipment

Salem Valley Veterinary clinic, 12 Center Street, Salem, CT 06420, USA
E-mail address: rbaratt1dvm@gmail.com

Vet Clin Equine 29 (2013) 367–395
http://dx.doi.org/10.1016/j.cveq.2013.04.001
0749-0739/13/$ – see front matter © 2013 Elsevier Inc. All rights reserved.

is significantly more expensive and does not presently have sensors that can be used intraorally for imaging the cheek teeth. Most portable CR systems can process small plates that can be used for intraoral imaging of the equine teeth.

PATIENT PREPARATION AND EQUIPMENT CONSIDERATIONS
Sedation

Adequate standing sedation is a prerequisite for obtaining diagnostic dental radiographs. When working in the field, a quiet, clean, and dry area of the barn is preferred. The practitioner is encouraged to use sedative-analgesic agents that provide profound sedation without inducing significant ataxia. For intraoral views, the tongue motion is reduced with the administration of either butorphanol or diazepam. Typically, the longer acting α-agonists romifidine (0.05–0.10 mg/kg) or detomidine (0.01–0.02 mg/kg) are used in combination with butorphanol (0.005–0.01 mg/kg). When performing long procedures, most practitioners will use these drugs in a constant-rate infusion (CRI), ensuring that the horse can be maintained in an even plane of sedation.

Ancillary Equipment

Various devices can be used to obtain open-mouth projections of the cheek teeth. Some full-mouth speculums permit placement of the plate or sensor between the speculum and the horse's face, and do not interfere with the image. In some cases it is sufficient to place a bite block made of wood between the incisors; a small section of polyvinylchloride (PVC) plumbing pipe can also be used (**Fig. 1**).

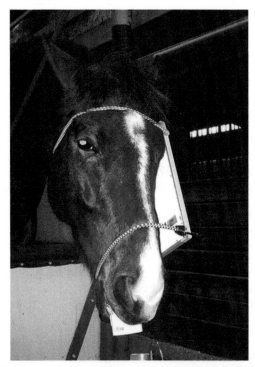

Fig. 1. The sedated patient tolerates the attachment of the computed radiography (CR) cassette to the head with bungee cords. The mouth is held open with a small section of 2-in (5-cm) polyvinylchloride (PVC) pipe. In most cases an assistant would not have to be near the horse's head when the radiograph is obtained in this manner.

With the CR systems, the cassette can often be attached to the horse's head with an elastic cord (Bungee cords, http://www.target.com) or simply held in position between the speculum strap and the horse's head (see **Fig. 1**). This action helps reduce scattered radiation exposure to assistants who do not need to hold the plate, and eliminates motion artifact not associated with chewing. With the DR systems the assistant should hold the sensor, and, when possible, the horse's head should be supported so that the head and the sensor both rest on the support (**Fig. 2**). Again, this minimizes motion artifact.

A radiographic marker that incorporates lead beads (Universal Medical, http://www.universalmedicalinc.com/) is useful for determining the orientation of the horse's head relative to the ground, and the identification of fluid lines within the sinuses (**Fig. 3**). Some form of instrument for holding the intraoral cassette in the mouth is needed. A simple holder can be fabricated from a short length of ½- to ¾-inch (1.3–1.9-cm) diameter PVC pipe that is slotted at one end (**Fig. 4**).

RADIOGRAPHIC VIEWS AND PRESENTATION CONVENTIONS
Presentation

The most common convention for presenting dental radiographs is labial mounting.[1] The radiographs are positioned so the viewer is looking at the images as if looking

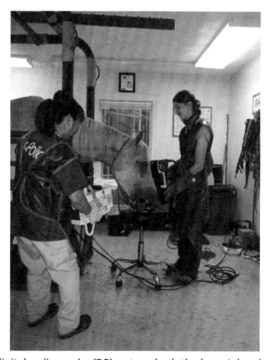

Fig. 2. With the digital radiography (DR) system, both the horse's head and the sensor are rested on the same support, thus minimizing motion artifact. Positioning is for the extraoral left maxillary lateral ventrodorsal (VD) oblique and the left mandibular lateral VD oblique views. The mouth is kept wide open with the Stubbs speculum, and the x-ray beam is directed from 45 to 60° ventral to the position for a straight lateral.

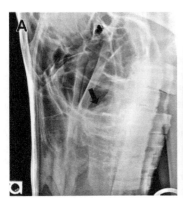
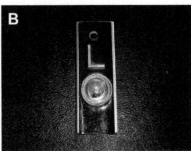

Fig. 3. (*A*) Left straight lateral view after the right maxillary second molar (110) had been extracted. Note that the left marker has beads that are aligned parallel to the fluid lines in the caudal maxillary sinus (*arrow*). (*B*) The left marker is backward owing to the horizontal flip of the image for correct presentation. To the right is an example of a left marker with lead beads.

into the patient's mouth. The right cheek teeth would be presented with the horse's nose on the viewer's right (**Fig. 5**). The maxillary incisors would be crown down, and the mandibular incisors presented crown up; the horse's left incisors would be to the viewer's right (**Fig. 6**). The dorsoventral (DV) views of the skull are usually presented with the nose down, and the horse's right side on the viewer's left (**Fig. 7**). These conventions become important when the radiographic label cannot be readily affixed to the intraoral cassette or the label is cropped out of the image, and the presentation is used to determine right-left orientation. The imaging software with the CR or DR system may not always comply with this convention, and it will be necessary to horizontally flip and or rotate some digital images, or make changes to the imaging software.

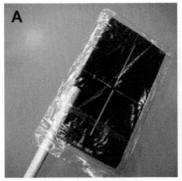
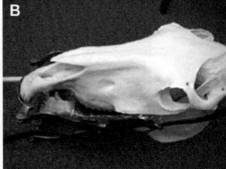

Fig. 4. (*A*) The intraoral cassette, which in this photograph measures 4 × 8 in (10 × 20 cm), is held in the horse's mouth with a section of 0.5-in (1.3-cm) PVC pipe that has been slotted at one end. (*B*) The cassette, protected with a plastic bag, is placed against the palate and held in position with the PVC holder. Excessive tongue movement or chewing will result in a blurred image. Additional administration of butorphanol or diazepam may eliminate tongue movement.

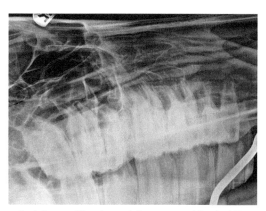

Fig. 5. The open-mouth right maxillary lateral dorsoventral (DV) oblique view. Note that the image required a horizontal flip for correct presentation (which is why the R marker is backward). The Stubbs speculum does not interfere with the image of the right maxillary arcade. This image was obtained with a 10 × 12-in (25 × 30-cm) cassette using the ScanX CR scanner and Metron software.

Radiographic Views

Straight lateral

The lateral view is obtained by placing the cassette on the side of the head, and the x-ray beam is centered on the rostral end of the facial crest, perpendicular to the sagittal plane. If the plate or sensor is on the horse's left side of the head, the image is presented with the nose to the viewer's left. However, owing to the magnification of the right cheek teeth, which are closer to the x-ray generator, the apices of the cheek teeth that are imaged on the straight lateral view are of right cheek teeth (**Fig. 8**). This

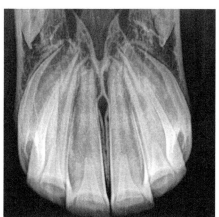
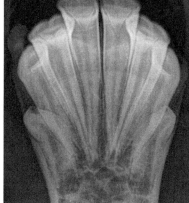

Fig. 6. The maxillary incisors are presented with the crowns down and the mandibular incisors with the crowns up. These intraoral images are of a 5-year-old Quarter Horse gelding, using a 4 × 4-in (10 × 10-cm) cassette and CR plates. Right-left markers are usually not used, as the software presents these images in the correct orientation: The horse's right is to the viewer's left.

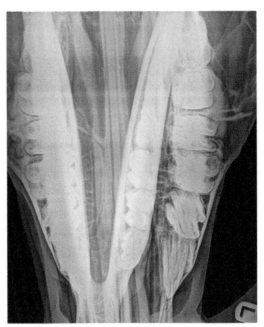

Fig. 7. This CR image, an offset mandible DV view of a 5-year-old Quarter Horse gelding, is presented nose down, with the horse's right to the viewer's left.

view is used primarily to image the paradental structures (sinuses and bones of the skull), especially fluid lines within the sinuses, but is also important for evaluation of gross dental deformities and abnormal tooth numbers. The mouth does not need to be open for this view, and a speculum is thus not necessary.

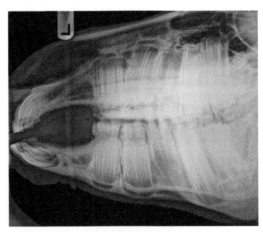

Fig. 8. Straight lateral radiograph of the head of a 1- to 2-year-old donkey. Because the left side of the head was closest to the x-ray imaging plate, the image is labeled left and presented with the horse's nose to the viewer's left. However, owing to magnification of the right cheek teeth (because they are closer to the x-ray generator), the apical detail is of the right cheek teeth.

Straight DV

The DV view is best obtained when the horse is heavily sedated and the head is allowed to rest on a low support. This placement allows the clinician to position his or her head directly over the x-ray generator, which greatly facilitates obtaining a true DV view. In this view the maxillary and mandibular cheek teeth are largely superimposed; however, one can evaluate the medial cortex of the mandibles and the lateral aspect of the maxillary cheek teeth, and the associated maxillae and sinus structures (**Fig. 9**). The nasal septum (vomer) should be on the midline in this view. Deviation of the nasal septum and soft-tissue filling defects of the nasal passages can also be appreciated on the DV projection. The intraoral DV or ventrodorsal (VD) projection can also be obtained with a vinyl cassette and CR plate of the appropriate size, and the use of a mouth speculum (**Fig. 10**). This projection eliminates the arcade overlap, and provides better detail of the nasal passages and vomer bone.

Offset mandible DV

This view is obtained by using either ties or a speculum (Juliuster, http://equinespecialties.highwire.com/product/juliuster) designed for this purpose (**Fig. 11**). Right and left offset mandible DV projections should be obtained so that the images can be compared and the pathologic situation more readily appreciated (**Fig. 12**).

Maxillary lateral DV oblique, extraoral

The positioning for this projection is obtained by setting up as for the straight lateral view, then raising the generator in the dorsal direction with the x-ray beam directed at the maxillary arcade, which is closest to the sensor/cassette (**Fig. 13**). As already noted, the lateral DV oblique view of the right maxillary arcade is obtained with the

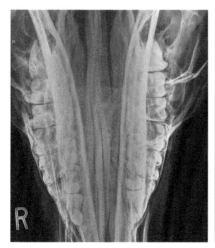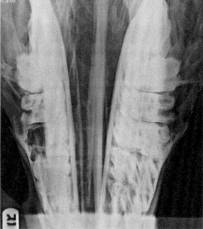

Fig. 9. Straight DV projection of a geriatric horse (*left*). In centric occlusion the palatal aspect of the maxillary cheek teeth are superimposed on the buccal aspect of the mandibular cheek teeth. The image on the left was obtained with a 200-mA generator at a focal distance of 26 in (66 cm). The image on the right (4-year-old, after oral extraction of 109) is a DV view obtained with a portable 15-mA generator, which requires a short tube-cassette distance for adequate technique; this results in some obliquity of the rostral cheek teeth. (*Courtesy of* Jennifer Rawlinson, DVM, Ithaca, NY.)

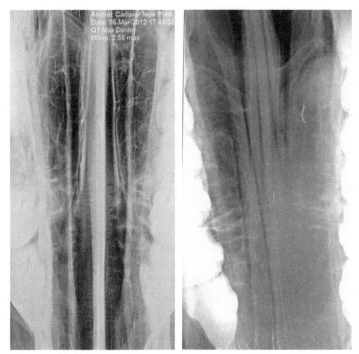

Fig. 10. The left image is an intraoral DV (4-year-old cadaver). This technique may be helpful in identifying subtle changes in the midline structures of the head. The image on the right is an intraoral DV view of a horse with a left ethmoidal hematoma.

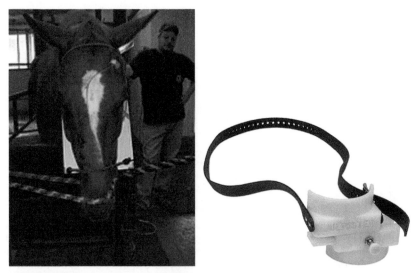

Fig. 11. The offset mandible DV projection can be obtained with 2 ropes and assistants applying a gentle pull in opposite directions (*left*) or with a speculum designed for this purpose (*right*).

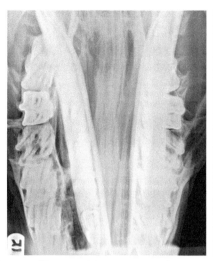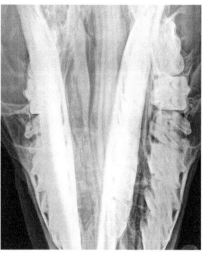

Fig. 12. Offset mandible DV views of an 11-year-old warmblood with a 109 crown fracture. There was no radiographic evidence of apical abscessation in any of the intraoral or extraoral views. There does appear to be a reduced opacity of the 109 infundibulae, indicating infundibular cemental hypoplasia.

right side of the head next to the sensor/cassette. For a survey view of the entire arcade, the beam is perpendicular to the long axis of the head, centered dorsal to the rostral end of the facial crest, and is about 30° to the horizontal plane. The image is presented with the horse's nose to the viewer's right (**Fig. 14**). This view is generally obtained in an effort to image the apical aspect of the maxillary arcade that is adjacent to the sensor/plate. By obtaining this projection with a bite block or speculum in place to hold the mouth open, the amount of arcade overlap is reduced, providing an image with more useful information that is easier to interpret.

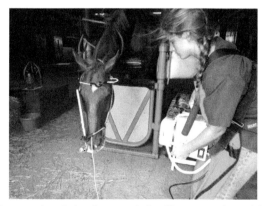

Fig. 13. The Stubbs speculum is in place, and the CR cassette is positioned between the speculum strap and the horse's head on the right side. The horse is positioned for the open-mouth right maxillary lateral DV oblique view; the x-ray beam is about 30° dorsal from the straight lateral.

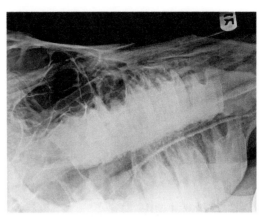

Fig. 14. Open-mouth lateral DV maxillary oblique view, as positioned in **Fig. 13**. In this view the left maxillary cheek teeth are projected, with magnification, into the interarcade space.

Maxillary lateral VD oblique, extraoral

This view is particularly important when an intraoral projection of the maxillary cheek teeth is not possible (either when using a DR system or if the amount of chewing precludes imaging with a CR intraoral plate). For this projection, the mouth must be held wide open with a speculum, and the beam is directed through the interarcade space at the maxillary cheek teeth on the side of the head next to the sensor/plate (see **Fig. 2**). The lateral VD angle is about 40° to 60° to the cassette/sensor, and the beam remains perpendicular to the long axis of the head. To obtain the correct projection one starts with the straight lateral positioning, then the x-ray generator is lowered without moving it in a caudal direction, which would result in caudorostral obliquity. When properly executed, this image will give apical detail similar to that obtained with intraoral plates (**Fig. 15**).

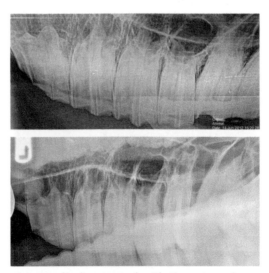

Fig. 15. The intraoral image (*top*) compared with the extraoral open-mouth lateral VD maxillary oblique image (*bottom*). The patient was a 10-year-old Hanovarian gelding. Note the similarity in apical detail that can be obtained with the extraoral technique. The apex of 211, which was not imaged in the intraoral view, was imaged on the extraoral view.

The presentation of the maxillary lateral VD view is consistent with the method outlined previously for the lateral projection. For the right maxillary lateral VD view, the sensor or plate is placed on the right side of the horse's head, and the image is presented with the horse's nose to the viewer's right.

Mandibular lateral VD oblique, extraoral

The positioning for this view is similar to that used for the maxillary lateral VD oblique view (see **Fig. 2**). Owing to the narrower space between the mandibles, there is generally considerable overlap of the mandibular arcades. In the mandibular lateral VD oblique projection, the roots of the mandibular arcade closest to the generator are superimposed on the crowns of the target mandibular cheek teeth. For example, in the lateral VD projection of the right mandibular cheek teeth, with the sensor/plate on the right side of the horse's head, the left mandibular cheek teeth reserve crowns/roots are superimposed on the crowns of the right mandibular cheek teeth (**Fig. 16**).

To image the crowns of the right mandibular cheek teeth, the positioning is similar to that used for the right maxillary (open-mouth) lateral DV view (see **Fig. 13**), but the x-ray beam is centered on the crowns of the mandibular cheek teeth in the interarcade space (**Fig. 17**).

Mandibular lateral DV oblique, extraoral

This view is an alternative projection of the mandibular cheek teeth, whereby the sensor/plate is placed ventrally, as for the straight DV view. The bisecting-angle technique is used, which in this case means an x-ray beam angle that is about 45° off the sagittal plane, with the beam centered on the mandibular cheek teeth closest to the generator (**Fig. 18**). The image is fairly similar to that obtained with the mandibular lateral VD technique.

Canine teeth

The maxillary and mandibular canine teeth can be imaged with either intraoral or extraoral techniques, using both DR and CR systems. For the extraoral view of the maxillary canine teeth the sensor/plate is positioned on the side of the head, and the x-ray beam is directed in a slightly caudorostral oblique angle with the x-ray beam centered on the canine teeth. Owing to the proximity of the mandibular incisors,

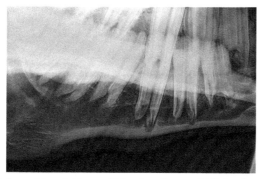

Fig. 16. Lateral VD view of the right mandible of an 8-year-old Holsteiner gelding presented for right mandibular swelling. There was a complicated crown fracture of the right mandibular fourth premolar (408). The DR sensor was placed on the right side of the horse's head. Note the apical bone lysis ("halo") and thickening of the ventral mandibular cortex, and soft-tissue swelling apical to 408.

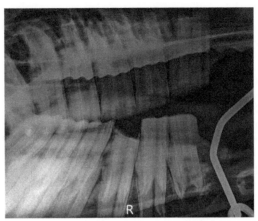

Fig. 17. This open-mouth lateral DV oblique view of the right mandibular cheek teeth is positioned similarly to the extraoral lateral DV maxillary oblique (see **Fig. 13**), with the x-ray beam centered on the interarcade space. (This is the horse with a complicated crown fracture of 408; the right mandibular lateral VD oblique is shown in **Fig. 16.**)

it is not generally possible to image both mandibular canines in one extraoral view (**Fig. 19**).

Alternatively, the sensor or plate can be placed in the mouth, although this requires sufficient sedation to prevent chewing (an aluminum full-mouth speculum [eg, Alumi-Spec Equine Speculum; Harlton's Equine Specialties. Elmwood, WI]). The occlusal DV view of the maxillary canines is obtained with the same technique used to image the maxillary incisors described next (**Fig. 20**). In the oblique intraoral views the target tooth is the canine closest to the x-ray generator. Thus, the DV oblique intraoral view of the left maxillary canine tooth would be obtained with the generator held on the horse's left side, with a DV angle of about 45° to the sensor/plate (**Fig. 25**).

The mandibular canine teeth are also readily evaluated with the intraoral technique used for the mandibular incisors. Both mandibular canine teeth can be imaged with the occlusal view (**Fig. 21**).

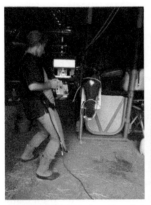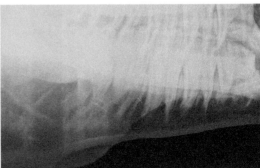

Fig. 18. Positioning for the right lateral mandibular DV oblique view. The x-ray beam is directed about 45° to the cassette/sensor, perpendicular to the long axis of the head and centered on the rostral end of the facial crest.

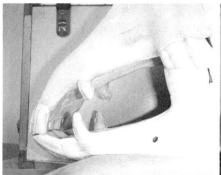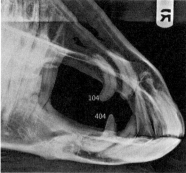

Fig. 19. This dry skull is used to demonstrate the extraoral positioning for imaging of the canine teeth. With a slightly caudorostral oblique lateral position, the canines are separated. In this case the right maxillary and mandibular canines (104, 404) are imaged caudally to the left canines. Because of the proximity of the roots of the mandibular canines to the incisors in most horses, both right and left mandibular canines are usually not imaged well in a single view.

Incisors

Incisors are imaged with a bisecting-angle, intraoral technique with both DR and CR systems (**Fig. 22**). Sedation sufficient to eliminate chewing is required; however, an aluminum speculum can be used to protect the cassette or sensor. The straight VD (mandibular occlusal) and DV (maxillary occlusal) views (**Fig. 23**) can be complemented with oblique views that separate the third incisors (**Fig. 24**). In geriatric horses the teeth and incisive bones are angled so that the x-ray beam can be almost

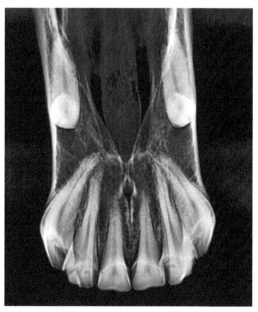

Fig. 20. DV intraoral view of the maxillary canine teeth. The positioning is the same as for the maxillary incisors (see **Fig. 25**).

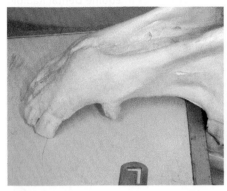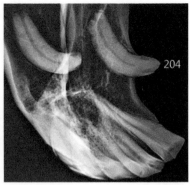

Fig. 21. Intraoral DV oblique view of the maxillary canines. The x-ray beam is at about a 45° angle to the plate, and perpendicular to the long axis of the head. Both canines are imaged; the target tooth in this instance was the left maxillary canine tooth (204).

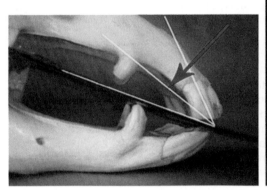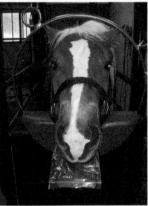

Fig. 22. The left photograph demonstrates the bisecting-angle technique for imaging the maxillary incisors. The x-ray beam (*red arrow*) is aimed at a 90° angle to the plane that bisects the angle formed by the tooth and the cassette. With adequate sedation, the horse will tolerate the placement of imaging plate in the mouth without chewing (*right*).

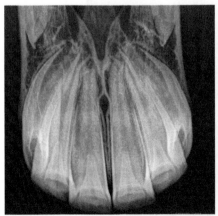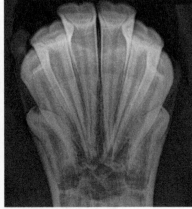

Fig. 23. Intraoral occlusal DV view of the maxillary incisors (*left*) and VD view of the mandibular incisors (*right*) of a 4-year-old gelding; the third incisors are erupted but not in wear. Note the wide-open apices of the third incisors and mandibular canine teeth. The conical, enamel-lined infundibulae are more apparent in the maxillary incisors.

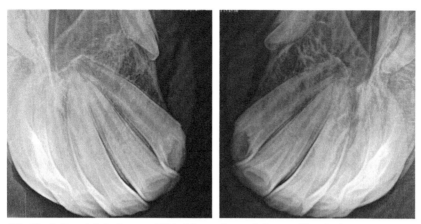

Fig. 24. The left and right intraoral DV oblique views of the maxillary incisors; compare with the straight DV view of the same horse in **Fig. 23**.

perpendicular to the sensor/plate, whereas this positioning will result in foreshortening of the incisors in the young horse.

Maxillary cheek teeth, intraoral

The bisecting-angle technique is used to image the maxillary cheek teeth with the CR plate placed intraorally. The CR plate, when placed on the palate, is almost at a 90° angle to the long axis of the maxillary cheek teeth. Therefore, the x-ray beam is directed at about a 45° angle to the plate, centered on the apical aspect of the cheek tooth (see **Fig. 25**; **Fig. 26**). This positioning must be modified by slightly more DV angle (50°–60°) in the young horse with a very long reserve crown, as the apical aspect may be projected off of the plate (**Fig. 27**). Intraoral imaging of the third maxillary molar is also challenging, as it tends to be projected off the caudal aspect of the plate (see

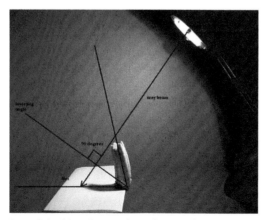

Fig. 25. Demonstration of the bisecting-angle technique for imaging the cheek tooth. The x-ray beam (represented by the tensor light) is directed perpendicular to the plane that bisects the angle between the tooth and the CR plate. The image (represented by the shadow of the tooth) is equal in length to the actual tooth.

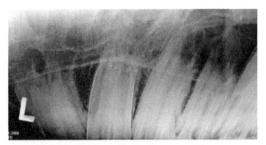

Fig. 26. Intraoral radiograph of the left maxillary cheek teeth in a 6-year-old horse. In this instance the beam is centered on the rostral end of the facial crest. Note that in the young horse the intraoral view will often only image the rostral 4 cheek teeth.

Figs. 26 and **27**). In some cases, the alternative extraoral views (maxillary VD oblique) will provide a better image of the third maxillary molars (see **Fig. 15**).

Mandibular cheek teeth, intraoral

To obtain this projection, the CR plate with 2.5 × 8.0-in (6.35 × 20.3-cm) dimensions is placed between the tongue and the lingual aspect of the mandibular cheek teeth. This action requires profound sedation, and even then, some horses will not tolerate this positioning of the plate. The x-ray beam is directed perpendicular to the plate; however, a slight lateral VD projection will usually result in capturing more of the reserve crown without significant lengthening artifact (**Fig. 28**). In a young horse, only the clinical crown and a portion of the reserve crown will be imaged (**Fig. 29**), whereas in the geriatric horse almost the entire tooth can be captured. As noted earlier, the open-mouth, mandibular DV oblique can also be used to image the crowns of the mandibular cheek teeth (see **Fig. 17**).

RADIOGRAPHIC ANATOMY AND PATHOLOGY

The equine hypsodont dentition has a unique gross, ultrastructural, and radiographic anatomy that reflects the adaptive evolution of this herbivore species.

Incisors

The radiographic anatomy of the incisor teeth is similar in both the deciduous and permanent dentition. The cementum extends supragingivally, and the enamel can be identified on the lengthy extent of the reserve crown (**Fig. 30**). The enamel-lined

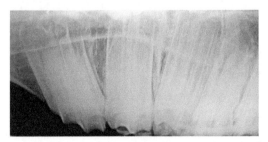

Fig. 27. In this intraoral radiograph of the left maxillary cheek teeth of a 3-year-old horse, the apices are projected off of the imaging plate. Intentional foreshortening of the image is required.

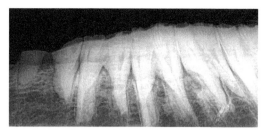

Fig. 28. Intraoral view of the left mandibular cheek teeth in a geriatric horse. Lateral slight VD obliquity helps capture the apices of some of the teeth.

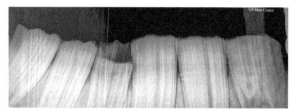

Fig. 29. Intraoral image of the right mandibular cheek teeth of a 7-year-old Lusitano gelding, presented with a complicated crown fracture of the first molar (409). Imaging of the apices of the mandibular cheek teeth with the intraoral technique is not possible in the young horse.

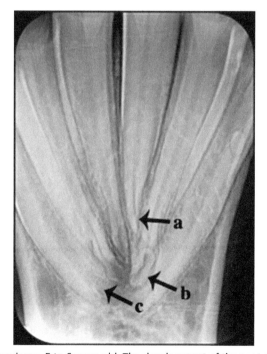

Fig. 30. Cadaver specimen, 5 to 6 years old. The development of the root of 301 has resulted in lateralization of the apical foramen (a). End-on view of the apical foramen of 302 illustrates that what appears to be a narrow circular apical foramen in the occlusal view is actually a flattened oval (b). The wide-open apex of the less mature third incisor, 403 is apparent (c). Note that the enamel defines the length of the reserve crown.

infundibulum is readily identified, and the pulp chamber is compressed labially by this structure (**Fig. 31**). Although not readily apparent on intraoral radiographs, serial sectioning of incisors or computed tomography (CT) studies reveal a complex pulp-chamber anatomy, which in cross section varies from oval just apical to the infundibulum, becoming compressed in the mesiodistal dimension and often dividing into 2 root canals apically. For most of the horse's life, normal coronal attrition is compensated for by continued eruption of the incisor and lengthening of the root, such that the overall length of the tooth in the radiographs appears relatively constant until the horse is older than 25 years.

Complicated crown fractures are those fractures of the clinical crown that result in pulp exposure. These fractures are relatively common in the horse, in both the incisors and cheek teeth. In brachydont species this type of fracture invariably results in pulp necrosis and often in apical abscessation. The horse, perhaps because of the hypsodont nature of the dentition, appears to be capable of mounting a pulpal response to injury, which maintains a viable pulp. The odontoblastic response to injury appears to be production of reparative (tertiary) dentin, similar in nature to that laid down at the occlusal aspect of the pulp horns during normal attrition.[2] Evidence of a "dentinal bridge" can sometimes be seen radiographically in incisors, and radiographic evidence of apical abscessation of incisors is rare (**Figs. 32** and **33**). Occasionally apical abscessation of incisors is evident radiographically as apical bone lysis (**Fig. 34**).

Equine odontoclastic tooth resorption and hypercementosis (EOTRH) is increasingly recognized as a form of periodontal disease involving the incisors and canine teeth of horses.[3] The degree to which both tooth resorption and hypercementosis occurs is variable; some horses exhibit primarily tooth resorption with very little

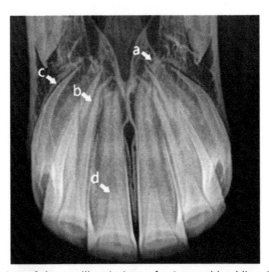

Fig. 31. Intraoral view of the maxillary incisors of a 4-year-old gelding. There is little root development of the third incisor, which has a very large apex (a). The second incisor, 1 year more mature, has some root development and a root canal (b). The periodontal ligament space (c) is represented radiographically as a radiolucent line between the tooth and the alveolar bone (the cribriform plate). The infundibulum is conical in shape and enamel lined (d). The pulp chamber is flattened in the area of the infundibulum, and on the occlusal surface would be represented by stained tertiary dentin (dental star) labial to the infundibulum (cup).

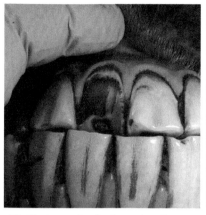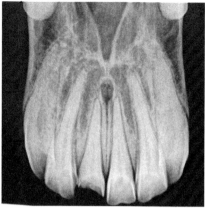

Fig. 32. Photograph of a long-standing complicated crown fracture of the right maxillary first incisor (*left*). The intraoral radiograph (*right*) reveals no evidence of apical bone lysis.

hypercementosis, whereas in others hypercementosis is the predominant feature (**Fig. 35**). Tooth resorption frequently occurs initially in the canine teeth and third incisors, and involves the second and first incisors sequentially over time. The tooth resorption most frequently involves the middle one-third of the tooth, with pathologic fracture occurring just apical to the free gingival margin (**Fig. 36**). Another common pattern is hypercementosis and labial tooth extrusion, with labial exposure of the entire reserve crown and root (**Fig. 37**). Radiographs of these extruded incisors generally exhibit a widened periodontal ligament space and a foreshortened reserve crown, attributable to the change in the angulation of the incisor as it is extruded.

Canine Teeth

Unlike the incisors, the canine tooth has a brachydont response to injury: pulp exposure usually does result in apical abscessation (see **Fig. 21**). Osteomyelitis with intrabony abscess formation may occur in the absence of fistulation (**Fig. 38**). As already

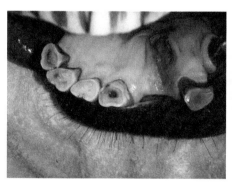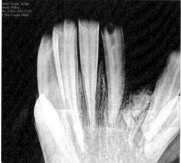

Fig. 33. In this geriatric pony, the left mandibular first incisor (301) has a pulp exposure evident clinically as an occlusal defect (photo, *left*). The intraoral radiograph (*right*) revealed a "dentinal bridge" that had formed about 8 mm apical to the occlusal surface. When this tertiary dentin was removed with a high-speed bur, bleeding pulp was encountered, indicating that this tooth was viable.

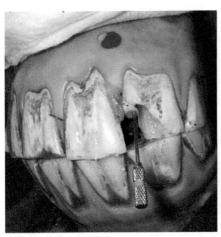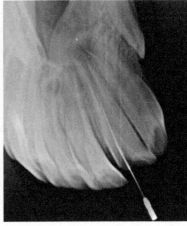

Fig. 34. The photograph on the left shows placement of a 60 mm endodontic file in the pulp exposed by the clinical crown fracture of 202 in a 5-year-old Morgan stallion; the injury occurred about 10 days previously. There is fistulation at the mucogingival line, apical to 201. The intraoral radiograph on the right reveals the file within the pulp chamber of 202. Treatment in this instance was with pulpectomy and placement of calcium hydroxide, and a composite restoration.

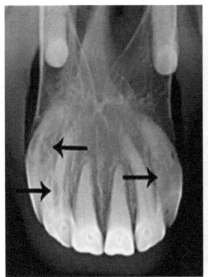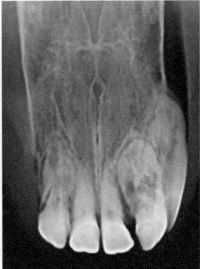

Fig. 35. Two examples of equine odontoclastic tooth resorption and hypercementosis (EOTRH) in geriatric horses. The radiograph on the left is typical of those horses that present with predominantly tooth resorption that affects the third incisors initially, and then involves the second and first incisors sequentially over several years (*arrows*). The radiograph on the right exemplifies those geriatric horses in which there is more predominant hypercementosis and extrusion of the incisors, again affecting the lateral incisors initially and progressing medially.

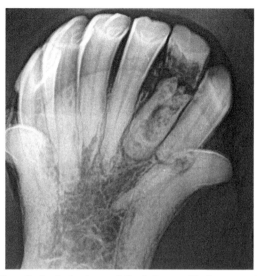

Fig. 36. EOTRH with pathologic fracture of the left mandibular second incisor (302). Note that the left mandibular third incisor may also be fractured at the junction of the middle and apical one-third in this view.

noted, EOTRH affects the canine teeth; however, tooth resorption in the canine teeth tends to occur in the coronal one-third, and bony replacement is more commonly observed in the distal two-thirds (**Fig. 39**). Spontaneous fracture of the crown may be followed by resorption and bone replacement of the root, with normal gingival healing by second intention (**Fig. 40**).

Maxillary Cheek Teeth and Sinuses

The infolding enamel obscures the anatomy of the cheek teeth in both intraoral and extraoral radiographs (**Fig. 41**). Although the infundibulum of the maxillary cheek teeth

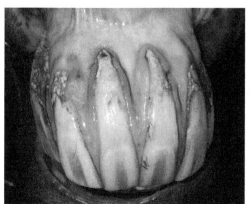
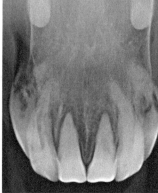

Fig. 37. EOTRH in a geriatric Thoroughbred gelding, in which extrusion is a predominant feature (*left*). The intraoral radiograph of this horse (*right*) reveals foreshortened central maxillary incisors and pathologic fracture of the third incisors caused by extensive tooth resorption.

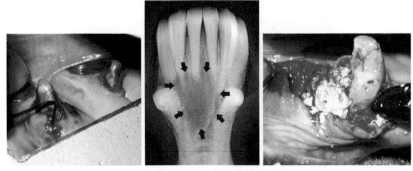

Fig. 38. Oral photograph (*left*) of a right mandibular canine tooth with a deep periodontal pocket. The radiograph in the center reveals a large area of mandibular bone lysis (*arrows*). The photograph on the right was obtained intraoperatively, and reveals the large amount of caseous purulent material present. (*Courtesy of* Edward Earley, DVM, Cogan Station, PA.)

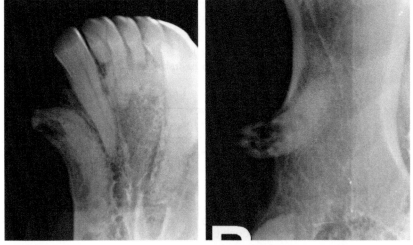

Fig. 39. Tooth resorption of the left mandibular canine (*left*) and the right maxillary canine (*right*) teeth. Loss of the periodontal ligament space around the root of this tooth indicates tooth resorption with bony replacement.

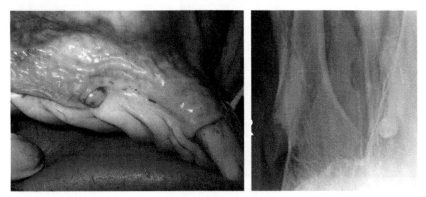

Fig. 40. There is intact gingival covering of the site where the right maxillary canine tooth crown had fractured (*left*), and the retained tooth root has undergone resorption with bone replacement (*right*).

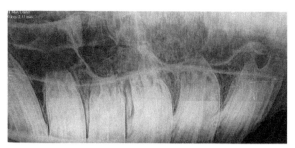

Fig. 41. Intraoral radiograph of the right maxillary arcade; although the anatomy of the crown is obscured by the infolding enamel, the apical anatomy can be evaluated, recognizing that the 3 individual roots are usually not distinguishable.

is enamel lined, even this structure is difficult to appreciate in radiographs. However, the area of interest is often the apical aspect of the cheek teeth and surrounding alveolus, and these structures can be readily evaluated with conventional radiography. It must be kept in mind that significant alveolar bone lysis (probably about 40% bone loss) must occur before it can be appreciated radiographically as a periapical "halo" (**Figs. 42** and **43**).

Other signs of apical infection of cheek teeth are blunting ("clubbing") of the tooth roots, widening of the periodontal ligament space, sclerosis (condensing osteitis) of apical alveolar bone, thickening of the lamina dura, and the apical deposition of cementum (**Fig. 44**). The radiographic sensitivity (ability to diagnose apical abnormality when present) and specificity (ability to identify patients who do not have the disease) have been shown to be low for the diagnosis of apical disease in people.[4] A recent study has demonstrated similar results in horses; periapical halo and apical sclerosis were the radiographic signs of apical disease with the highest sensitivity and specificity.[4]

The practitioner must be familiar with the radiographic appearance of "eruption cysts" that are a normal finding in juvenile horses presented with unilateral or bilateral facial swelling over the apices of premolars. These cases lack nasal discharge or malodorous breath; radiographically the apical anatomy is well defined and there is thinning of the alveolar bone, rather than condensing osteitis (sclerotic bone).

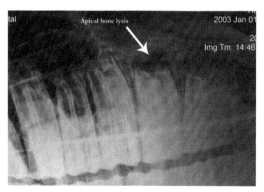

Fig. 42. Apical bone lysis (halo) and condensing osteitis associated with the right maxillary third premolar (107) in a 5-year-old warmblood gelding. This horse presented with right facial swelling rather than nasal discharge.

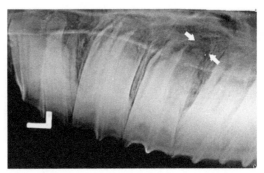

Fig. 43. Intraoral view of the left maxillary arcade with blunting and periapical bone lysis (halo) indicated by the arrows.

Radicular cysts that are associated with abnormal permanent maxillary premolar development are frequently associated with clinical signs such as obstruction of the nasal passage and nasal discharge, in addition to facial swelling (**Fig. 45**).

Sinusitis secondary to apical disease of the maxillary molars is relatively common, usually presenting as a fetid unilateral nasal discharge. Fluid lines within the compartments of the maxillary and conchal sinuses are a frequent radiographic finding (**Figs. 46** and **47**). Overt dental disease is not always readily apparent radiographically, and differentiating primary sinusitis from that of dental etiology can be challenging. Careful oral examination for the presence of exposed pulp horns, crown fractures, abnormal periodontal pocket depths, and infundibular decay may direct the practitioner to the diseased tooth responsible for the sinusitis. Some cases will require CT for identification of the diseased cheek tooth, as the sensitivity and specificity of identification of apical disease is better with CT than with DR. On the other hand, most pulp exposures discovered on routine oral examinations will not have radiographic evidence of apical abscessation. In these cases, either the pulp has succeeded in producing a protective layer of tertiary dentin, or the apical abnormality has not progressed to the point of being radiographically detectable. Radiographic examination is indicated to confirm

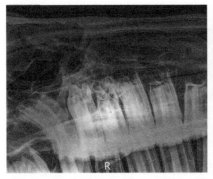
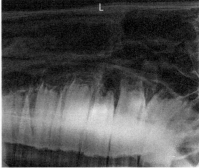

Fig. 44. Extraoral lateral DV maxillary oblique radiographs of a 4-year-old Clydesdale gelding presented for right nasal discharge. There is periapical bone lysis (halo) and condensing osteitis and widened periodontal ligament space of the right first and second molars (109, 110). Compare with the radiograph on the right, the extraoral lateral DV view of the left maxillary arcade.

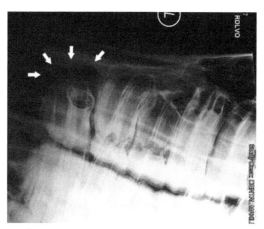

Fig. 45. Radicular cyst (*arrows*) involving the left maxillary second premolar (206) in a 2-year-old horse. (*Courtesy of* Jennifer Rawlinson, DVM, Ithaca, NY.)

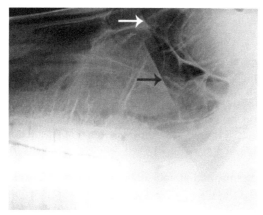

Fig. 46. Fluid lines within the conchal (*white arrow*) and maxillary (*black arrow*) sinuses in a geriatric horse.

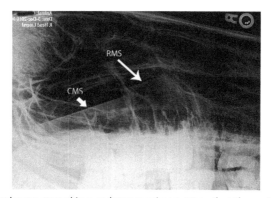

Fig. 47. Fluid lines demonstrated in a cadaver specimen. Note that the rostral maxillary sinus (RMS) and caudal maxillary sinus (CMS) are separated by a bony septum and drain into the nasomaxillary orifice into the middle nasal meatus. The RMS and the ventral conchal sinus share a common space dorsal to the infraorbital canal, and are enclosed dorsally by the bulla of the ventral conchal sinus.

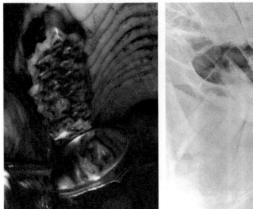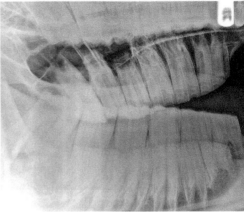

Fig. 48. Oral examination of an 11-year-old Morgan gelding revealed a complicated crown fracture of the right maxillary second molar (110) involving the buccal pulp horns #1 and #2. The lateral VD oblique view of the right maxillary cheek teeth revealed no radiographic evidence of apical disease of this tooth.

the absence of apical pathosis (**Fig. 48**) and for comparison with follow-up radiographic examinations.

The presence of an oroantral fistula may allow packing of feed material in the maxillary sinus. In these cases, the radiographic appearance of the sinus may be of a soft-tissue density with an irregular radiopacity caused by the presence of feed material, purulent fluid, and gas (**Fig. 49**). Osteomyelitis accompanying severe sinusitis may allow communication of the right and left sinuses, resulting in a bilateral nasal discharge.

Sinus cysts, neoplasms, and ethmoidal hematomas are causes of unilateral nasal discharge that are not of dental origin, but which may be identified radiographically (**Figs. 50** and **51**).

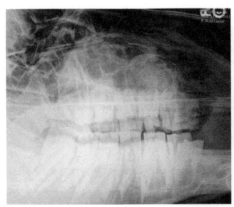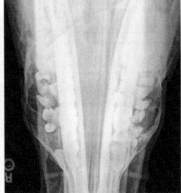

Fig. 49. Right lateral and DV view of a 25-year-old warmblood mare with bilateral facial swelling and fetid nasal discharge. Oral examination revealed bilateral oronasal fistulae and a right oroantral fistula. The right maxillary sinus was packed with feed and purulent material. There is bony expansion of the maxillae around the second and third premolars, also found to be packed with feed and purulent material.

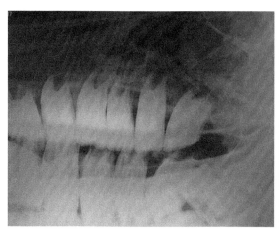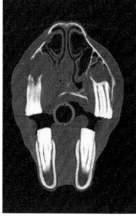

Fig. 50. Right lateral DV oblique view (*left*) of the maxillary cheek teeth in a geriatric horse with dysphagia, weight loss, and bilateral nasal discharge. Note the absence of normal alveolar bone detail and periodontal ligament space associated with the cheek teeth. A computed tomography scan (*right*) confirmed the presence of a large invasive mass (paranasal adenocarcinoma). (*Courtesy of* Jennifer Rawlinson, DVM, Ithaca, NY.)

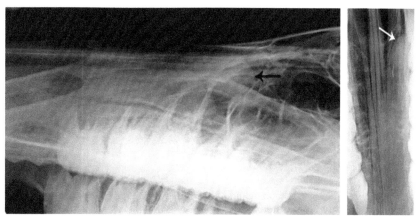

Fig. 51. Lateral DV oblique radiograph (*left*) and DV radiograph (*right*) demonstrating an ethmoidal hematoma in the left dorsal nasal conchus and nasal meatus (*arrows*).

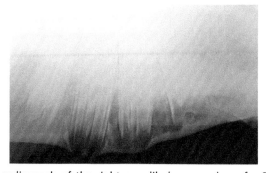

Fig. 52. Extraoral radiograph of the right mandibular premolars of a 3-year-old Arabian mare. There is thinning of the ventral mandibular cortex and enlargement of the dental sac of the third and fourth right mandibular premolars (407, 408), with normal appearance of the developing tooth roots.

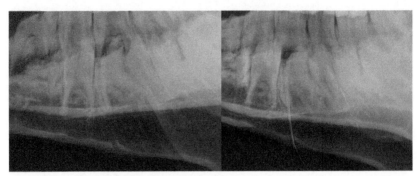

Fig. 53. Complicated crown-root fracture of the left mandibular fourth premolar (308) and ventral drainage (*left*). A radiopaque probe was placed in the draining tract (*right*). (*Courtesy of* Leah E. Limone, DVM, Hamilton, MA.)

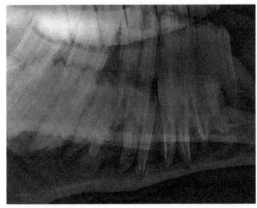

Fig. 54. This 8-year-old warmblood gelding has bilateral complicated crown fractures of the mandibular fourth premolars. There is apical bone lysis (halo) evident, as well as thickening of the underlying cortical bone.

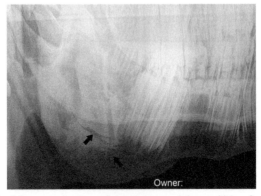

Fig. 55. Lateral VD oblique projection of the right caudal mandible of a 2-year-old donkey (see also **Fig. 8**). Arrows point to fracture lines.

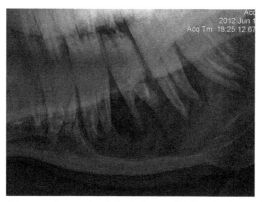

Fig. 56. Lateral VD oblique radiograph of the left mandibular cheek teeth. A large radicular cyst involves the caudal 4 cheek teeth.

Mandibular Cheek Teeth

The absence of infundibulae and associated sinus structures, and the presence of only 2 roots make radiographic interpretation of the mandibular cheek teeth somewhat more straightforward than the maxillary counterparts. Eruption cysts and apical abscessation both can present as firm swellings of the ventral mandible. As in the case of the maxillary cheek teeth, the eruption cysts tend to exhibit normal radiographic appearance of the apical aspect of the developing roots, with a surrounding cystic structure and thinning of the cortical bone ventrally (**Fig. 52**). Apical abscessation of the mandibular cheek teeth often presents with fistulation and purulent ventral drainage. The draining tract can be probed and radiographically imaged to identify the diseased tooth (**Fig. 53**). The apically diseased mandibular cheek tooth may present with a radiographic halo and condensing osteitis in the absence of ventral drainage (**Fig. 54**). Other causes for mandibular swelling, such as fracture (**Fig. 55**), tooth impaction, radicular cysts (**Fig. 56**), and neoplasia, can be diagnosed with standard radiographic techniques, but may require CT imaging for accurate 3-dimensional assessment and treatment planning.

REFERENCES

1. Wiggs RO, Loprise HB. Veterinary dentistry, principles & practice. Philadelphia: Lippincott-Raven; 1997. p. 155.
2. Dixon PM, duToit N. Dental anatomy. In: Easley J, Dixon PM, Schumacher J, editors. Equine dentistry. 3rd edition. Edinburgh (United Kingdom): Saunders Elsevier; 2010. p. 51–76.
3. Stazick C, Bienert A, Kreutzer R, et al. Equine odontoclastic tooth resorption and hypercementosis. Vet J 2008;178:372–9.
4. Townsend NB, Hawkes CS, Rex R, et al. Investigation of the sensitivity and specificity of radiological signs for diagnosis of periapical infection of equine cheek teeth. Equine Vet J 2011;43(2):170–8.

Advanced Imaging in Equine Dental Disease

Kurt Selberg, MS, DVM[a],*, Jeremiah T. Easley, DVM[b]

KEYWORDS

- Imaging • Dental • Advanced • Equine • Disease

KEY POINTS

- Magnetic resonance imaging and computed tomography are becoming more widespread in availability.
- Advanced imaging of the skull in dental disease allows for more accurate diagnosis with targeted treatment of the disease process.
- Advanced 3-dimensional imaging may be vital to the successful diagnosis and outcome.

INTRODUCTION

Dental and sinus disorders are relatively common and of major clinical importance in equine medicine. Routine radiographs are often implemented as an initial diagnostic test when horses present with signs of dental- or sinus-related disease. Clinical signs may include purulent nasal discharge, facial swelling, dropping feed, eye discharge, or weight loss. Radiographic sensitivity and specificity for dental disease have a wide range, ranging from 52% to 69% and 70% to 90%, respectively.[1,2] Obtaining quality skull radiographs can be difficult. In addition, the complexity and overlap of anatomic structures can make interpretation challenging. Patients that are recalcitrant to medical therapy, with normal or equivocal radiographic findings with clinical signs, require surgical intervention; previous dental surgery with persistent signs, disease that involves multiple areas, or extensive disease may require additional advanced imaging. Advanced imaging such as computed tomography (CT), magnetic resonance imaging (MRI), and nuclear scintigraphy may be employed to help better characterize the extent and identify the exact location of the disease, and allow for more effective treatment.

NUCLEAR SCINTIGRAPHY

The availability of nuclear scintigraphy has become widespread. Costs associated with nuclear scintigraphy can vary depending on region and the clinic's breakdown

[a] Department of Biosciences and Diagnostic Imaging, University of Georgia, 501 DW Brooks Drive, Athens, GA 30602, USA; [b] Preclinical Surgical Research Laboratory, Colorado State University, 300 W Drake, Fort Collins, CO 80524, USA
* Corresponding author.
E-mail address: selberg@uga.edu

Vet Clin Equine 29 (2013) 397–409
http://dx.doi.org/10.1016/j.cveq.2013.04.009
0749-0739/13/$ – see front matter © 2013 Elsevier Inc. All rights reserved.

of body parts included in an examination. A focused examination of the skull can be performed for $400 to $700 in cases of suspected dental disease.

Nuclear scintigraphy uses radionuclides attached to different molecules specific for the body system of interest. In the case of bone scans, methylene diphosphanate (MDP) and hydroxymethylene disphosphanate (HDP) are the most common bone tracers. Nuclear scintigraphy camera design incorporates a thallium-doped sodium iodine crystal that scintillates in response to gamma photons emitted during decay after intravenous injection of the radioisotope. Small flashes of light are produced at the crystal. The photomultipliers pick up the light and convert it to electrical signals. The electrical signals are converted by the attached computer to create an image. The image matrix is generally set to 256 × 256, with image counts between 200–300,00.

When performing scintigraphy on the skull, a minimum of dorsal and lateral views should be obtained. The head and axial spine generally have more movement during image acquisition. Dynamic capture (motion correction) is recommended when obtaining images of the skull. Most, if not all, images are acquired under no or standing sedation. The normal scintigraphic appearance of the dental arcades changes with age (**Fig. 1**).[3] As the horse ages, the radiopharmaceutical uptake pattern changes from well-defined arches, to less definition of the arches, to a more linear-continuous pattern. This is due to increased uptake in the interdental bone.[3] This may make differentiating age-related changes from periodontal disease challenging. In these cases, clinical signs and intraoral findings are paramount to making the correct diagnosis.[4] Indications for nuclear scintigraphy include suspected dental disease recalcitrant to medical therapy, normal radiographs with clinical signs, previous dental surgery with persistent signs, and disease that involves multiple areas.

Scinitgraphic images reflect physiologic rather than anatomic structure and are sensitive to bone turnover.[5] Dental disease often involves the surrounding alveolar bone, periodontal ligament, and paranasal sinus, with associated bony turnover and

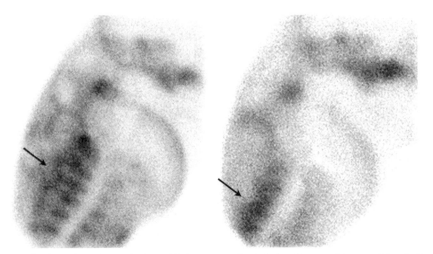

Fig. 1. The lateral nuclear scintigraphic image on the left is a 3 year-old warm blood; the image on the right is of a 15 year-old warm blood with no history of dental disease. The young horse has well defined arches along the tooth root and delineation between the teeth. The older horse has increased radiopharmaceutical in the interdental space, blending with the cheek teeth into a linear pattern of uptake.

inflammation.[6] In small studies,[4,7,8] scintigraphy illustrates areas of dental and sinus disease well. In these studies, some of the patients had minimal or equivocal changes on radiographic images. The additional scinitgraphic images allowed for better, more targeted treatment. The sensitivity and specificity of scitigraphy have been reported at 95% and 86%, respectively.[1] When clinicians had both radiographs and scintigrams to evaluate concurrently, sensitivity and specificity for detection of dental disorders increased to 97.7% and 100%.[1] Additionally, a negative nuclear scintigraphic scan in an area of suspicion may direct the clinician to seek other diagnostic tests or anatomic areas for similar presenting signs.[8]

Abnormalities detected on bone scan show up as focal or diffuse areas of increased radiopharmaceutical uptake (RU) associated with the affected anatomic area. Periapical tooth abscesses often have focal uptake (**Fig. 2**), where sinus disease is more often diffuse and often follows the outline of the paranasal sinus.[4,9] There may be overlap of abnormal RU in cases of diffuse disease and when both the tooth root and sinuses are affected. In these cases, radiographic images offer the added benefit of being an anatomic study. Additionally, nuclear scintigraphy images differentiate sinus from apical dental disease well when orthogonal views are available.[10]

COMPUTED TOMOGRAPHY

CT is cross-sectional images of structures in a body plane reconstructed by the computer from differential radiograph absorption collected from the tube detector. The tube detector rotates around the longitudinal axis of the body, collects data, and assigns gray scale values based on attenuation, thus producing an image free from superimposition. Most CT scanners today are based on third-generation technology, Meaning that the radiograph tube and detectors are rigidly linked so that they rotate together around the patient (a motion called rotate–rotate).

Multislice CT machines are widely available. The most common in veterinary medicine are 4- and 16-slice machines. The only real difference is the number of slices collected per rotation, and thus the speed. The minimum slice thickness and resolution remain unaffected. All other factors being equal, the 16-slice system is 4 times faster. However, only a small proportion of the time spent in the scanner is actually

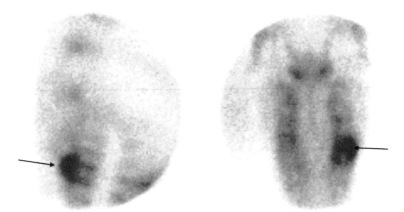

Fig. 2. Lateral and dorsal skull nuclear scintigraphic images of a 10 year-old warm blood. Focal marked radiopharmaceutical is present at the apex of the left first maxillar molar (*arrows*), consistent with apical tooth root abscess.

used for image acquisition. Most time is spent on patient positioning and anesthesia setup/monitoring.

CT examination of the skull in the horse is generally done under general anesthesia. The horse is positioned in dorsal recumbency. The weight of the[11–13] body is supported by a supplemental table, generally designed to move in unison with the existing CT table. CT machines with a moving gantry are also available. This allows for standing sedated CT examination of the skull (**Fig. 3**).[14] These systems are not as widely available and require a recessed area in the back of the gantry to allow for the horse's head into the CT. The gantry or floor must be able to be raised or lowered to fit the height of the horse.

The native images are acquired in the transverse plane in the horse. Postacquisition reconstruct images can be made in any plane (**Fig. 4**). Additionally, 3-dimensional images for surgical planning and owner/client education can be made (**Fig. 5**). CT anatomy has been reviewed previously,[11,15] and is briefly described here (see **Fig. 4**).

Once acquired, the images can be optimized to evaluate bone, soft tissue, and brain. This manipulation (window width/window level) is important to fully evaluate the skull. An important function of CT is the measure of tissue attenuation (radiopacity) in Hounsfield units (HUs) (**Table 1**). This can help differentiate pure fluids from soft tissue masses. In general, HUs for soft tissue are approximately 60, and fluid should be less than 20. However, as fluid becomes inspissated, mucosa becomes edematous, or as tumors become necrotic, there is overlap in these values. In 18 horses undergoing CT for dental-related reasons, it was not possible to differentiate exudate from swollen sinus lining.[16]

The widespread acceptance of CT for dental and skull disorders has progressed the knowledge base. CT has played a pivotal role in the diagnosis and effective treatment

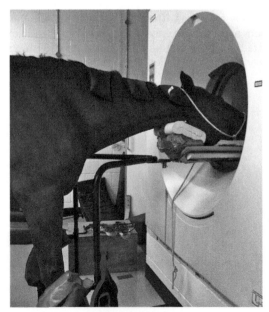

Fig. 3. Example of a standing CT. Note that the CT gantry is elevated from the floor to accommodate the standing sedated patient. (*Courtesy of* Sarah Powell, VetMB, MA, MRCVS, Newmarket, United Kingdom.)

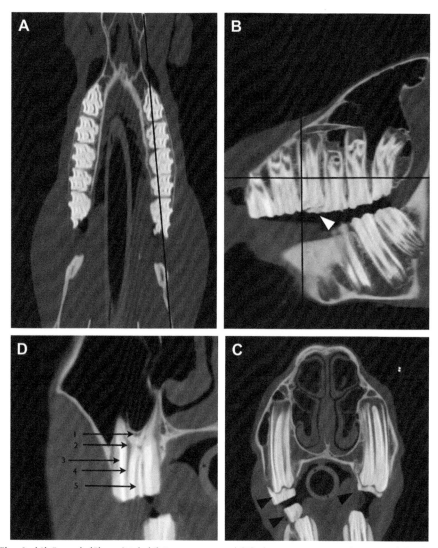

Fig. 4. (A) Dorsal, (B) sagittal, (C) transverse, and (D) closeup transverse images of the first maxillary molar. Reference lines have been applied for the approximate level of the recon on the dorsal (*line* of sagittal image) and sagittal (*lines* for dorsal and transverse images). The arrowheads are highlighting the residual deciduous teeth (caps). 1. Periodontal space. 2. Dental pulp. 3. Enamel folds/dentin. 4. Pulp canal. 5. Infundibulum.

of equine dental and sinonasal disorders.[12,16–19] Common CT features of dental disease include widening of the periodontal space, tooth root lysis/blunting, tooth root fragmentation, alveolar bone sclerosis, and apical tooth root gas.[12,16] The most common tooth affected is the first maxillary molar with or without concurrent involvement of the adjacent molar and premolar.[16] Because of the close association of the fourth premolar, and first and second molar with the maxillary sinus, there is often a secondary sinusitis. Gas within the maxillary teeth infundibulum leading to tooth decay (caries) has been implicated in tooth root fracture and apical tooth root infection.[12,16]

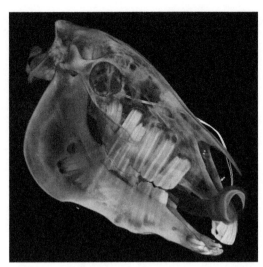

Fig. 5. 3-dimensional surface rendering CT image of the equine skull. With viewing software, this can be manipulated to see every angle of the skull and cut away anatomy to visualize internal structures.

However, gas can be seen in normal and abnormal teeth and has not been linked with apical tooth root infection.[12]

Sinusitis can be either primary or secondary (dental) in origin. Sinusitis CT characteristics include thickening of the mucosa, reduced air filling, fluid within the sinus, and expansion of the sinus (**Fig. 6**). Inspissated pus is a common finding in sinus disease, and may be difficult to resolve with medical treatment.[10] Inspissated purulent material is usually soft tissue attenuating and may have small gas pockets internally. Disease can affect any of the sinuses. The most commonly affected sinuses are the rostral and caudal maxillary sinuses, and ventral conchal sinus.[10] The ventral conchal sinus seems to have the greatest affinity to harbor inspissated pus.[10]

MAGNETIC RESONANCE IMAGING

This can be a confusing subject, and it is beyond the scope of the article to review MRI acquisition. A review of the subject is available.[20] It is helpful to realize that MRI is unlike CT, and radiographs are images are based on attenuation (ie, bone is white; air is black, and soft tissues are shades of grays). Magnetic resonance images are based

Table 1 Hounsfield units of tissues	
Tissue	**Hounsfield Unit**
Bone	1000
Soft tissue	40–60
Brain	30–40
Water	0
Fat	−100
Air	−1000

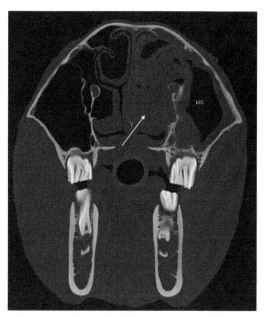

Fig. 6. Transverse CT image at the level of the second maxillary molar in a 20 year-old quarter horse. There is soft tissue attenuating material in the left ventral conchal sinus (*arrow*). Centrally in the material is focal gas pocketing. This is consistent with inspissated material. The septae of the ventral conchal sinus are expanded. The mucosa of the left rostral maxillary sinus is thickened. This horse has concurrent fractures of the upper first molar and fourth premolar.

signal measured from spinning magnetic moments of the hydrogen nuclei. Images are described in signal intensity, often relative to muscle or normal areas of the same tissue. Several sequences exist and produce an image with distinct characteristics and diagnostic value. In general, cortical bone, teeth, air, tendons, ligaments, and some stages of hemorrhage are black. Fat is generally of high signal on sequences that do not have fat suppression. Other soft tissues are shades of gray, depending on their magnetic properties (**Table 2**).

Similar to CT, images of the skull are generally made while recumbent under general anesthesia. Magnetic resonance hardware comes in a variety of field strengths (Tesla).

Table 2
Examples of tissue appearance on common imaging sequences

	T1 Weighted	T2 Weighted	STIR
Bone cortex	Very low signal (black)	Very low signal (black)	Very low signal (black)
Bone marrow	High signal (white)	High signal (white)	Low signal (gray-black)
Fluid (low protein)	ISO-signal (gray)	High signal (white)	High signal (white)
Fluid (high protein)	High signal (white)	Low signal (gray)	High signal (white)
Acute hemorrhage	Low to ISO-signal (black to gray)	Low to ISO-signal (black to gray)	Low to ISO-signal (black to gray)
Subacute hemorrhage	High signal (white)	High signal (white)	Various signal
Fat	High signal (white)	High signal (white)	Low signal (gray-black)

This may vary the scanning protocol and time required for the anatomic area to be scanned as optimized for the machine. Scan protocols can range from 45 to 120 minutes, depending on the scanner and sequences used. Magnetic resonance images can be obtained in infinite body planes to suit the anatomic area. Pricing may vary on geographic location, scanner available, and body part(s) images. A rough average is $2500 for the skull to be imaged. Not all magnetic resonance gantries can accommodate the equine skull, and whether this can happen depends on the gantry diameter, length, and patient size.

MRI has been well received by the equine community for musculoskeletal images due to its superior soft tissue contrast resolution.[21–24] Little has been published regarding dental disease diagnosed with MRI. The literature that is available includes normal anatomy of structures of the skull to pathologic change in the brain and pharynx.[25–28] The list of publications for use in skull pathologic change continues to grow. Information about periodontal disease, sinusitis, and endodontal disease can be extracted from MRI (**Fig. 7**) in great detail.

In people, work is underway to use MRI as a noninvasive and nonionizing way of imaging the teeth with a suitable clinical scan time.[29] Although MRI provides great soft tissue contrast, teeth are void of signal in conventional MRI. A new technique allows both the solid and soft tissue components to be imaged for dental and

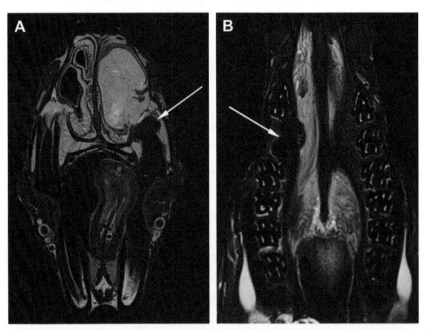

Fig. 7. (*A*) Transverse T2 weighted magnetic resonance image at the level of the third maxillary premolar. (*B*) Dorsal short-tau inversion recovery magnetic resonance image at the level of the apex of teeth. The apex of right third maxillary premolar is malformed (*arrow*). The periodontal space is widened with intermediate signal tissue. There is complete loss of dental pulp in the right third maxillary premolar. This is linear intermediate-to-high signal centrally located in the normal left third maxillary premolar compared with the affected premolar. A large mass with intermediate-to-high signal mass is immediately dorsal to the abnormal apex of the right third maxillary premolar. This fills the rostral maxillary sinus, ventral conchal sinus, and dorsal conchal sinus with associated expansion of the conchae.

maxillofacial applications.[30] The same study, using ex vivo equine teeth, showed great detail of the tooth.[30] This will allow for more accurate diagnosis of endodontal disease.

SUMMARY

Advanced diagnostic imaging has become essential in equine veterinary medicine, most notably in the diagnosis and treatment of dental- and sinus-related diseases. Veterinarians' understanding of dental disease has drastically improved in recent years since access to nuclear scintigraphy, CT, and MRI services has spread. Although conventional and digital radiography will always be considered the first-line diagnostic modality for dental- and sinus-related disorders, as a clinician it is important to realize the value of advanced diagnostic imaging.

Dental-related disease is classically difficult to diagnose and treat with a high potential for complications. Diseases can have an effect localized to the tooth alone, or impact the sinuses, oral cavity, nasal cavity, or even result in systemic effects. With this in mind, it is important to utilize all diagnostic tools available until a definitive diagnosis is obtained. Performing dental surgery without an accurate diagnosis can lead to long-term complications. Complications such as chronic oronasal, orosinus, or orocutaneous fistulas are extremely difficult to resolve and often lead to frustration to the clinician and client, excess financial burdens to the client, and high morbidity or even destruction of the horse. Because of this, it is imperative when treating dental disease that actions are appropriate and accurate and that complications are overall unavoidable. Advanced diagnostic imaging through nuclear scintigraphy, CT imaging, and MRI in most scenarios provides an accurate diagnosis leading to a well-constructed and precise treatment plan for the horse. It is the authors' opinion that invasive surgical treatment of dental-related disorders not be performed until there is high confidence in the diagnosis.

Three-dimensional imaging via CT or MRI has revolutionized capabilities to accurately understand anatomy in vivo and diagnose dental- and sinus-related disease. The authors have experienced numerous cases where 3-dimensional imaging was vital to the diagnosis. Although CT and MRI are both significantly more expensive compared with other diagnostic tools, the financial cost of inaccurate diagnosis and treatment can often result in higher overall costs.

An 11-year-old Jenny was referred for evaluation after a 6 month history of purulent discharge from the left nasolacrimal duct. Previous diagnostics and treatments included retrograde flushing of the nasolacrimal duct, culture of the discharge, multiple examinations by the referring veterinarian and ophthalmologist, and successive courses of antibiotic therapy throughout the 6 month time period. There were no dental-related clinical signs that could be identified on oral examination. No cause of the dacryocystits could be identified, and there was no resolution of clinical signs. CT examination of the skull and contrast dacryocystorhinography revealed soft tissue swelling within and surrounding the left nasolacrimal duct at the level of the third maxillary premolar, and a small communication was noted between the rostral medial tooth root and the nasolacrimal duct along with narrowing of the contrast column. Irregular soseeous lysis of the alveolar bone was present axial to the left third maxillary premolar (**Fig. 8**). Periapical infection of premolar and exclusive drainage via the nasolacrimal duct were diagnosed. Oral extraction of third premolar resulted in resolution of clinical signs.[31]

A 5-year-old Lusitano stallion with a 7 week history of right-sided maxillary swelling at the level of the right second maxillary premolar was evaluated. An oral examination was unremarkable, and radiographs revealed mild increased radiopacity or sclerosis

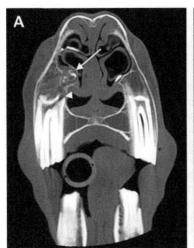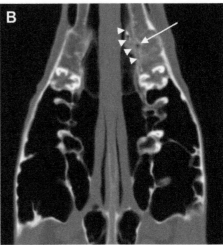

Fig. 8. (*A*) Transverse CT image at the level of the third maxillary premolar in an 11 year-old donkey. Focal gas is present in the mesial medial tooth root (*arrowhead*). The nasolacrimal duct has positive contrast infused. This is surrounded by soft tissue-attenuating material and malformation of the conchal scrolls (*arrow*). (*B*) Dorsal CT image of the equine skull immediately dorsal to the apex of the maxillary teeth. There is focal gas secondary to a periapical abscess in the mesial medial tooth root of the left maxillary second premolar (*arrow*). Note the close proximity of the mesial medial tooth root of the left maxillary premolar to the nasolacrimal duct (*arrowheads*).

at the level of tooth roots of right maxillary second and fourth premolar and first molar. Broad-spectrum antibiotic therapy resulted in short-term resolution of the maxillary swelling. Prior to CT examination, the tentative diagnosis was periapical abscess of the right second maxillary premolar, with possible pathologic change of fourth premolar and first molar. The CT examination revealed increased soft tissue swelling at the apex of the first molar, gas in the mesial–medial tooth root of the first molar, and thickening with erosion through the bony concha of the infraorbital canal (**Fig. 9**). This horse was diagnosed with periapical tooth root abscess of the right first maxillary molar, with erosion and drainage into the infraorbital canal.

Dentigerous cysts are easily diagnosed via radiography. However, radiography does not provide complete understanding of the cyst's location and its intimate relationship to the calvarium. Successful surgical removal of a dentigerous cyst is commonly performed without 3-dimensional imaging. However, case reports of horses recovering from anesthesia with permanent neurologic dysfunction as a result of fracture to the calvarium exist.[32] In the authors' opinion, 3-dimensional imaging should always be recommended, and owners should be warned of the risk of performing surgery if they decline advanced imaging prior to removal of a dentigerous cyst. A 6-year-old pony presented with a 6-month history of a draining tract from the base of the right ear pinna. A dentigerous cyst was diagnosed on radiographs, and owners elected to evaluate further via CT imaging prior to surgical removal (**Fig. 10**). CT examination revealed dental tissue immediately dorsal and caudal to the right temporomandibular joint, connected to the calvarium and pressing against the brain (see **Fig. 10**). Surgical removal was not recommended due to the location of the cyst and the risk of death or permanent neurologic damage to the pony.

MRI is not as commonly used in cases of dental- and sinus-related disease. It is often assumed that MRI is not as useful for evaluating bone or dental tissue in

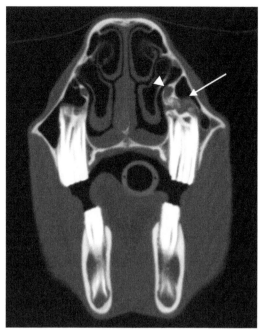

Fig. 9. Transverse CT image at the level of the third maxillary premolar of a 5-year-old Lusitano stallion. Soft tissue-attenuating material at the apex of right maxillary third premolar (*arrow*) intimately associated with the infraorbital canal. There is thickening of the concha surrounding the infraorbital canal and widening of the infraorbital canal (*arrowhead*).

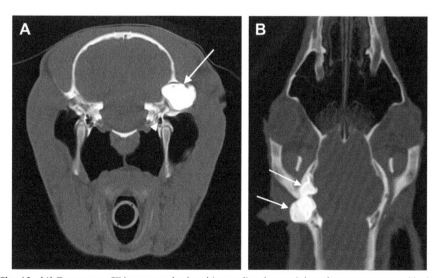

Fig. 10. (*A*) Transverse CT image at the level immediately cranial to the temporomandibular joint and through the tympanic bulla (*arrowhead*) of a 6-year-old pony. (*B*) Dorsal CT image at the level of the eye. A smooth well-demarcated dense mineral-attenuating structure (dental origin tissue) is present in the left temporal bone and extends into the calvarial cavity (*arrows*).

comparison to CT imaging. Both imaging modalities are capable of providing similar findings if the clinician/radiologist is comfortable with interpretation of either modality.

Advanced 3-dimensional imaging was vital to the successful diagnosis in afore mentioned cases. Dental disease results in a variety of clinical signs, and diagnosis prior to surgical treatment is difficult to impossible without the aid of advanced imaging. As clinicians, it is important to weigh the pros of advanced imaging against the cons of an inaccurate diagnosis and potentially inappropriate and harmful surgical treatment.

REFERENCES

1. Weller R, Livesey L, Maierl J, et al. Comparison of radiography and scintigraphy in the diagnosis of dental disorders in the horse. Equine Vet J 2001;33(1):49–58.
2. Townsend NB, Hawkes CS, Rex R, et al. Investigation of the sensitivity and specificity of radiological signs for diagnosis of periapical infection of equine cheek teeth. Equine Vet J 2011;43(2):170–8.
3. Archer DC, Blake CL, Singer ER, et al. The normal scintigraphic appearance of the equine head. Equine Vet Educ 2010;15(5):243–9.
4. Archer DC, Blake CL, Singer ER, et al. Scintigraphic appearance of selected diseases of the equine head. Equine Vet Educ 2003;15(6):305–13.
5. Weaver MP. Twenty years of equine scintigraphy—a coming of age? Equine Vet J 1995;27(3):163–5.
6. du Toit N. Aetiology and diagnosis of periapical dental disease in equids. Equine Vet Educ 2011;23(11):559–61.
7. Boswell JC, Schramme MC, Livesey LC, et al. Use of scintigraphy in the diagnosis of dental disease in four horses. Equine Vet Educ 1999;11(6):294–8.
8. Semevolos SA, Hackett RP, Scrivani PV. Nuclear scintigraphy as a diagnostic aid in the evaluation of tooth root abscessation. Proc Am Ass equine Practnrs 1999; 45(5):103–4.
9. Barakzai S, Tremaine H, Dixon PM. Use of scintigraphy for diagnosis of equine paranasal sinus disorders. Vet Surg 2006;35(1):94–101.
10. Dixon PM, Parkin TD, Collins N, et al. Equine paranasal sinus disease: a long-term study of 200 cases (1997–2009): ancillary diagnostic findings and involvement of the various sinus compartments. Equine Vet J 2011;44(3):267–71.
11. Kinns J, Pease A. Computed tomography in the evaluation of the equine head. Equine Vet Educ 2009;21(6):291–4.
12. Veraa S, Voorhout G, Klein WR. Computed tomography of the upper cheek teeth in horses with infundibular changes and apical infection. Equine Vet J 2010;41(9): 872–6.
13. Morrow KL, Park RD, Spurgeon TL, et al. Computed tomographic imaging of the equine head. Vet Radiol Ultrasound 2000;41(6):491–7.
14. Townsend NB, Barakzai SZ, Nelson AH. An investigation into the sensitivity and specificity of standing computed tomography in the diagnosis of dental associated sinusitis in 27 horses. In: Proceedings of the 48th BEVA Congress. Fordham, Ely, Cambridgeshire: Equine Veterinary Journal Ltd; 2009. p. 240.
15. Windley Z, Weller R, Tremaine WH, et al. Two- and three-dimensional computed tomographic anatomy of the enamel, infundibulae and pulp of 126 equine cheek teeth. Part 2: findings in teeth with macroscopic occlusal or computed tomographic lesions. Equine Vet J 2010;41(5):441–7.
16. Henninger W, Mairi Frame E, Willmann M, et al. CT Features of alveolitis and sinusitis in horses. Vet Radiol Ultrasound 2003;44(3):269–76.

17. Chalmers HJ, Cheetham J, Dykes NL, et al. Computed tomographic diagnosis—stylohyoid fracture with pharyngeal abscess in a horse without temporohyoid disease. Vet Radiol Ultrasound 2006;47(2):165–7.

18. Gibbs C, Lane JG. Radiographic examination of the facial, nasal and paranasal sinus regions of the horse. II. Radiological findings. Equine Vet J 1987;19(5): 474–82.

19. Tietje S, Becker M, Böckenhoff G. Computed tomographic evaluation of head diseases in the horse: 15 cases. Equine Vet J 1996;28(2):98–105.

20. Murray RC. Equine MRI. Oxford (UK): Wiley-Blackwell; 2011.

21. Dyson SJ, Murray R, Schramme MC. Lameness associated with foot pain: results of magnetic resonance imaging in 199 horses (January 2001–December 2003) and response to treatment. Equine Vet J 2005;37(2):113–21.

22. Werpy N. Magnetic resonance imaging for diagnosis of soft tissue and osseous injuries in the horse. Clin Tech Equine Pract 2004;3(4):389–98.

23. Zubrod C, Schneider R, Tucker R, et al. Use of magnetic resonance imaging for identifying subchondral bone damage in horses: 11 cases (1999–2003). J Am Vet Med Assoc 2004;224(3):411–8.

24. Selberg K, Werpy N. Fractures of the distal phalanx and associated soft tissue and osseous abnormalities in 22 horses with ossified sclerotic ungual cartilages diagnosed with magnetic resonance imaging. Vet Radiol Ultrasound 2011;52(4): 394–401.

25. Jakesova V, Konar M, Gerber V, et al. Magnetic resonance imaging features of an extranodal T cell rich B cell lymphoma in the pharyngeal mucosa in a horse. Equine Vet Educ 2008;20(6):289–93.

26. Oto C, Haziroglu RM. Magnetic resonance imaging of the guttural pouch (diverticulum tubae auditivae) and its related structures in donkey (*Equus asinus*). Ankara Üniversitesi Veteriner Fakültesi 2011;58(1):1–4.

27. Rodriguez MJ, Agut A, Soler M, et al. Magnetic resonance imaging of the equine temporomandibular joint anatomy. Equine Vet J 2010;42(3):200–7.

28. Tucker RL. Magnetic resonance imaging of the equine head and neck region. Equine Vet Educ 2008;20(6):294–6.

29. Idiyatullin D, Corum C, Moeller S, et al. Dental magnetic resonance imaging: making the invisible visible. J Endod 2011;37(6):745–52.

30. Hövener JB, Zwick S, Leupold J, et al. Dental MRI: imaging of soft and solid components without ionizing radiation. J Magn Reson Imaging 2012;36(4):841–6.

31. Cleary OB, Easley JT, Henriksen MD, et al. Purulent dacryocystitis (nasolacrimal duct drainage) secondary to periapical tooth root infection in a donkey. Equine Vet Educ 2011;23(11):553–8.

32. Hunt RJ, Allen D, Mueller PO. Intracranial trauma associated with extraction of a temporal ear tooth (dentigerous cyst) in a horse. Cornell Vet 1991;81(2):103–8.

Advances in the Treatment of Diseased Equine Incisor and Canine Teeth

Jennifer T. Rawlinson, DVM[a],*, Edward Earley, DVM, Fellow EQ AVD[b,c]

KEYWORDS

- Equine • Teeth • Extraction • Endodontic • Periodontal • Odontoplasty • Incisor
- Canine

KEY POINTS

- The single most important factor in performing successful dental therapy is an accurate diagnosis. Therefore, practitioners should focus on performing a complete oral examination and perfecting dental image acquisition and interpretation before focusing on treatments.
- Almost all dental work performed on the incisor and canine teeth can be performed using standing-sedation constant-rate infusion combined with regional and local nerve blocks; this includes extensive surgical extraction of all incisor teeth.
- Dental overgrowths involving pulp horns should be reduced by only 3 mm every 3 to 4 months to avoid the risk of pulp damage, and incremental motorized reduction should not exceed 15 seconds per tooth before cooling with water.
- Treatment of advanced periodontal disease, pockets larger than 5 mm, involves the removal of debris, pocket debridement, decontamination of the site, and possible placement of regenerative materials.
- Splinting of teeth severely affected by periodontal disease and/or equine odontoclastic tooth resorption and hypercementosis is not recommended, as it creates more surface area for debris entrapment and unnecessarily elongates the period the animal will be in pain.
- The use of a surgical or dental drill for surgical extractions dramatically increases the practitioner's ability to precisely remove bone, avoid damage to adjacent tooth and bone, work quickly and efficiently, respond to extraction complications (reserve crown or root fracture), and handle cases that are more challenging in an exacting manner.
- Successful vital pulp therapy needs to be performed shortly after the inciting trauma.
- Mineral trioxide aggregate is proving to be the superior material for direct pulp capping and vital pulp therapy.

[a] Department of Clinical Sciences, Cornell University College of Veterinary Medicine, C3 512 Clinical Programs Center, Ithaca, NY 14850, USA; [b] Department of Clinical Sciences, Cornell University Hospital for Animals, Ithaca, NY 14853, USA; [c] Laurel Highland Farm and Equine Services LLC, 2586 Northway Road Extension, Williamsport, PA 17701, USA
* Corresponding author.
E-mail address: jee2@cornell.edu

Vet Clin Equine 29 (2013) 411–440
http://dx.doi.org/10.1016/j.cveq.2013.04.005
0749-0739/13/$ – see front matter © 2013 Elsevier Inc. All rights reserved.

INTRODUCTION

In the last 2 decades there has been a tremendous increase in literature regarding the equine oral cavity and dental structures. Emphasis has been placed on establishing normal equid dental structure, histology, and physiology, and describing and exploring equid dental pathophysiology. A broader understanding of scientifically supported general dental principles and their applicability to the equid is developing. It is this new understanding of normal and abnormal within the equid oral cavity that has driven continued investigation into improving equine dental therapeutic techniques.

Specific research into the structure, function, pathology, and treatment of equine incisor and canine teeth is relatively limited when compared with literature published on the premolar and molar teeth; this is a testament to the relative infrequency of abnormality associated with the incisors and canines.[1] When incisor or canine tooth abnormality is present, the rostral positioning of these teeth allows for quicker recognition by attentive owners and easier examination, imaging, and treatment by the veterinarian. Examination with a bright light, dental explorer, periodontal probe, and/or an incisor speculum will reveal clinically visible abnormality, while easily obtainable intraoral radiographs will give excellent diagnostic images of underlying dental and surrounding hard and soft tissue structures. Once a diagnosis is reached, the anatomic positioning, the brachydont-like nature of the canine tooth, and the singular endodontic structure of the incisor and canine tooth expands treatment options, improves the realization of optimal dental and surgical techniques, and increases the capacity for and likelihood of necessary rechecks and home care.

Even with advances in the understanding of incisor and canine physiology and pathology, the most important goals of treatment are comfort and function. A clinician should always be wary of performing dental treatments based on tradition and/or anecdotal evidence. A thoughtful treatment plan will critically evaluate the diagnosis, mastication mechanics, future demands on the oral cavity, pathologic progression, animal comfort, and owner compliance. Treatments should be aimed at maximizing function and eliminating pain. If a treatment does not improve the patient's ability to prehend food in a comfortable manner or to perform required tasks painlessly and efficiently, the clinician needs to assess the reason for performing a procedure. Critical evaluation of whether any treatment is necessary at all will find that the equid oral cavity has an impressive ability to adapt to normal variation in individual and breed anatomy, chronic pathologic conditions, and environmental influences. Therefore, a clinically supported diagnosis and full appreciation of the patient's health and environment is necessary in prescribing an appropriate treatment plan.

ODONTOPLASTY

The removal of tooth structure to achieve a more normal tooth shape and occlusion has been practiced for hundreds of years in the horse. Many terms have been used to describe the removal of dental structure including floating, oral equilibration, occlusal adjustment, and dental corrective procedure. Odontoplasty is a commonly used human and veterinary dental term defined as "the adjustment of tooth length, size, and/or shape, includes the removal of enamel projections"[2] and "the surgical contouring of tooth surface to enhance plaque control and gingival morphology."[3] Odontoplasty can include the removal of enamel, cementum, dentin, and/or restorative material, and the definitions accurately describe the removal of dental structure to treat malocclusions, sharp enamel/dental overgrowths, crowding, periodontal disease, and diastemata. In the interest of trying to simplify and standardize veterinary and equid dental terminology, the term odontoplasty is used in this article to describe the removal of equine dental structure.

Malocclusions of any type may require odontoplasty of the incisors. Using the classification system for malocclusions established by Edward Angle[4] and later modified by Martin Dewey,[5] it is found that class I, II, and III malocclusions are the most common incisor malocclusions requiring incisor odontoplasty (**Table 1**). The 5 most common incisor malocclusions in the horse are increased tooth height caused by lack of occlusal contact present in class II and III malocclusions, dorsal curvature of the incisors (smile), ventral curvature of the incisor arcade (frown), a diagonal incisor arcade, and a stepped or irregular arcade caused by an abnormal number or malpositioning of the incisors.[6,7]

It should be noted that an incisor dorsocurvature has been established as a normal geriatric presentation for donkeys.[8] Not all of the incisor malocclusions will require odontoplasty; in fact, many require very little adjustment. Determination of whether incisive odontoplasty is necessary at all comes after a full oral examination, deliberation of mastication mechanics, completion of all cheek teeth reductions, and reexamination of the incisors. Consideration for odontoplasty of all dental overgrowths requires familiarity with the positioning of pulp horns and critical evaluation of whether reduction of dentin overlying a pulp horn will be necessary. Minor malocclusions and resulting dental overgrowths may include only peripheral cementum and enamel, in which case full reductions can be completed without risk of pulpal injury.

Reduction Recommendations

Over the last decade, a couple of major changes in thinking have occurred regarding the treatment of incisor malocclusions. A wave of research into the thickness and production of equine secondary and tertiary dentin has established scientifically supported guidelines for "safe" reduction of equid tooth height. Although the data currently published focus on cheek teeth, extrapolation of the findings to incisor teeth

Table 1			
Angle's modified malocclusion classification with common terms and presentation for equine incisor malocclusions			
Class	**Clinical Description**	**Equine Term**	**Overlong Incisors**
I	Maxilla and mandible normal length but tooth malpositioned (crowded, over-/undererupted, rotated, tipped, etc)	Dorsal curvature, smile	101, 201, 302, 303, 402, 403
		Ventral curvature, frown	102, 103, 202, 203, 301, 401
		Diagonal	101–103/301–303 or 201–203/401–403
		Step, irregular	Variable
II	Mandible positioned distally relative to the maxilla; mandibular brachygnathism	Overjet, overbite, parrot mouth	If minor, maxillary labial and mandibular lingual surfaces. If major, all maxillary incisors
III	Mandible positioned mesially relative to the maxilla; maxillary brachygnathism	Underbite, sow or monkey mouth	If minor, maxillary palatal and mandibular labial surfaces. If major, all mandibular incisors
IV	Asymmetrical length (usually shortened) of 1 of the 4 oral quadrants	Wry bite	Variable depending on position

is logical until incisor-specific research is published. One study reported that nearly 50% of overgrown teeth had less subocclusal secondary dentin than control matched teeth, and the height of dental overgrowth exceeded the thickness of subocclusal secondary dentin in 58% of overgrown teeth.[9] On average, the mean thickness of subocclusal secondary dentin in cheek teeth was 9 to 11 mm.[9,10] Another key fact when considering reduction is knowing that over the equid lifetime of 30 years an equine tooth will need to deposit roughly 100 mm of subocclusal secondary dentin, which translates to roughly 3 mm/y (0.3 mm/mo) of subocclusal secondary dentin deposited.[11] Recognizing normal and abnormal subocclusal secondary dentin thickness and the projected rate of subocclusal secondary dentin deposition provides the practitioner with an estimate in appropriate occlusal height reduction. With regard to pulpar temperatures during odontoplasty, prolonged grinding (>30 seconds) and the absence of water cooling significantly placed a tooth at risk for thermal damage.[12] This same study also found that the mean amount of dental material removed for teeth exceeding a critical temperature increase of 5.5°C was 5 mm, whereas the mean amount of dental material removed that did not exceed the critical temperature threshold was 3 mm. Therefore, considering all this new information, the current recommendation is that dental overgrowths involving pulp horns are reduced by only 3 mm every 3 to 4 months to avoid the risk of pulp damage, and incremental motorized reduction should not exceed 15 seconds per tooth before cooling with water.[13]

Incisor Diagonal Arcade

Imaging and evaluation of the equine maxilla in horses with a diagonal bite have demonstrated consistent deviation of the incisive bone to the left and right.[14] Whether the skeletal malformation is the cause or effect of the diagonal is unknown, but it is apparent that in adult horses complete correction and maintenance of an incisor diagonal bite is limited by the incisive bone malformation (**Fig. 1**). What, then, is a "normal" bite for an anatomically abnormal skull? The horse holds the answer. A predominance of horses examined with a diagonal bite maintained a cheek teeth occlusal angle between 15° and 35°, considered normal,[15] or slightly less on the ipsilateral side to the maxillary overlong incisors, and the cheek teeth occlusal angle contralateral to the overlong maxillary incisors was greater than normal.[14] Cheek teeth occlusal angles were directly influenced by the deformation of the hard palate and maxillary bone.

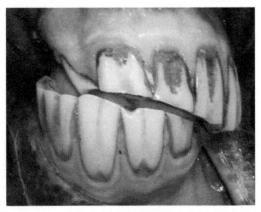

Fig. 1. A 200/400 diagonal in a 15-year-old horse with incisive bone deviation to the left.

Odontoplasty of diagonal bites should be conservative, taking into consideration the most normal masticatory motion the patient will be able to achieve with an anatomically malformed skull and asymmetrically conditioned muscles of mastication. The goal of dental reduction should be to maximize the patient's excursion of mandible and reduction of enamel points. Maximizing excursion can be done by conservatively reducing the height of the overlong lateral incisors; reduction of overlong middle incisors may be necessary for severe cases. It is unclear if the excursion to molar contact (EMC) formula can be used to assist in estimating reduction in horses with skeletal abnormalities.[16,17] No attempt should be made to change the cheek teeth occlusal angles or completely reduce overlong incisors unless the diagonal and skeletal malformation is very mild, as most horses with diagonals masticate with high efficiency and display few clinical signs of discomfort.

Equid canine tooth odontoplasty should be reserved for malpositioned or malformed teeth if the amount of reduction does not threaten the pulp. Canine tooth pulp can lie as close as 5 mm to clinical crown enamel.[15] If further reduction is medically necessary, the veterinarian should be prepared to perform vital pulp therapy in the case of pulp exposure.

PERIODONTAL THERAPIES

Periodontal disease in equid incisors and canines can result from age-related anatomic changes, local gross dental abnormalities, foreign-body entrapment, lack of routine dental care, and equine odontoclastic tooth resorption and hypercementosis (EOTRH). Periodontal disease is inflammation and infection of the periodontium compromising the gingiva, periodontal ligament, cementum, and alveolar bone. The first sign of periodontal disease is gingivitis, seen clinically as hyperemia, edema, ulceration, and/or spontaneous bleeding of the gingiva. Gingivitis is the tissue's inflammatory response to periodontopathogenic bacteria in dental plaque accumulated on the tooth surface. The cellular inflammatory infiltrate and bacterial by-products, such as collagenase, hyaluronidase, protease, chondroitin sulfatase, and endotoxin, destroy connective tissue and gingival epithelium. These elements lead to increased tissue vulnerability and deeper infection.[18–20] Untreated gingivitis can progress to periodontitis, the infection of the nongingival components of the periodontium. The transition from gingivitis to periodontitis is caused by changes in the pathogenic potential of dental plaque, inappropriate or inadequate host response to gingival infection, and various risk factors (eg, systemic disease, stress, age, lack of routine oral care, diet).[21] Periodontitis can progress slowly with periods of quiescence, or rapidly, but it always results in some degree of regional destruction of the periodontium.

Gingival inflammation, gingival recession, subgingival calculus accumulation, degradation of the dental papillae, feed entrapment between tooth and tissue, decreased alveolar bone height, prominent juga with associated age-inappropriate incisor angle, gingival fistulas, and subgingival eroded cementum are signs of periodontal disease in equid incisors and canine teeth (**Fig. 2**). To fully evaluate a periodontal lesion, gross calculus is removed either with a hand scaler or extraction forceps, gingival sulcus depth is measured with a periodontal probe, and intraoral radiographs are acquired of the diseased region. The normal depth of the equine gingival sulcus has not been scientifically reported, but estimates have ranged from 3 to 5 mm.[22] Radiographs are necessary for treatment planning when gingival sulcus depth exceeds 5 mm, as this finding indicates loss of the periodontium. Extensive research is available regarding periodontal disease associated with equine cheek teeth and diastema formation. One significant and extensive study found that feed

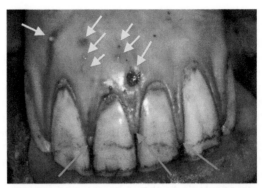

Fig. 2. A 15-year-old Thoroughbred gelding with signs of severe periodontal disease. There is marked loss of the gingival papillae (*blue arrows*), and multiple gingival fistulas (*yellow arrows*) draining purulent material. EOTRH should be suspected and radiographs acquired.

entrapment within the interproximal space of cheek teeth was associated with the development of periodontitis in 89% of horses studied, and that gingival recession with loss of interproximal tissues and cemental erosion resulted in an abnormal interproximal space with consequent accumulation of food material.[23] This degradation of the periodontium allows for accumulation of food material, which leads to further loss of the periodontium, perpetuating the negative feedback cycle. The best way to prevent the development of severe periodontal disease is early recognition with appropriate dental therapy and prevention of disease progression. Fortunately, the rostral positioning of equid incisor and canine teeth allows for easy examination and access for treatment.

Basic Dental Cleaning

Accumulation of calculus associated with the canine and incisor teeth, particularly the mandibular canine teeth, is common.[1] Calculus accumulation can be so severe that large, deep labial contact ulcers can develop. Large deposits of calculus can be removed with small extraction forceps by firmly grasping the side of the calculus with the instrument tips and applying a quick rotational force away from the tooth. Care should be taken to avoid grasping the tooth and applying excessive force, as tooth fracture may result. Once the gross calculus is removed, dental scalers and curettes are used to remove the remainder of the calculus and smooth the tooth surface (**Fig. 3**). As peripheral cementum coats the outer surface of the equid tooth, achieving a glassy smooth finish is not expected, but the surface of the tooth should be smooth to the touch. Only curettes should be used subgingivally because the heel, back, and toe of the instrument are rounded and will not inadvertently damage gingival tissue and attachments. Gingiva and soft tissue contacting the removed calculus will be inflamed when exposed. Sometimes coronal degeneration or abnormalities are discovered under calculus; exposing regions of degeneration can be painful (**Fig. 4**). Teeth with coronal abnormalities need to be radiographed to rule out EOTRH and assess the overall health of the tooth. Some teeth may require further treatment such as extraction, endodontic therapy, and/or restoration. If no coronal degeneration and periodontal pocketing (probe measurement >5 mm) exist, the site should be flushed with an antimicrobial solution (0.12% chlorhexidine) and left. The inflamed gingiva and mucosa will heal quickly. Owners can be advised to use a soft-bristled toothbrush with water (no tooth paste necessary) to brush the incisor and canine teeth daily to prevent future formation of calculus.

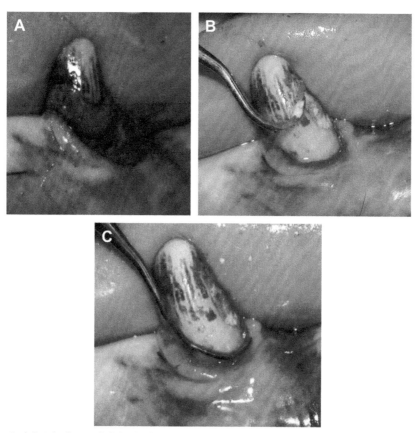

Fig. 3. (*A*) Calculus and debride deposition on a mandibular canine tooth. (*B*) Calculus is removed from the clinical crown with a scaler that has a sharp point and 2 sharp cutting edges. (*C*) A curette with a rounded heel, back, and toe is used for subgingival cleaning to avoid damaging normal gingiva and gingival attachments. (*Courtesy of* Dr. Stephen Galloway, DVM, Fellow AVD EQ in Fayetteville, TN.)

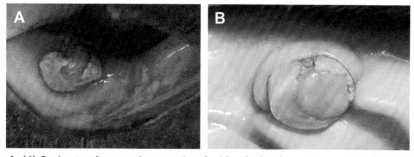

Fig. 4. (*A*) Canine tooth resorption associated with calculus deposition and gingival inflammation. (*B*) Canine tooth resorption with no calculus or gingival inflammation, but infiltration of gingiva and granulation tissue into the tooth in regions of severe resorption.

Advanced Periodontal Therapy

Treatment of advanced periodontal disease (pockets >5 mm) involves the removal of debris, pocket debridement, decontamination of the site, and possible placement of regenerative materials. Access to the lesion can be either closed, if the apical region of the pocket is visible, or open, via the surgical creation of a periodontal flap for deeper defects. Foreign material, plaque, and calculus can be removed from the lesion with irrigation, dental curettes, and/or ultrasonic dental scalers, if available. Debridement of the pocket epithelium, infiltrated connective tissue, and infected cementum can be performed with a scalpel, dental curette, ultrasonic scaler, and/or high-pressure dental air-abrasion unit using sodium bicarbonate (Equine Dental System; Harlton's Equine Specialties, Elmwood, WI). Methods for the removal of soft tissue via scalpel incisions are well described and illustrated.[21] Dental curettes can be used to debride pocket epithelium by engaging the cutting surface on the soft tissue, applying digital pressure to the exterior portion of the pocket if necessary, and using a singular, swift up-stroke. This motion is repeated until the pocket is completely debrided. The use of a high-pressure air-abrasion unit with sodium bicarbonate has been reported for the debridement of periodontal pockets.[24] Although this may seem like a quick, easy way to clean a pocket, its use requires some caution. This instrument has been shown to be as effective as dental curettes for debris, biofilm, and plaque removal and debridement of hard and soft tissue, but if used improperly, extensive loss of gingiva, soft tissue, bone, and dental structures, as well as air emphysema may occur.[25,26] Air abrasion is not effective nor designed for calculus removal. An air-abrasion unit removes hard and soft tissue structure rapidly without instantaneous tactile or visual operator feedback; therefore, the risk for iatrogenic trauma is present. The dental curette allows for both gross and fine removal of calculus, debris, and tissue with instantaneous tactile feedback as a guide; consequently, it is the preferred instrument. The use of air abrasion is not necessary in the rostral oral cavity, where access allows for detailed use of the dental curette.

Physical pocket debridement removes a large portion of the periodontopathogenic bacteria and detrimental bacterial by-products. Further decontamination can be achieved with sterile saline, 0.12% chlorhexidine, 3% hydrogen peroxide, or 0.5% betadine syringe irrigation.[21] Placement of a perioceutic, an absorbable antimicrobial gel (Doxirobe; Pfizer, Exton, PA), into the pocket can enhance healing. Following the material directions, the material is mixed and placed with a syringe deep into the pocket and filled to the gingival margin. The material polymerizes on contact with gingival crevicular fluid and is fully resorbed or lost around 3 weeks after insertion. Systemic antibiotics can be used for cases of severe periodontal disease, but this is less common in equid incisors and canines. The use of bone-regenerative materials such as calcium sulfate (plaster of Paris), bioactive ceramic granules (Consil; Nutramax Laboratories Inc, Edgewood, MD), and real bone allograft (Equine Osteoallograft Periomix; Veterinary Transplant Services Inc, Kent, WA) in appropriate lesions can lead to regeneration of hard tissue. These materials are placed in vertical bony pockets to encourage regrowth of alveolar bone, and their use has been described.[27]

Periodontal Disease and EOTRH

Periodontal disease is commonly present with EOTRH. The cause of EOTRH has not yet been determined, but it is clear that the loss of dental and regional structure resulting from EOTRH opens the door for severe periodontal infection. The inflammation resulting from periodontal disease causes further degradation of both hard and soft periodontal structures. Treatment of periodontal disease will not stop EOTRH, but will break the negative feedback cycle between EOTRH and periodontal disease temporarily. In the early stages of EOTRH whereby loss of the dental papillae and periodontium lead to regional feed accumulation, both veterinarian and owner can work together to keep the incisors and canines free of debris through daily tooth brushing and oral irrigation, and frequent professional periodontal therapy (every 3–6 months). Antibiotic therapy can also be used to temporarily decrease the build-up of periodontopathogenic bacteria and regional infection. As EOTRH progresses, visual examination, radiographic findings, and the patient's signs of pain will determine when both owner and veterinarian need to consider extractions. Splinting of mobile teeth severely affected by periodontal disease and/or EOTRH is not recommended, as it creates even more surface area for debris entrapment and unnecessarily elongates the period the animal will be in pain.

Tooth Luxation and Avulsion

Periodontal splinting is appropriate for emergency situations whereby trauma has led to either severe mobility or avulsion of an incisor or canine tooth. In cases of avulsion, the lost tooth should be placed in either Hanks Balanced Salt Solution (Life Technologies, Grand Island, NY) or milk to maintain the viability of periodontal ligament fibers and cells, and reimplantation should be performed within a few hours. Fracture of the rostral maxilla and mandible involving the incisors is well known, especially in younger horses. Delicate regional debridement before fracture repair involving avulsed or partially avulsed teeth is necessary. The region should be rinsed copiously, not under pressure, with sterile saline, and visible debris particles removed. The anatomy is realigned as best as possible and stabilized with wires, wire-mesh periodontal splints (Ribbond; Dentsply, Mannheim, Germany), and/or self-cure, nonexothermic composite resin material (Protemp Garant; 3M ESPE, St Paul, MN), depending on the severity of the fracture. Exothermic acrylics should be avoided because of the potential for thermal damage to already traumatized tissue. Fully avulsed teeth will need endodontic therapy in 3 weeks. Partially avulsed teeth will need frequent radiographic monitoring, every 3 months, to determine whether the tooth remains vital. This monitoring is particularly important for management of deciduous dental trauma, as apical infection of deciduous teeth can cause severe damage or death to developing permanent teeth.

OPERCULECTOMY

Equid canines are the teeth most likely to benefit from an operculectomy. An operculectomy is the surgical excision of the gingiva or mucosa, the operculum, lying over an unerupted tooth.[28,29] Unerupted and malpositioned canine teeth causing headshaking, biting problems, and abnormal head carriage are reported.[13] Malpositioned, supernumerary, submucosal, unerupted, and vestigial canine teeth can be of tremendous discomfort with some forms of bits. Unerupted deciduous canine teeth are spicule-like structures 0.5 to 1.0 cm long and are commonly referred to as vestigial canine teeth in the horse (**Fig. 5**).[15] Problematic actively erupting and unerupted canine teeth can usually be palpated in the bar region, and localized swelling and inflammation may be present in some cases. Radiographs of the problematic tooth are recommended. Unerupted teeth can be either embedded or impacted. Embedded teeth lack the eruptive force necessary to move through surrounding tissue; this lack of eruptive force may be due to dental malformation or systemic disease. Impacted teeth are unerupted owing to obstruction by a physical barrier (eg, adjacent teeth, thickened alveolar bone, scarred gingiva).[30] Radiographs help determine the source

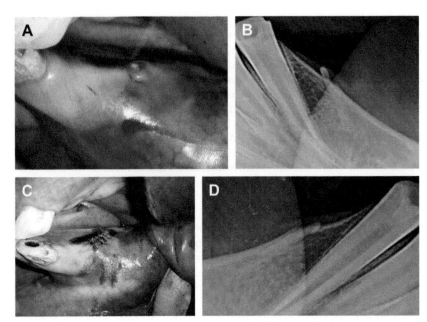

Fig. 5. Mandibular vestigial canine teeth in a mare. The left mandibular canine tooth (*A, B*) was causing regional inflammation, edema, and discomfort for the mare; therefore, the tooth was extracted in a simple manner (*C*). The unerupted right mandibular vestigial canine tooth was causing no regional inflammation or discomfort; consequently, no treatment was recommended (*D*). (*Courtesy of* Dr Robert Baratt, DVM, Fellow AVD SA EQ in Middletown, CT.)

of maleruption, the location of the clinical crown, and the treatment plan. Published material describing the frequency and nature of unerupted canine teeth in the horse is scarce. In the author's experience, problematic impacted canine teeth usually involve overlying soft tissue with or without a thin layer of alveolar bone. Rarely, horses will present with vestigial canine teeth in the submucosal tissue. Pain is caused when pressure either builds within a normal eruption cyst or when applied pressure results in pinching of the gingiva, mucosa, or thin alveolar bone into the unerupted clinical crown of the tooth. Unerupted teeth solidly encased in bone rarely cause discomfort for the horse. It should be noted that normal erupting canine teeth causing mild regional swelling will be the source of short-lived discomfort for the horse until the clinical crown pierces the gingiva, releasing internal pressure; these canine teeth do not need to be treated. In addition, unerupted teeth causing no regional discomfort, inflammation, or swelling do not need to be prophylactically treated, as most teeth will remain quiescent. Problematic deeply impacted, angled, embedded, or malformed teeth will most likely require surgical extraction by an experienced veterinarian.

Superficially impacted teeth or inflamed actively erupting canine teeth can be treated by an operculectomy. Remarkably, an operculectomy procedure performed nearly 150 years ago has recently been republished.[13] To perform an operculectomy, the overlying soft tissue is blocked with lidocaine, and either a scalpel or cutting bur on a water-cooled high-speed drill is used to remove the gingiva and mucosa. The overlying soft tissue is incised in an oval pattern to match the shape of the clinical crown. The incised oval portion of tissue is removed down to the level of the crown or periosteum. In some cases, alveoloplasty, the removal and reshaping of alveolar bone, may need to be performed to expose the full circumference of the clinical crown at its largest diameter. This bone can be removed and smoothed with either small rongeurs or the drill. Once the full circumference of the clinical crown is visible, the procedure is complete. No attempt is made to fully expose the clinical crown, as the tooth is expected to erupt into the mouth after the removal of the obstructing tissues. The site should be monitored for healing and complete eruption of the tooth. In some cases the tooth may not fully erupt, but these cases rarely require further treatment because the source of discomfort, pinched tissue, is removed. It is usually easiest to simply extract problematic vestigial teeth (see **Fig. 5**).

EXTRACTION

Advances over the last decade in canine and incisor extraction techniques have involved improvements in patient management during extraction, the surgical approach to extraction, and the equipment used. Little has changed regarding simple extraction techniques to remove singular incisors and persistent deciduous incisors. Because of their location in the mouth, equine incisor and canine teeth are prone to trauma including dental fracture, supporting bone fracture, avulsion, and excessive abrasion resulting from behavioral or environmental conditions. Supernumerary and malpositioned teeth can cause traumatic malocclusions and/or feed entrapment, leading to periodontal disease. Iatrogenic pulp exposure caused by overzealous reduction can lead to apical abnormality, and EOTRH can cause severe pain, dental and regional anatomic destruction, and infection. All of these conditions may necessitate the extraction of 1 or more teeth. Before extraction, presurgical radiographs should be obtained to clearly identify or confirm the tooth to be extracted, evaluate the health of regional hard and soft tissue, determine the extent of dental abnormality, appraise the health of adjacent dental structures, and establish the anatomic conformation of the tooth or teeth to be extracted. Radiographs are critical for appropriate treatment planning and execution of precise surgical technique.

Sedation and Regional Anesthesia

Because of the risks associated with general anesthesia, extraction procedures should be performed standing when possible. Standing extractions even with extensive surgical involvement can be performed with a constant-rate infusion of detomidine (Dormosedan; Pfizer, New York, NY) with or without the addition of an opioid and regional/local nerve blocks. Techniques for multimodal pain control and constant-rate infusions for prolonged surgical procedures (>1 hour) have improved and are well described.[31–34] Even with excellent sedation and systemic pain control, extensive and/or surgical extractions require regional and local anesthesia via nerve blocks. Maxillary (via the extraperiorbital fat body insertion)[35] and mental nerve blocks theoretically should anesthetize the region of the incisor and canine teeth.[36] An inferior alveolar nerve block can also be used to anesthetize the ipsilateral mandible if a mental nerve block is unattainable.[37] In some horses, especially those with EOTRH, additional local nerve blocks may be necessary to provide acceptable surgical-site anesthesia. Performing involved extractions without regional and/or local anesthesia will prove frustrating for the practitioner and horse, and it is not advised.

Anatomic Considerations

To perform extractions successfully, dental and regional anatomy of the equine tooth needs to be considered. Both incisors and canine teeth are single rooted. Incisors are radicular, hypsodont teeth with long reserve crowns, 7 to 10 cm, which erupt continually throughout the life of the horse. Therefore as a horse ages, incisor extraction should theoretically become easier. The interproximal bone between the incisors on the maxilla and mandible is relatively thin, which is significant when considering extraction, as the interproximal bone will be easier to deform and/or remove. This thin bone allows for easier instrument placement, in contrast to the thick cortical bone encasing the canine tooth. The dental structure of the equine canine tooth is less complex than the incisors and cheek teeth, but its formidable size and surrounding bone make it challenging to extract. The average length of a canine tooth from crown tip to apex is 5 to 7 cm, and only one-quarter to one-third of this is clinical crown.[15] Canine teeth do not continually erupt like the incisors and cheek teeth, so the length of the tooth within the alveolus changes minimally. Therefore, extraction of the equine canine tooth requires a surgical approach if the pathologic condition has not already caused significant degradation of the periodontium and loosening of the tooth.

Equipment

Incisor and canine extractions require a mix of basic surgical tools and specialized dental equipment. A basic surgical pack with scalpel, forceps, Metzenbaum and Mayo scissors, and a needle driver is always good to have on hand, as even planned simple extractions may require some unplanned incisions, freshening of tissue edges, and site closure. Simple extractions involve the use of dental elevators and extraction forceps. Elevators and forceps used to extract wolf teeth (Harlton's Equine Specialties, Elmwood, WI) can be used[38] in addition to winged dental elevators size 5 to 8 mm (Miltex Inc, York, PA), the author's preference. Lane bone-holding forceps with ratchet, 13 in/33 cm (OrthoMed Inc, Portland, OR), have been found to be particularly useful for grasping incisors solidly to allow for application of avulsion and rotational force. Bone curettes, bone files, and small double-action rongeurs are used to debride debris from alveoli and smooth jagged bone margins after extraction. Sterile saline or 0.12% chlorhexidine can be used to flush the alveolus before formation of the final blood clot.

Surgical extractions entail the use of more specialized equipment. The Selden periosteal elevator (I.R.H. Surgical Co., Sialkot, Pakistan) is used for the elevation of gingival and mucogingival surgical flaps. Bone removal will require the use of a drill or osteotome. A pneumatic surgical drill, high-speed water-cooled dental drill (iM3 Dental Unit; iM3, Vancouver, WA), or an electric low-speed high-torque dental drill can be used to remove bone. All drills require some form of water irrigation during use to prevent thermal injury to healthy tissue. In the past, bone removal was performed mostly with an osteotome or chisel and mallet. The drill dramatically increases the practitioner's ability to precisely remove bone, avoid damage to adjacent tooth and bone, respond to extraction complications (reserve crown or root fracture), and handle cases that are more challenging in an exacting manner. Each drill type will have its own specific burs. Carbide cutting burs 4 to 6 mm in diameter work well for equine bone removal. In cases where multiple neighboring incisors are to be extracted, small, fine osteotomes or chisels can be used with a mallet to luxate teeth, but these should not be used next to healthy teeth. Small blood vessels encased in bone are located in regions surrounding the incisors, and can cause decreased visualization at the surgical site if disturbed. Bone wax (Ethicon, Princeton, NJ) works well for hemostasis in these situations. Finally, suture material should be a quick absorbing monofilament such as 2-0 or 3-0 poliglecaprone 25 (Monocryl; Ethicon, Princeton, NJ) on a cutting needle. Some horses have developed labial ulcers from the use of stiff monofilament; therefore, the option of using 2-0 polyglactin 910 (Vicryl; Ethicon, Princeton, NJ) on a cutting needle may be considered.

Simple Extraction

Incisor extraction can be accomplished in 2 ways depending on the nature and severity of the pathologic disorder associated with the tooth or teeth. Extraction of persistent deciduous and uncomplicated singular incisors not involving EOTRH can be accomplished simply by gingival elevation and periodontal ligament avulsion or transection. Either a sharp dental elevator or scalpel blade, vertically placed in the gingival sulcus and advanced 3 to 4 mm, will break down the gingival attachments to the tooth. Advancement of a sharp dental elevator or luxator into the periodontal ligament space will start to break down the periodontal ligament. Controlled, sustained rotational force is applied to the elevator once it is well seated. With time, the ligament starts to fatigue and the tooth becomes mobile. At this point, the wolf-tooth or incisor-extraction forceps can be used to apply continued rotational and avulsion force until the tooth is extracted. The use of fine, flexible osteotomes and chisels for periodontal ligament destruction has been described.[39] The use of these instruments is effective, but use between a healthy and diseased tooth may result in damage to the periodontium and dental structure of the healthy remaining tooth. Therefore, these tools should be used carefully and with forethought to the surrounding anatomy. Another interesting technique, described by Galloway,[40] places a positive thread Steinman pin into the center of the incisor to be extracted. When the pin is solidly placed it can be used to apply lateral, labial, and palatal forces to the tooth until it becomes mobile enough to extract with forceps. Regardless of the way the tooth has been extracted, the alveolus is debrided and bone margins are smoothed. The site is either left open or partially closed in a cruciate pattern to help maintain the blood clot. Owners are asked to flush accumulated feed from the surface of the wound daily for 1 to 2 weeks pending healing.

Surgical Extraction

In cases of the extraction of complicated singular incisors, multiple incisors, EOTRH-affected incisors, and canine teeth, a surgical approach allows for improved visualization, reduced accidental damage to healthy teeth and tissue, meticulous debridement of diseased tissue and dental remnants, and primary closure. In addition, a surgical approach increases the surgeon's ability deal with complicated extractions whereby reserve crowns and roots have fractured as a result of initial trauma or resorption.

A surgical approach to incisor extraction involves the creation of a gingival or mucogingival flap to reveal underlying tooth and bone. Flap creation depends on the teeth being extracted, but usually entails the creation of a mesial and distal releasing incision extending 2 to 6 cm. Incisions are made with a scalpel blade and cut through the periosteum. The overall structure of the flap is trapezoid, with the base being larger than the gingival margin. The flap is elevated off the bone by working the periosteal elevator between bone and periosteum. Once exposed, roughly 30% to 60% of labial bone overlying the reserve crown is removed, with the drill making sure to extend bone removal to the mesial and distal periodontal ligament space. Removing this bone allows for easier access to the periodontal ligament space for instrument placement and decreases supporting structures, allowing for a cleaner and quicker extraction. Dental elevation and extraction are performed as previously described, and the area is debrided, flushed, and smoothed. The gingival or mucogingival flap can be partially or completely closed depending on the nature of the extraction and abnormality. If primary closure is desired, wound edges are freshened, and if the flap has extended past the mucogingival junction, the periosteum is transected to allow for greater flap mobility. Sutures are placed in either a simple interrupted or simple continuous pattern.

Extraction of a canine tooth follows all the steps previously detailed with a few specific additional considerations (**Fig. 6**). A mucogingival flap will be created to remove this tooth. The mesial releasing incision should extend 3 to 4 cm toward the vestibule from the mesial aspect of the tooth. The distal releasing incision runs directly caudal 3 to 4 cm from the distal aspect of the tooth. The periosteum is undermined and the flap elevated. Owing to the length and curve of the reserve crown and root, attention during drilling needs to focus on following the path of the tooth, continually defining the mesial and distal periodontal ligament margins. For most canine teeth, 60% to 80% of the labial bone plate will need to be removed with the drill to allow for elevation. Note that the mental foramen will be located in the apical region of the canine tooth in some horses, and care must be taken not to damage this structure. Once the reserve crown and root are uncovered, a dental elevator is used to fatigue the periodontal ligament, and the tooth is removed with extraction forceps. All bone margins should be smoothed, and the site should be debrided and flushed clean. The flap is closed in a tension-free manner; therefore, the periosteum underlying the mucosa is transected. The flap is closed by suturing in a simple interrupted pattern.

Postoperative radiographs are recommended for every extraction procedure to ensure that no dental fragments have been left behind, and to provide documentation of the procedure and lack of adjacent hard-tissue damage. Postoperative pain medication and antibiotics may be indicated, depending on the extent of the extraction technique. Postoperatively patients are fed a pelleted or bran mash for 12 hours, and soft soaked hay is reintroduced over 24 hours to allow for increased gastrointestinal motility after extended sedation. Once manure is produced, first-cut hay is recommended for the extent of the healing period for incisor extractions. Canine tooth extraction requires no alteration to the diet after the first 24 hours.

Complications

Mucogingival flaps in the incisor and canine region of the horse are notorious for dehiscence (**Fig. 7**). The reason behind this is not exactly known, but time devoted to mastication, frenulum attachment, gravity, tongue action, and devitalization of the flap during creation have all been considered. In the author's experience, dehiscence, if present, usually occurs between days 5 and 10, when granulation tissue, partial primary closure, and wound contraction have already started to occur at the surgical margin. Sutures involved with the dehiscence are removed, and the owner is instructed to flush debris from the wound daily with warm water until complete healing has occurred by second intention (usually 2–5 weeks).

The removal of all or most of the incisors can lead to extrusion of the tongue beyond the labial margin (**Fig. 8**). The tongue appears to protrude most when horses are at rest, but there is wide variation between individuals. Tongue protrusion can be a problem for horses in show where this is considered a violation, but horses appear to suffer no physical or mental trauma as a result of this complication.

If performed correctly, complications associated with heavy bleeding, fracture, adjacent tooth trauma, and postoperative inappetance should not be encountered.

EOTRH Extractions

Tooth resorption associated with EOTRH is well documented to be associated with the canine and incisor teeth.[41] Therefore in cases of EOTRH, radiographs of both the incisors and canines should be taken. Severe cases of EOTRH require staged or complete extraction of the affected incisor and canine teeth to alleviate infection and pain caused by this disease (**Fig. 9**). Resorptive lesions in older horses can be found under excessive calculus deposition on the mandibular and maxillary canine

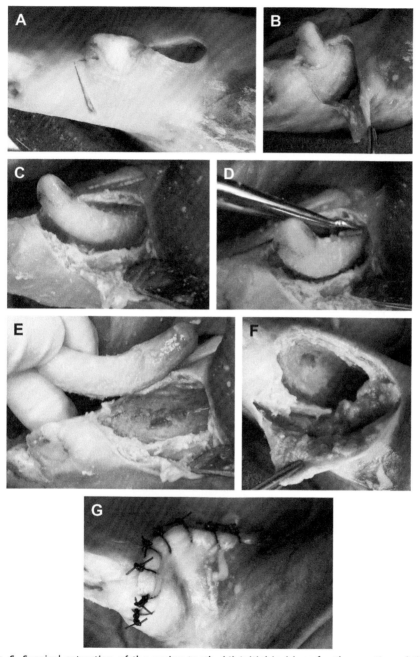

Fig. 6. Surgical extraction of the canine tooth. (*A*) Initial incisions for the creation of the mucogingival flap. (*B*) Elevation of the mucogingival flap including the periosteum. (*C*) Removal of roughly 60% of buccal alveolar bone. Note complete bone removal to the mesial and distal margins of the tooth. (*D*) Proper placement of the dental elevator into the peri-odontal ligament space. (*E*) Completely extracted canine tooth. (*F*) Extraction site curetted clean of debris and bone margins smoothed. (*G*) Closure of extraction site with simple inter-rupted suture pattern.

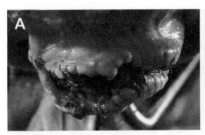
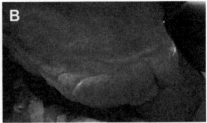

Fig. 7. (*A*) Surgical-site dehiscence (day 8 postextraction) of all maxillary incisors with primary closure. (*B*) Same horse 4 weeks later at recheck with full healing of site.

teeth. Exposing these lesions after removal of calculus will cause discomfort for the horse, and the practitioner should be prepared to address the problem either through extraction under primary care or referral to an equine veterinary dental specialist. In severe cases of EOTRH requiring extraction of all incisors, owners will need extensive presurgical counseling regarding the surgery, postoperative care, nutrition, possible complications (as discussed above), and anticipated outcome. It is also highly recommended that horses requiring extraction of all incisors be referred to a veterinary dentist or surgeon experienced in this procedure, as retrieval of all infected dental material and extraction of severely resorbed teeth can be technically challenging.

Horses with severe EOTRH display little discomfort after extraction of all incisors. Postoperative pain is controlled with nonsteroidal anti-inflammatory medication, and an antibiotic is given to prevent infection for 7 to 10 days. An evaluation of 22 horses undergoing partial or complete extraction demonstrated low morbidity postoperatively.[39] The most severe complication encountered was one case of sensitivity during eating in the postoperative period (1 week) that was resolved with administration of phenylbutazone. Horses with no incisors are able to eat hay, and many owners and

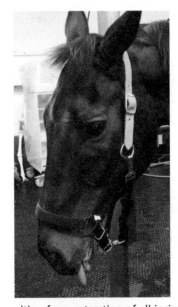

Fig. 8. Tongue protrusion resulting from extraction of all incisors.

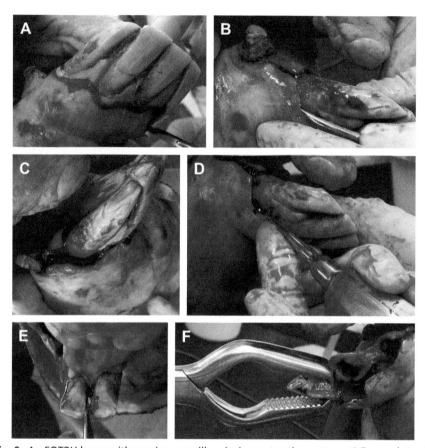

Fig. 9. An EOTRH horse with previous maxillary incisor extractions returns 1.5 years later to have mandibular incisors extracted. (*A*) Initial incision runs 3–4 mm from free gingival margin and eliminates dental papillae. (*B*) Elevation of gingival flap. (*C*) Gingival flap elevated. (*D*, *E*) Placement of dental elevator is between teeth into periodontal ligament space. (*F*) Once the tooth is mobile, Lane bone-holding forceps are used to apply rotational and avulsion forces. (*G*) Continued elevation of gingival flap into mucosa is allows for tension free flap and bone contouring. (*H*) Bone rongeurs are used to smooth bone margins and remove all diseased bone. (*I*) The alveoli are curetted to remove all remaining dental material and infected tissue. (*J*) Tissue margins are trimmed and freshened. (*K*) The extraction site is closed. (*L*) Wound closure from a different horse with both maxillary and mandibular incisors extracted.

veterinarians report that these horses can graze by grasping forage with the lips and pulling. Although it is impressive that these horses can graze, it should be assumed that they cannot maintain themselves on pasture alone until proven otherwise. Therefore, owners will need to be aware that supplementation with hay, hay stretchers, senior feed, or similar feed will be necessary for pasture horses. Once healed, horses will be able to return to full work, and many owners report improved disposition and increased energy.

Sometimes severely resorbed teeth make complete extraction particularly challenging, and there has been discussion within the dental community as to whether clinical crown amputation is acceptable for these teeth. There is no study

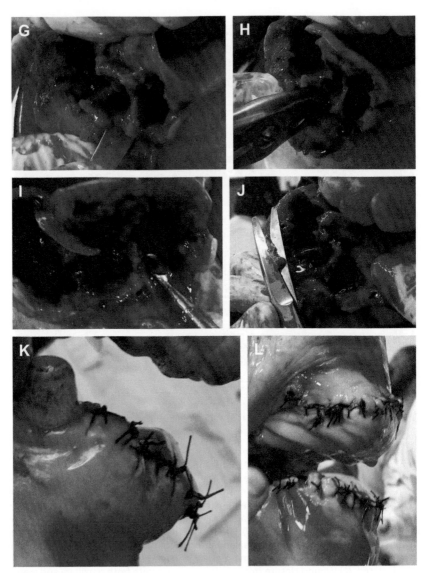

Fig. 9. (continued)

documenting the long-term success of this procedure in horses; however, in cats with severe tooth resorption, crown amputation is acceptable and successful if no periodontal ligament or regional bone abnormality or infection is visible on radiographs.[42] Whether horses are similar to cats in this manner is unknown. The author suspects that the degree of regional/dental necrosis, bulbous hypercementosis, and inflammatory tissue reported by Staszyk and colleagues[41] in 2008 would lead to postoperative regional inflammation and infection if portions of an incompletely resorbed tooth were purposefully left in the alveolus. The practitioner and the owner should carefully weigh the pros and cons of this approach if resorption is severe enough for this procedure to be considered.

VITAL PULP THERAPY

Pulp exposures in horses can occur as a result of traumatic incident, severe or rapid abrasion, or dental therapy. Accidental pulp exposure is possible during routine reductions of overgrowths, owing to the variable thickness of subocclusal secondary dentin separating the pulp horn from the occlusal surface. Conservative reductions in crown height provide the best defense for iatrogenic pulp exposures, as already described. When pulp exposure does occur there is a small window of opportunity to keep the tooth vital. Tooth vitality is essential to maximizing long-term tooth performance, as the tooth will be more resilient to occlusal forces and wear and less prone to resorption and apical infection. Maintaining vitality in young teeth is particularly important, as it will allow the tooth to continue laying down dentin, thus increasing its strength over time.

Two major types of dental fractures can occur. An uncomplicated crown fracture refers to loss of a portion of tooth involving cementum, enamel, and/or dentin without obvious pulp exposure. Near or indirect pulp exposures can occur in these cases. Indirect pulp exposure involves dentinal loss to within 1 to 2 mm of pulp tissue. The decreased length and unmineralized oral aperture of exposed dentinal tubules compromises the tooth's ability to prevent contamination of the pulp, and the exposure of nerve fibers within the tubules can lead to significant discomfort. Depending on the severity of the fracture, the treatment plan could range from conservative (with no treatment) to dentinal bonding or restoration. Complicated crown fracture refers to a fracture through the cementum, enamel, and dentin with direct pulp involvement and exposure. Treatment options for these fractures are extraction, root canal therapy, or vital pulp therapy, depending on the timing and extent of the fracture. Past literature has suggested that no treatment may be necessary for pulp exposures in the horse because of an exuberant odontoblastic response to trauma, but close follow-up will reveal that at least 25% of these cases develop apical swellings.[43] Finally, pulp can be exposed directly or indirectly from rapid tooth wear termed abrasion. Abrasion is the pathologic wearing down of tooth structure by an external mechanical force (chewing on stall doors, trees, watering systems, cribbing, iatrogenic reduction). If the rate of dental tissue loss exceeds the deposition of secondary and tertiary dentin, a pulp exposure will result.

Research-based guidelines for successful vital pulp therapy for human and canine teeth are well established.[44–46] Research-supported guidelines for vital pulp therapy in equine teeth have not yet been established, although there are discussions of success using various techniques and timing in the literature.[22,47,48] Although pulpal response to insult in horses has been suggested to be more resilient than in human and canine dentition, it is wise to adhere to the more conservative human/canine guidelines to maximize the success of therapy. Teeth that are good candidates for vital pulp therapy are those within 48 to 72 hours of injury that involve mostly the clinical and coronal reserve crown. Young teeth with large quantities of pulp have been shown to survive longer periods of exposure, up to 1 week, with no decrease in success rates.[45] Performing vital pulp therapy past these timelines significantly reduces success rates in dogs and humans. Therefore, owners need to be informed of possible decreased success rates in horses if an extended or unknown period of time has elapsed between exposure and vital pulp therapy. If an extended period of time has passed, pulpal bleeding can be elicited, and if an owner opts for vital pulp therapy, close radiographic follow-up of the treated tooth is highly recommended (every 3–6 months for a minimum of 2–3 years).

Performing Vital Pulp Therapy

Successful vital pulp therapy requires the adherence to 3 basic dental principles: treatment of a noninflamed pulp, application of a pulp dressing, and creation of a bacteria-tight seal.[44] To achieve these 3 goals of treatment one must remove inflamed pulp, apply an acceptable pulp dressing (calcium hydroxide or mineral trioxide aggregate [MTA]), and create a bacteria-tight seal with a high-quality restoration. To maximize results the procedure needs to be performed in as sterile a manner as possible, meaning that all equipment used to work with the pulp should be sterilized and only sterile saline should be used to irrigate the pulp during the pulpotomy. Once a seal has been created over the pulp dressing, nonsterile instruments and techniques can be used. Vital pulp therapy has a high rate of success (95%) in humans and dogs if these principles are followed.[44-46]

Four techniques have been described for treating exposed pulp: pulp capping, partial pulpotomy, full pulpotomy, and pulpectomy. Pulp capping is the direct application of a pulp dressing onto the exposed pulp with minimal restoration. These procedures are of marginal long-term success. Pulp capping can be implemented in emergency situations when the veterinarian is either unprepared or unable to perform a more appropriate procedure for long-term success. Partial removal of coronal pulp is a partial pulpectomy with application of a pulp dressing and restoration, and is the treatment of choice for vital pulp therapy. Full pulpotomy refers to the removal of all coronal pulp to the level of the crown-root junction with restoration; this is not indicated for use in horses, owing to the crown to root length ratio. Finally, a pulpectomy is the complete removal of all pulp tissue to the apical delta with subsequent root canal treatment.

Considerations for Vital Pulp Therapy

Pros	Cons
• Tooth remains vital and continues to mature and strengthen	• Repair may fail in future
• Vital tooth responds to insult in more resilient manner than nonvital tooth	• Annual radiographic follow-up is recommended
• Easier and quicker to perform than extraction or root canal therapy	• Procedure requires knowledge of basic endodontic and restorative principles
• Fracture site in horse will wear away with age and tooth may appear normal in future	• Procedure requires materials and instrumentation not commonly carried by general practitioner
• Relatively inexpensive	• Time limitations from exposure to repair should be respected to maximize success

Equipment

Equipment needed to perform vital pulp therapy is specialized but within the scope of general practice. Hand curettes and scalers are needed to initially clean the tooth of debris and tartar. An antimicrobial irrigant such as 0.12% chlorhexidine solution is used to flush the tooth surface after cleaning. As the procedure is initially performed in a sterile manner, a sterile vital pulp pack should be kept on hand; the contents of this pack are shown in **Fig. 10**. A pneumatic or electric surgical or dental drill (see extraction equipment) with a carbide cutting bur (2–4 mm diameter) is used to enlarge the pulp access site, recontour the tooth, and perform the pulpectomy. Only a drill should be used for the pulpectomy, as hand instruments may cause avulsion of

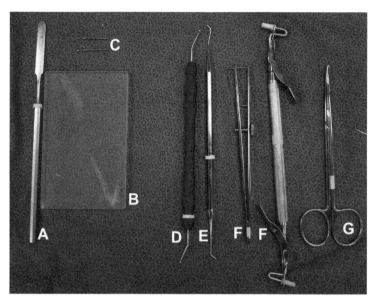

Fig. 10. Contents of a sterile vital pulp therapy surgical pack. Metal mixing spatula (A), glass slab (B), cutting burs (C), mineral trioxide aggregate (MTA) working instrument (D), condenser (E), amalgam carriers (F; 2 sizes), and Metzenbaum scissors (G).

healthy remaining pulp. A large syringe (60 mL) delivers sterile saline to the drill site during the pulpectomy. Sterile X-coarse paper points (Henry Schein, Bartlett, TN) provide hemostasis and dry the canal after drilling; college pliers (Henry Schein, Bartlett, TN) are used to hold the paper points. Either MTA (Dentsply, Tulsa, OK) or calcium hydroxide powder (Pulpdent; Watertown, MA) can be used as a pulp dressing, and an amalgam carrier (Hu-Friedy Dental, Leimen, Germany) is used to deliver the material to the pulp surface. A glass slab and metal cement spatula will be necessary to mix these materials. Choice of restorative materials is wide, and directions and ancillary equipment will vary greatly depending on the material chosen. Materials commonly used on pulp medicants as intermediate layers to support a final restoration include calcium hydroxide cement (Dycal; Dentsply), intermediate restorative material (IRM; Dentsply), glass ionomer cement (Ketac-Fil; 3M ESPE), and a resin reinforced glass ionomer cement (Ionosit Microspand; Patterson Dental, St Paul, MN). A final restoration with a microhybrid composite material is recommended. Standard equipment for a composite restoration includes 37% phosphoric acid, unfilled resin, excavators, flowable or microhybrid composite, and restorative finishing burs (**Fig. 11**). Depending on the type of restorative materials used, a dental light-cure unit and amalgamator may be necessary.

Patient Preparation

The patient is adequately sedated and a regional nerve block placed. A preoperative radiograph is taken to evaluate if vital pulp therapy is appropriate. Traumatized soft tissue surrounding the exposed tooth is managed appropriately if necessary. The tooth is cleaned with a hand scaler and curette (or ultrasonic equipment if available), and irrigated with antimicrobial flush. Antimicrobial soaked gauze is placed on the tooth for roughly 5 minutes to enhance site preparation.

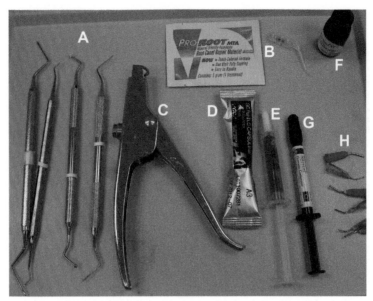

Fig. 11. The nonsterile restorative tray contains: excavators (A; 4 types shown), MTA and sterile saline (B), glass ionomer capsule activator (C), glass ionomer capsule (D), 37% phosphoric acid (E), unfilled resin (F), flowable composite (G), and composite applicator tips (H).

Sterile Partial Pulpectomy

1. Sterile gloves are donned and the sterile tray prepped (**Fig. 12**).
2. Using sterile irrigation (assistant applies with syringe) and drill, the tooth surface is smoothed.
3. Using sterile irrigation and drill, exposed pulp is removed to minimal depth of 7 to 10 mm.
4. College pliers are used to gently place sterile paper points onto the remaining bleeding pulp, and left in place until hemostasis is achieved (3–5 minutes). A small amount of epinephrine (1 drop) can be placed into the access if bleeding is persistent. One must never blow compressed air onto exposed pulp, as air embolism and desiccation of pulp may result.
5. Once the site is free of blood, the pulp dressing is prepared and applied. According to the manufacturer's directions, either the MTA or calcium hydroxide is mixed with sterile saline on the glass slab with the spatula to create a dry paste. The paste is packed into the amalgam carrier and deposited onto the pulp. The pulp dressing should be roughly 2 to 3 mm thick. The material is lightly packed with the condenser. The walls of the access site are cleaned with the spoon excavators (not pictured) until no debris is visible.
6. Following the manufacturer's directions, an intermediate restorative layer roughly 2 to 3 mm thick is placed, and the walls of the access site are cleaned in preparation for the final restoration.

Final Restoration

Now that the canal is sealed, work can continue in a nonsterile fashion. If composite or glass ionomer is used for final restoration, no undercut is necessary for cavity preparation.

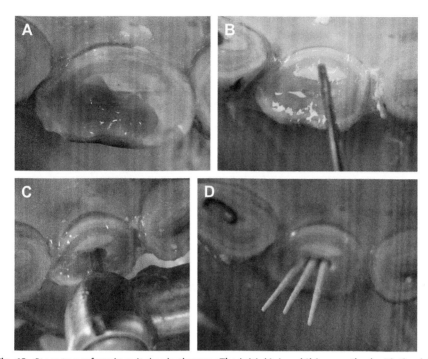

Fig. 12. Steps to performing vital pulp therapy. The initial injury (*A*) is smoothed with the drill (*B*). Once the tooth surface contour is shaped, 7 to 10 mm of pulp are removed from the pulp horn with the bur (*C*). Sterile paper points are placed on the pulp until hemostasis (*D*). Paper points are removed, and the pulp medicant is prepared. The pulp medicant is packed into an amalgam carrier that is placed either within or at the pulp horn access site, and the plunger depressed (*E*). The pulp medicant is lightly packed with a condenser to achieve a 2- to 3-mm thickness (*F*). The walls of the access site are cleaned with sterile excavators. An intermediate layer is placed on top of the pulp medicant to allow for final restoration (*G*). The walls of the site are etched, and a thin layer of unfilled resin is dropped and lightly blown around the site (*H*). The site is light-cured, and flowable composite material is placed into the site for complete restoration. The composite is cured (*I*). The restoration is smoothed with a white-stone bur (*J*), and a final layer of unfilled resin is applied and cured.

1. Walls of the access site are cleaned with the spoon excavator. The walls must be pristine to maximize bonding of the final restorative materials.
2. Access walls are etched with 37% phosphoric acid for 15 seconds.
3. The acid is carefully rinsed from the tooth structure and caught on gauze for proper disposal.
4. Access sites are dried using paper points or the air source on the dental unit.
5. A small amount of unfilled resin is dropped or brush-dripped onto cavity walls. Air is used to thin and coat the walls of the site, and curing with a light-gun is done for 15 seconds.
6. Using a plastic working instrument, composite material is placed into the access site. Depth of composite should be a minimum of 3 mm to allow for best retention. Light-curing for minimum for 45 seconds is performed.
7. Finishing burs or a fine diamond bur are used to shape and smooth restoration. Step 5 is repeated to ensure complete filling of dentinal tubules and microdefects in the composite.

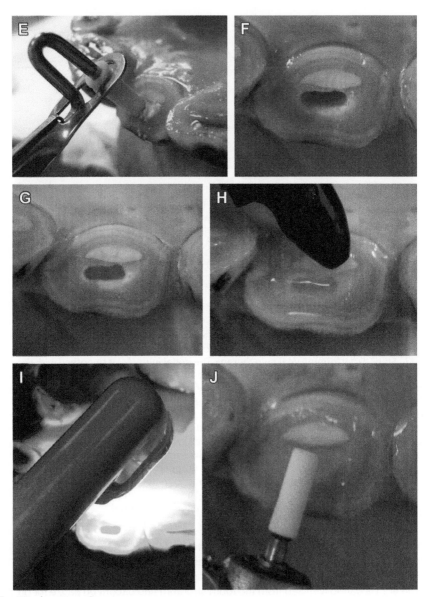

Fig. 12. (continued)

8. A postoperative radiograph is necessary for tracking and documenting the response of the tooth to therapy.

Considerations

Radiographic recheck examinations of the treated tooth 6 months postoperatively and then annually is highly recommended to ensure long-term treatment success. The formation of a dentinal bridge, continued formation of secondary dentin, and lack of periodontal and apical abnormality determine radiographic success. The treated tooth should be kept out of occlusion for the initial healing period (6 months) to prevent disturbance to the restorative material. Either the loss of crown height resulting from the traumatic incident or crown height reduction of the opposing tooth, about 1 to 2 mm, will result in loss of occlusal contact. Although this is not normally recommended for humans and dogs, the use of restorative materials is still relatively novel in the horse, and scientific literature establishing a restorative material that reliably withstands equine occlusal forces has yet to be published. Once the tooth erupts back into occlusion, the restorative material can be worn eventually to the level of the dentinal bridge, and the cycle of normal wear reestablished.

An ideal pulp dressing should stimulate healing of pulp tissue and formation of reparative dentin while being nontoxic, noncarcinogenic, biocompatible, insoluble in tissue fluids, antibacterial, antifungal, and dimensionally stable. The 2 main choices for pulp dressing are calcium hydroxide powder and MTA.[49,50] Calcium hydroxide has a long record of successful use for vital pulp therapy, although it does not meet all ideal requirements. Its advantages are that it is antibacterial and antifungal, disinfecting the superficial pulp. Because of its extreme alkalinity (pH 12.5), it will cause roughly 1.5 mm of pulp necrosis on placement,[51] which could be considered beneficial as it allows for additional debridement of inflamed pulp tissue. The toxicity of calcium hydroxide dissipates with depth, and only mild inflammation will be present below the region of tissue necrosis. This mild inflammation will initiate hard-tissue healing (tertiary dentin formation) in the absence of bacteria.

MTA is composed mainly of calcium, silica, and bismuth. This material was developed to meet all of the aforementioned ideal characteristics.[52,53] MTA is made of hydrophilic fine particles that harden in the presence of dampness or blood. It too has a high alkalinity that is regionally antimicrobial, but on setting the material neutralizes and becomes biocompatible.[54] It is radiopaque, and it is more difficult for external bacteria to infiltrate MTA than hard-setting calcium hydroxide cements. In addition, hardened MTA has excellent sealing capacities. It requires a working time of about 5 minutes and a hardening time that varies from 3 to 6 hours according to the density of the air entrapped during mixing and the dampness of the receiving site. The extended setting time can be considered a disadvantage. An extensive literature review demonstrates that MTA is a material of choice for pulp capping in addition to many other endodontic applications because of its biocompatibility, excellent sealing capacity, cellular adherence, and dentinal regenerative ability.[55–57]

In emergency situations, it has been suggested that either calcium hydroxide powder or IRM[22] should be used for a pulp-capping procedure until complete vital pulp therapy is performed. Calcium hydroxide powder becomes soluble with saliva and would be washed away in the first few minutes after application; IRM should not be used directly on pulp as stated in the package insert.[58] If an emergency situation arises, MTA can be used as a temporary direct pulp-capping material. Once placed, the horse should not be allowed to eat or drink until it is fully set. MTA has been proved to be less cytotoxic and superior to IRM as a primary pulp-capping medicant.[59–61]

ROOT CANAL THERAPY

The efficacy of performing root canal therapy in equine teeth is still questionable. Two major obstacles, canal shape and continuous occlusal wear, inhibit the long-term success of equine root canal therapy. Although the incisor tooth has only one pulp cavity, the shape of the pulp horn and root canal of the tooth varies considerably. The pulp horn of the coronal third of the tooth is compressed in a labiolingual direction by the infundibulum, and on transection resembles the shape of a barbell. In the middle third of the tooth, the pulp horn becomes cylindrical for roughly 2 to 3 cm, and in the apical third compresses laterally into a barbell shape once again (**Fig. 13**).[22] The unique shape of the pulp cavity in the apical and coronal third can sometimes lead to a complete central, longitudinal separation of the pulp, effectively creating 2 pulp cavities for a short distance. Both the changing shape and the potential division of the equine incisor pulp cavity can lead to complications and inadequacy during the instrumentation and obturation steps of root canal therapy. In addition, the apical foramen of equine incisor roots can vary in number and position, making a high-quality, leakproof obturation very challenging to achieve.[22]

Continuous occlusal wear of equine teeth makes obturation with softer traditional materials (a sealer cement and gutta percha) suboptimal because of eventual exposure. Orthograde endodontic therapy for equine incisors has been reported,[22,62] but a scientific study documenting long-term success beyond 18 months is unavailable. Apicoectomy with retrograde endodontic treatment of equine cheek teeth has been well described, and success has been evaluated from 3 to 49 months postoperatively depending on the tooth.[47] Of 17 teeth treated in this manner, 35% needed extraction, 17% had continued periodontitis, and 47% were considered successful.[63] A major complication encountered in the previous study was eventual exposure of the soft endodontic obturation materials resulting from occlusal wear. These materials quickly deteriorated, and the exposed pulp cavity became contaminated with feed. Feed contamination led to further deterioration of the tooth's structural integrity. The use of novel obturation materials (eg, MTA) that harden and resist wear on the occlusal surface could potentially remedy this problem, but currently no published equine research exists in this area. Finally, when all pulp material is removed, the tooth partially desiccates and loses the ability to internally respond to environmental challenges. Both of these conditions lead to demineralization and fragility of the tooth with resultant repeated dental fracturing and/or crumbling. Because of anatomic limitations, lack of evidence for long-term success, continued wear of the tooth, and the risk for continued tooth degeneration, endodontic therapy for equine incisor teeth remains controversial, and prudent case selection and client education is critical when considering this procedure.

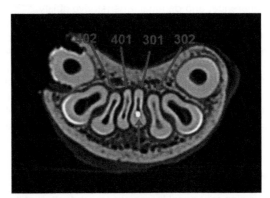

Fig. 13. Computed tomography scan of a mandibular rostral mandible at the apical third of the central incisor teeth (teeth 301 and 401) demonstrating the lateral compression of the teeth and the labiolingual attenuation of the canal. Note the discrepancy between a snugly placed gutta percha cone and the remaining root canal needing to be obturated (*pink arrow*). (*Courtesy of* Dr Stephen Galloway, DVM, Fellow AVD EQ in Fayetteville, TN.)

Equine canine teeth are more similar to the brachydont teeth; therefore, routine end-odontic techniques and equipment can be used to treat this tooth. A description of an orthograde or retrograde root canal procedure is beyond the scope of this article. There are many sources that clearly describe the scientifically supported steps for successful root canal therapy in dogs and humans.[64,65] Performing successful root canal procedures takes extensive training and practice, and it is recommended that only veterinary dental specialists perform these procedures. Root canal therapy is not a procedure that can be learned at a weekend course or by reading an article.

SUMMARY

Treatment of the incisor and canine teeth in the horse can be rewarding, but the single most important factor in performing successful dental therapy is an accurate diagnosis. Therefore, practitioners should concentrate on performing complete oral examinations and perfecting dental image acquisition and interpretation before focusing on treatments. Odontoplasty, periodontal therapy, uncomplicated extractions, and vital pulp therapy are all procedures that can be learned and mastered by general practitioners willing to spend the money to acquire the specialized equipment and invest the time required to learn and practice the techniques. Dental therapies in horses have advanced significantly over the last 20 years. Continued modernization of equine dental therapies should be based on all available and applicable scientific literature, cadaveric experimentation, and well-documented experience. The foundation for treatment should be based on scientifically proven general dental principles, and tailored to species-specific differences and challenges.

REFERENCES

1. Dixon PM, Tremaine WH, Pickles K, et al. Equine dental disease part 1: a long-term study of 400 cases: disorders of the incisor, canine, and first premolar teeth. Equine Vet J 1999;31(5):369–77.
2. Pediatric dental dictionary 2007. Available at: dentaldictionary.info. Accessed October 18, 2012.
3. Lathrop T. Stedman's medical dictionary. 28th edition. Philadelphia: Hubsta Ltd; 2008.
4. Angle EH. Treatment of malocclusion of the teeth and fracture of maxillae, Angle's system. Philadelphia: SS White Dental MFG Co; 1900.
5. Proffit WR, Fields HW. Contemporary orthodontics. 3rd edition. St Louis (MO): Mosby, Inc; 2000. p.185–7.
6. Scrutchfield WL. Incisors and canines. American Association Equine Practitioner Proceedings 1991;37:117–21.
7. Rucker BA. Incisor and molar occlusion: normal ranges and indications for incisor reduction. American Association Equine Practitioner Proceedings 2004;50:7–12.
8. duToit N, Burden FA, Dixon PM. Clinical dental examination of 357 donkeys in the UK: part 1—prevalence of dental disorders. Equine Vet J 2009;41(4):390–4.
9. Marshall R, Shaw DJ, Dixon PM. A study of the sub-occlusal secondary dentin thickness in overgrown equine cheek teeth. Vet J 2012;193:53–7.
10. White C, Dixon PM. A study of the thickness of cheek teeth sub-occlusal secondary dentin in horses of different ages. Equine Vet J 2010;42:119–23.
11. Shaw DJ, Dacre IT, Dixon PM. Pathological studies of cheek teeth apical infections in the horse: 2 quantitative measurements in normal equine dentin. Vet J 2008;178:321–32.

12. O'Leary JM, Barnett TP, Parkin TD, et al. Pulpar temperature changes during mechanical reduction of equine cheek teeth: comparison of different motorized dental instruments, duration of treatments and use of water cooling. Equine Vet J 2012;21:1–6.

13. Easley J. Corrective dental procedures. In: Easley J, Dixon PM, Schumacher J, editors. Equine dentistry. 3rd edition. Philadelphia: WB Saunders; 2011. p. 272, 268.

14. Earley ET. Skeletal abnormalities in the equine skull associated with diagonal incisor malocclusion. American Association of Equine Practitioner Focus Proceedings 2011;131–3.

15. Dixon PM, duToit N. Dental anatomy. In: Easley J, Dixon PM, Schumacher J, editors. Equine dentistry. 3rd edition. Philadelphia: WB Saunders; 2011. p. 70 p. 68, 66–67, 67.

16. DeLorey MS. A retrospective evaluation of 204 diagonal incisor malocclusions. J Vet Dent 2007;24(3):145–9.

17. Rucker BA. Utilizing cheek teeth angle of occlusion to determine length of incisor shortening. American Association of Equine Practitioner Proceedings 2002;48:448–52.

18. Wiggs RB, Lobprise HB. Veterinary dentistry: principles and practice. Philadelphia: Lippincott-Raven Publishers; 1997. p. 685.

19. Carranza FA, Rapley JW, Haake SK. Gingival inflammation. In: Newman MG, Takei HH, Carranza FA, editors. Carranza's clinical periodontology. 9th edition. Philadelphia: WB Saunders Co; 2002. p. 263–8.

20. Kinane DF. Causation and pathogenesis of periodontal disease. Periodontol 2000 2001;25:8–20.

21. Wolf HF, Rateitschak KH, Hassell TM. Color atlas of dental medicine: periodontology. 3rd edition. New York: Thieme; 2005. p. 39–66, 309–22, 281–5.

22. Klugh DO. Principles of equine dentistry. London: Manson Publishing Ltd; 2010. p. 34–7, 180–201, 218–20, 211–8, 219–20.

23. Cox AL. Pathological studies of equine periodontal disease. University of Edinburgh, Master of Science Thesis; 2010.

24. Easley J, Rucker BA. Equine dental equipment, supplies and instrumentation. In: Easley J, Dixon PM, Schumacher J, editors. Equine dentistry. 3rd edition. Philadelphia: WB Saunders; 2011. p. 258–9.

25. Wenstrom JL, Dahlen G, Ramberg P. Subgingival debridement of periodontal pockets by air abrasion in comparison to ultrasonic instrumentation during maintenance therapy. J Clin Periodontol 2011;38:820–7.

26. Petersilka GJ. Subgingival air-polishing in the treatment of periodontal biofilm infections. Periodontol 2000 2011;55:124–42.

27. Galloway SS, Galloway MS. Dental materials. In: Easley J, Dixon PM, Schumacher J, editors. Equine dentistry. 3rd edition. Philadelphia: WB Saunders; 2011. p. 360–3.

28. Merriam-Webster medical dictionary 2012. Available at: http://www.merriam-webster.com/medical/operculectomy. Accessed October 25, 2012.

29. Blood DC, Studdert VP. Bailliere's comprehensive veterinary dictionary. London: WB Saunders; 1993. p. 645.

30. Neville BW, Damn DD, Allen CM, et al. Oral and maxillofacial pathology. 3rd edition. London: Saunders Elsevier; 2009. p. 74.

31. Valverde A. Alpha-2 agonists as pain therapy in horses. Vet Clin North Am Equine Pract 2010;26:515–32.

32. Clutton RE. Opioid analgesia in horses. Vet Clin North Am Equine Pract 2010;26:493–514.

33. Goodrich LR. Strategies for reducing the complication of orthopedic pain preoperatively. Vet Clin North Am Equine Pract 2009;24:611–20.
34. Goodrich LR, Clark-Price S, Ludders J. How to attain effective and consistent sedation for standing procedures in the horse using constant rate infusion. Am Assoc Equine Pract Proceedings 2004;50:229–32.
35. Staszyk C, Bierert A, Baumer W, et al. Simulation of local anesthetic nerve block of the infraorbital nerve within the pterygopalatine fossa: anatomical landmarks defined by computed tomography. Res Vet Sci 2008;85:399–406.
36. Rawlinson JE. Addressing pain: regional nerve blocks. Am Assoc Eq Practitioner Focus Proceedings 2011;74–81.
37. Harding PG, Smith RL, Barakzai SZ. Comparison of two approaches to performing an inferior alveolar nerve block in the horse. Aust Vet J 2012;90(4):146–50.
38. Tremaine W, Schumacher J. Exodontia. In: Easley J, Dixon P, Schumacher J, editors. Equine dentistry. 3rd edition. London: Saunders Elsevier; 2011. p. 319–23.
39. Baratt RM. Clinical management of equine odontoclastic tooth resorption and hypercementosis. American Association Equine Practitioner Focus 2011;112–6.
40. Galloway S. Presented in American Association Equine Practitioner Dry Laboratory. Maryland, December 4–8, 2010.
41. Staszyk C, Bienert A, Simhofer H, et al. Equine odontoclastic tooth resorption and hypercementosis. Vet J 2008;178:372–9.
42. DuPont GA. Crown amputation with intentional root retention for dental resorptive lesions in cats. J Vet Dent 2002;19(2):107–10.
43. Baker GJ. Endodontic therapy. In: Baker GJ, Easley J, editors. Equine dentistry. 2nd edition. Edinburgh (United Kingdom): Elsevier; 2005. p. 295.
44. Trope M, Chivian N, Sigurdsson A, et al. Traumatic injuries. In: Cohen S, Burns RC, editors. Pathways of the pulp. 8th edition. St Louis (MO): Mosby; 2002. p. 610–5.
45. Clarke DE. Vital pulp therapy for complicated crown fracture of permanent canine teeth in dogs: a three-year retrospective study. J Vet Dent 2001;18(3): 117–21.
46. Niemiec BA. Assessment of vital pulp therapy for nine complicated crown fractures and fifty-four crown reductions in dogs and cats. J Vet Dent 2001;18(3): 122–5.
47. Simhofer H. Endodontic therapy. In: Easley J, Dixon P, Schumacher J, editors. Equine dentistry. 3rd edition. London: Saunders Elsevier; 2011. p. 369–71, 371–75.
48. Rawlinson JE. Pulp happens: how to perform vital pulp therapy. American Association Equine Practitioners Focus Proceedings 2011;134–40.
49. Tabarsi B, Parirokh M, Asgary S, et al. A comparative study of dental pulp response to several pulpotomy agents. Int Endod J 2010;43(7):565–71.
50. Galloway S, Galloway M. Dental materials. In: Easley J, Dixon P, Schumacher J, editors. Equine dentistry. 3rd edition. London: Saunders Elsevier; 2011. p. 355–9.
51. Powers J, Wataha J. Dental materials: properties and manipulation. St Louis (MO): Mosby Elsevier; 2008. p. 141–67.
52. Parirokh M, Torabinejad M. Mineral trioxide aggregate: a comprehensive literature review—part I: chemical, physical, and antibacterial properties. J Endod 2010;36(1):16–27.
53. Danesh F, Vahid A, Jahanbani J, et al. Effect of white mineral trioxide aggregate compared with biomimetic carbonated apatite on dentine bridge formation and inflammatory response in a dental pulp model. Int Endod J 2012;45:26–34.

54. Parirokh M, Torabinejad M. Mineral trioxide aggregate: a comprehensive literature review—part II: leakage and biocompatibility. J Endod 2010;36(2):190–202.
55. Parirokh M, Torabinejad M. Mineral trioxide aggregate: a comprehensive literature review—part III: clinical applications, drawbacks, and mechanism of action. J Endod 2010;36(3):400–13.
56. Nair PR, Duncan HF, Ford TR, et al. Histological, ultrastructural and quantitative investigations on the response of healthy human pulps to experimental capping with mineral trioxide aggregate: a randomized controlled trial. Int Endod J 2008; 41:128–50.
57. Modena KC, Casas-Apayco LC, Atta MT, et al. Cytotoxicity and biocompatibility of direct and indirect pulp capping materials. J Appl Oral Sci 2009;17(6): 544–54.
58. Dentsply. IRM directions for use. Tulsa (OK): 2005.
59. Hirschman WR, Wheater MA, Bringas JS, et al. Cytotoxicity comparison of three current direct pulp-capping agents with a new bioceramic root repair putty. J Endod 2012;38(3):385–8.
60. Ma J, Shen Y, Stoijicic S, et al. Biocompatibility of two novel root repair materials. J Endod 2011;37(6):793–8.
61. Mozayeni MA, Milani AS, Marvasti LA, et al. Cytotoxicity of calcium enriched mixture cement compared with mineral trioxide aggregate and intermediate restorative material. Aust Endod J 2012;38(2):70–5.
62. Garcia F, Sanroman F, Llorens MP. Endodontics in horses. J Vet Med 1990;37: 205–14.
63. Simhofer H, Stoian C, Zetner K. A long-term study of apicoectomy and endodontic treatment of apically infected cheek teeth in 12 horses. Vet J 2008; 178:411–8.
64. Homstrom SE, Frost P, Eisner ER. Veterinary dental techniques. 2nd edition. Philadelphia: WB Saunders Company; 1998. p. 255–318.
65. Cohen S, Burns RC. Pathways of the pulp. 8th edition. St Louis (MO): Mosby; 2002.

Advances in the Treatment of Diseased Equine Cheek Teeth

Henry Tremaine, BVetMed, MPhi, Cert ES, MRVS

KEYWORDS

- Horses • Dentistry • Cheek teeth • Odontoplasty

KEY POINTS

- There have been significant advances in dental therapeutic techniques in recent years.
- The overzealous use of modern powered tools to perform routine rasping in inadequately restrained horses has been shown to be potentially harmful and the risks of iatrogenic damage when performing techniques, such as diastema widening (odontoplasty), have been revealed.
- The need for good-quality imaging to facilitate precise interventional techniques is inescapable, and refinement of traditional extraction techniques and the use of better analgesia and restraint have greatly reduced patient morbidity.
- Restorative techniques to salvage diseased teeth have shown some early promise but the complex anatomy and limited understanding of endodontic pathology are currently limitations to their success. Exciting developments in this field are anticipated in years to come.
- The absolute requirement for specialized training and instrumentation to perfume equine dental techniques safely and effectively is now realized, with an expansion in further education toward this goal.

INTRODUCTION

In recent years there have been numerous scientific publications on equine dentistry. These have mostly involved cadaver studies on dental anatomy, including pulp anatomy[1]; secondary dentine thickness mesially, distally, and occlusally[2]; dental pathology of pulp,[3,4] periodontium,[5,6] and caries[7–9]; and physiologic studies of forces of mastication in Equidae.[10] The findings of these works are to be found elsewhere in this issue. Although the outcome of the articles, if applied appropriately, inform present and future treatments, studies advancing treatments and evidence-based, safety, and efficacy studies are sparse. However, those studies that have been published have cast doubt on some historically popular and anecdotally evidenced practices that, although they may have been widespread, have little to merit their continued use. There are 2 goals of equine dental treatments. Firstly, to maintain the dentition as an effective organ for food mastication, and secondly, to treat appropriately any dental

Department of Clinical Veterinary Science, University of Bristol, Langford House, Langford, Bristol BS405DU, UK
E-mail address: henry.tremaine@bristol.ac.uk

Vet Clin Equine 29 (2013) 441–465
http://dx.doi.org/10.1016/j.cveq.2013.04.013
0749-0739/13/$ – see front matter © 2013 Elsevier Inc. All rights reserved.

disorder diagnosed from clinical signs, examination, and ancillary diagnostic data. A modern approach to all of these techniques is included in accompanying articles.

Maintenance of Masticatory Apparatus

The practice of routine odontoplasty by rasping (floating) has evolved through a cycle. At first this was performed occasionally in unsedated horses that were showing clinical disease, without sedation and using crude equipment, often without previously performing a thorough examination. More recently, rasping has been routinely practiced in asymptomatic horses with or without tranquillization, using potent mechanized equipment with little regard to the long-term consequences. Neither approach is comprehensive or fit for purpose in a modern evidence-based age. Understanding of dental occlusion is still primitive and the merits of extensive, routine peripheral occlusal odontoplasty (rasping of edges or occlusal surfaces) has yet to be validated robustly. Some studies involving small numbers have been inconclusive.[11] However, the presence of sharp dental prominences detected on examination with mirrors or dental endoscopes has been associated with gingival and mucosal ulceration, which can be painful and associated with dysmastication. Dysmastication associated with pain from disease such as periodontitis produces malocclusion and abnormal wear patterns and hence the removal of sharp dental foci causing soft tissue trauma is justified. It must be born in mind that horses grazing naturally sustain physiologic occlusal wear that results in sharp dental peripheries without accompanying soft tissue disorders, or dysmastication, suggesting that sharp dental peripheries are an effective profile for normal mastication in healthy horses. However, for horses managed indoors or fed a largely cereal diet from chest height, as is the practice in many riding or livery stables, dental occlusion and wear patterns may not follow the physiologic model, necessitating routine dental interventions.[12]

There is some evidence that the rasping of teeth is associated with stress in horses,[13] and this is exacerbated when using powered equipment for the creation of bit seats. This result alone is sufficient justification for the use of chemical sedation, especially when the additional benefits of analgesia, muscle relaxation, and increased tolerance are considered. The use of potent powered dental instruments, capable of damaging teeth irreparably in unsedated horses, is hard to justify in the modern age, regardless of the advances in instrument design. The benefits of chemical sedation have to be balanced against the costs incurred and any associated risks in horses with mitigating disease. However, the evidence for the safety of sedatives when used appropriately is overwhelming.

How Much Tooth is it Safe to Remove?

The answer to this is not clear and a more useful question is, "How much tooth is it necessary to remove." A scientific basis to answer this is currently lacking. Removal of peripheral buccal processes, which are prominent occlusally and can cause buccal mucosal trauma, is indicated.[14] Focal sharp prominences on the lingual aspect of the mandibular molars can similarly cause lingual laceration and merit reduction to a smooth surface. Excessive transverse ridges (ETR), which often occlude in the interproximal spaces of the opposing arcade, have been attributed to restricted mesiodistal temporomandibular movement, although evidence to support this is lacking. However, they can have a plunger-cusp effect to impact food into diastema and exacerbate accumulation of putrefying food, leading to chronic painful periodontitis. Reduction of such ETRs to a level that is consistent with the undulations on the occlusal surface of the other teeth in the row is appropriate.

The removal of excessive dental material from the occlusal surface of the teeth must be questioned. Dentine is composed of dentinal tubules, within which the odontoblast processes deposit concentric primary dentine in the developing tooth and secondary dentine at the coronal aspect to replace masticatory occlusal attrition.[15] The mechanisms of this complex process have yet to be understood but are likely to be under neurologic influence. Odontoblast processes contain nerves that are sensitive to forces on the dental surface and probably have a role in maintenance of the occlusal secondary dentine bridge. It has been speculated that normal attrition results in a smear layer of material that is spread across the occlusal surface and decreases the permeability of the occlusal dentine.[14] The rate of secondary dentine deposition occlusally has yet to be estimated, but it is probable that excessive occlusal rasping results in artificially excessive occlusal wear at an accelerated rate. This wear has the potential to expose the more porous occlusal dentine, and may be associated with increased sensitivity.

Modern instruments have the capacity to remove dental tissues rapidly, especially those instruments with diamond-coated discs or burrs. The use of these has been shown to produce potentially harmful aerosols of dental dust and oral bacteria, and, in addition, their use can be accompanied by heat generation.[16–18] The use of mechanical tools has been shown to have the potential to increase the temperature of the pulp by an amount that is potentially lethal to odontoblasts (up to 24°C). The heating effect can be ameliorated by using short contact times and is greatly reduced by the use of water cooling, whether integrated into the unit or applied separately to the grinding surface (**Fig. 1**). Despite the development of quiet instruments it is appropriate that all horses are sedated when using power dental instruments for them to be used safely and with precision. Mechanical rasping has been shown to increase heart rate and blood pressure significantly compared with controls, suggesting that it is associated with stress and sensitivity; this was most marked in the mandibular teeth, which seem to display increased sensitivity associated with this procedure.[13]

It remains to be conclusively shown whether reduction of overgrowths can assist with prevention of malocclusion and dental misalignment, although this has been suggested anecdotally.

PERIODONTAL DISEASE

Periodontal disease is widespread in horses and its prevalence increases with age in both horses and donkeys.[6,7,19,20] This syndrome, which comprises gingivitis, periodontitis, alveolar bone recession, and peripheral subgingival caries, is frequently

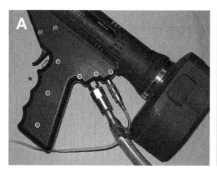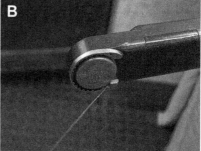

Fig. 1. (*A*) Water-cooled, vacuum-assisted dental burr (Flexi-Float, Veterinary Dental Products Ltd). (*B*) Rotating, diamond-coated disc with water cooling of the same instrument.

accompanied by moderate to severe oral pain, which can result in inability to ingest food effectively and significant loss of body condition. Clinical signs include those of oral pain, such as slow eating, dysmastication, oral dysphagia (quidding), selective appetite, hypersalivation, and weight loss. Other less obvious signs that can indicate oral pain are resistance to commands when ridden, harness resentment, and head shyness.

The predisposing feature to periodontitis in horses is food sequestration in the gingival sulcus (**Fig. 2**), which is usually predisposed by inappropriate interproximal diastemata.[6] The diastemata, which are most prevalent between mandibular dentition, especially at Triadan positions 09/10 and 10/11,[6,7] vary in configuration depending on the dental morphology and have been categorized as open diastemata, in which there is no occlusal contact with parallel interproximal mesial and distal dental surfaces, and valve diastemata,[21] in which there is actual or approximate occlusal dental contact and a wider interproximal space at the gingival margin, resulting in food accumulation in the space. In the latter case, the fibrous particles are forced into the diastema during mastication, which is exacerbated by transverse ridges, and subsequent entrapment of food because of the close interproximal contact. Food decomposition and the presence of oral bacteria in a carbohydrate substrate result in the release of acids. These factors combine to initiate a chronic inflammatory cascade afflicting the gingival bone, periodontium, and alveolar bone that contributes to demineralization of the interproximal peripheral cementum and enamel in a form of peripheral caries, particularly in chronic cases (**Fig. 3**).[6,21] The inflammatory changes present as hyperemia and recession of the gingiva, with severe focal pain, and ultimately destruction of the collagenous periodontal ligament fibers and lysis of the alveolar bone plate. Diagnosis is

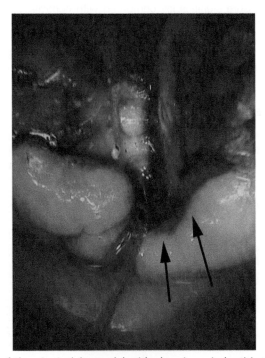

Fig. 2. Recession of the gingival (*arrows*) I with chronic periodontitis to produce a deep pocket.

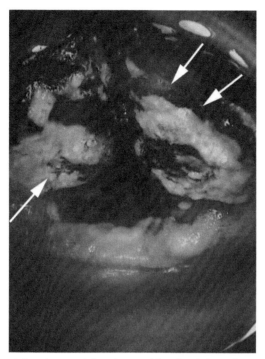

Fig. 3. Advanced peripheral cemental caries resulting in pitting of cementum and enamel (*arrows*) either side of a diastema affected by chroming periodontitis.

described elsewhere and is based on history and oral examination. Observation of the extent of the disorder can be greatly enhanced using oral endoscopy, which facilitates measurement of the depth of the periodontal pocket. Many of these inflammatory processes are reversible, although deep periodontal membrane destruction and alveolar lysis can result in permanent loss of mechanical stability and increased mobility of the tooth, which accelerates dental destruction. Advanced changes are shown on oral radiographs, especially open-mouthed oblique occlusal views, and alveolar sclerosis can extend apically as far as the roots in the most severe cases.[22]

The key maneuver in the management or treatment of this syndrome is the evacuation of entrapped food material in the diastema.[23] Removal of the food is essential before the inflammatory cascade can be arrested, which in turn enables healing of the periodontal lesion and gingival regrowth to partly obliterate the diastema. This process necessitates careful cleaning with high-pressure water and air, dental picks, and right-angled forceps (**Fig. 4**). Thorough removal of this food can be challenging, and even more challenging is prevention of ongoing food impaction. Therapy is further impeded by the focal pain associated with these periodontal pockets rendering the horses fidgety and intolerant to periodontal clearance.

Severe periodontal disease treatment is achieved most effectively with the horse restrained in stocks, well sedated, after administration of opioid and nonsteroidal analgesic, and frequently accompanied by the use of gingival and regional local analgesia. The mouth can be thoroughly washed with high-pressure water to remove any loose food material and start the evacuation of the diastema. Periodontal pocket debridement is then continued using picks, alligator forceps, and water jets. In cases

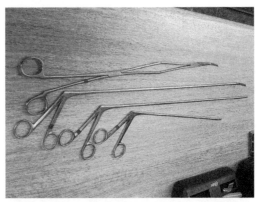

Fig. 4. Removal of entrapped fiber from diastema can be challenging. A range of specialized forceps including right-angled ones can be useful for this.

in which there is close interproximal contact or a valve configuration to the diastema, entrapped food cannot be freed. In such cases, widening of the diastema (odontoplasty) has been shown to be of short-term and long-term benefit (**Fig. 5**).[23] The principle of this treatment is that odontoplastic widening facilitates evacuation of the periodontal pockets and enables subsequent self-clearance by the horse's tongue during eating. In cases in which periodontal disease is caused by pathologic diastema secondary to a malerupted tooth, extraction of the misaligned tooth may assist with remission of the periodontal lesions.[24] After removal of entrapped food and debridement of the periodontal pocket and gingiva using high-pressure water or air abrasion (**Fig. 6**), deposition of topical antimicrobials is sometimes practiced, although long-term studies of these treatments are yet to be published. In addition, some clinicians place temporary polysiloxane stents in the widened space to impede further food entrapment (**Fig. 7**) and to maintain antimicrobial levels in the periodontal pocket. Anecdotal evidence suggests that these practices are helpful.

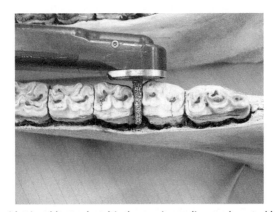

Fig. 5. Diastema widening (dentoplasty) is done using a diamond-coated burr such as this or high-speed handpiece placed in the interproximal space, parallel with the space. Good restraint and careful, accurate, controlled placement are needed to avoid inadvertent pulp penetration.

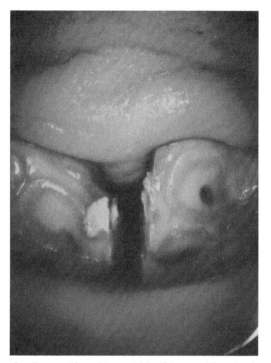

Fig. 6. This diastema has been widened to a width of 4 mm without pulp exposure, allowing effective periodontal debridement.

TREATMENT OF CARIES

The causes and development of caries involve the action of cariotic bacteria in a carbohydrate substrate to produce acids, which results in the progressive demineralization of dental tissues. The details are described elsewhere. The precise role of sequestration of food in contact with peripheral cement in the development of peripheral caries, interproximal caries, gingivitis, and periodontitis is still unclear, although there is a high prevalence of peripheral caries coinciding with periodontitis.[9,25] The importance of the presence of putrefying and impacted food in the development of caries is known.[26,27] Therefore, treatment measures to reduce oral food sequestration are likely to have preventative benefit. These measures include the rinsing of the mouth with water, rinsing with antibacterial mouthwash, correction of any dental overgrowths that contribute to dysmastication, and the manipulation of diets to assist masticatory action. Remedial benefits of interventional treatments to reduce peripheral caries have not been shown. In hypsodonts, exposed crowns with peripheral caries erupt continuously and, if the decay process is halted, it is conceivable that the diseased crown will be worn away as it erupts to be replaced by more recently erupted healthy tooth that has not undergone caries and periodontal disease, and hence at least the progression of decay can be delayed.

Infundibular Caries

Caries afflicting the occlusal infundibulum is a common finding in teeth of clinically asymptomatic horses and donkeys and preferentially afflicts the maxillary 09s.[28,29]

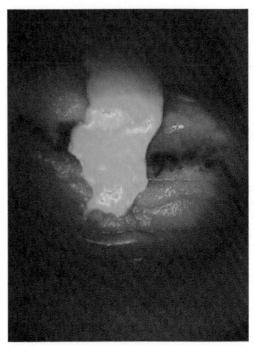

Fig. 7. After widening, pliable nonirritant stents are helpful to avoid food accumulation in the diastema while the inflammation heals.

Marked carious lesions have been examined histologically and lesions are considered to be a physiologic normal finding in horses as age advances.[30] Horses with infundibular caries were not over-represented in a study of maxillary teeth afflicted with pulpitis.[4] However, in a study reporting the location of dental fractures, fractures along a plane through infundibulae were prevalent.[30] This finding suggests that advanced caries (**Fig. 8**) can result in structural weakening predisposing to dental fracture along

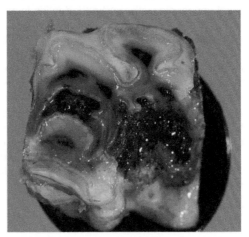

Fig. 8. The infundibular caries in the picture is advanced and has penetrated through the cementum, infundibular enamel, and into the primary dentine.

a stress concentration plane, when the normal masticatory forces and cyclical loading are applied. The maxillary 09s are the teeth most prevalently afflicted by advanced caries and this coincides with the teeth that present most commonly with sagittal plane fractures (**Fig. 9**).[31] The Honmer scale for grading carious lesions has been applied to horses, and teeth with grades 1 and 2 caries could be perceived as being within the limits of physiologic normality.[32] Carious lesions that have penetrated the infundibular enamel resulting in its demineralization and discoloration are probably pathologic even if clinically asymptomatic.

Treatment of caries remains largely anecdotal. Debridement of lesions using high-speed burrs followed by filling of the lesions and restoration using a variety of materials including flowable and light cured composites and glass ionomer have been reported (**Fig. 10**), but the efficacy of these treatments in arresting the progression of caries and delaying the subsequent fracture of teeth remain anecdotal, although encouraging pilot data have been reported.[33] Computed tomographic studies[34] showing the variation in pattern of normal infundibula in equine maxillary teeth amplify the challenge of attributing clinical significance to lesions. Furthermore, some teeth showed organic material sealed in apparently intact infundibulae by cementum deposited more occlusally, suggesting this finding to be a normal variation in Equidae. In addition, the profile of many infundibulae are curved, which makes their debridement using straight burrs and Hedstrøm files technically challenging.

Peripheral Caries

Peripheral caries has been reported in several studies in recent years and its prevalence may seem to be increased because of improvements in examination techniques

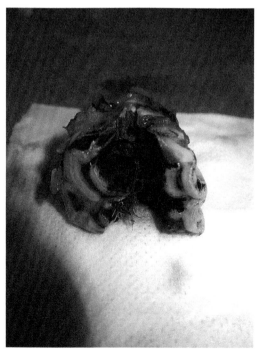

Fig. 9. This tooth has sustained a pathologic sagittal fracture coalescing 2 carious infundibulae and resulting in pulp exposure.

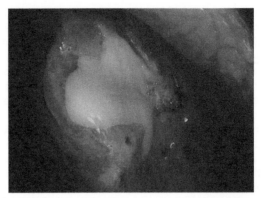

Fig. 10. This tooth has undergone occlusal restoration using flowable composite. This material has inferior hardness compared with some products but its convenience in inaccessible caudal teeth makes it useful.

with widespread use of mirrors and dental endoscopy.[26,27] Peripheral caries lesions are often associated with food retention in the gingival sulcus and reflection, and are often observed coincidentally with periodontitis that is often associated with food impaction in periodontal pockets. Peripheral caries results in marked pitting of the peripheral cementum and enamel (**Fig. 11**), which can facilitate the adhesion of food containing carious bacteria to the dental surface and in the gingival sulcus,

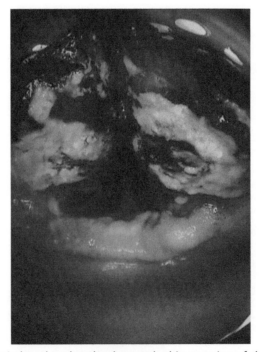

Fig. 11. A deep periodontal pocket that has resulted in recession of the gingival margin, accumulating inflammatory mediators and bacteria.

thus propagating the disorder. The role of this caries in perioendo transmission of bacteria leading to pulpitis remains unclear.[32] It has been suggested that diets high in fermented material, such as haylage, and diets with high components of digestible carbohydrates might accelerate peripheral caries, but this has yet to be validated.

Peripheral caries with food accumulation in the gingival sulcus is often associated with gingivitis, which can be painful and hence preventative treatments such as frequent mouth irrigation to remove food sequestration from the cheeks are likely to be beneficial.

PULPITIS

Pulpitis (including apical abscessation, apical necrosis, and suppurative apical infection) is significant both clinically and economically in horses and donkeys.[7,32] It afflicts maxillary and mandibular teeth that are young, at a stage when apical foraminae remain wide in patency, whereas there is ongoing increase in dental length that coincides with recent eruption of the secondary dentition.[3,35] It has been suggested that at this stage the confinement of the expanding tooth within the mandible of the upper jaw can lead to impaction of apical vasculature, which predisposes the pulp to ischemic compromise and predisposes to inoculation with anachoretic bacteria. Other suggested mechanisms include perioendo pulpal inoculation and pulp contamination via occlusal fissures or fractures.[31,32,35] Pulp inflammation leading to vascular compromise of odontoblasts at the occlusal end of the occlusal pulp horn could result in cessation of secondary dentine production, causing porosity or failure of the occlusal secondary dentine bridge and eventual exposure of the pulp cavity to oral bacteria. This hypothesis is supported by the presence of dentinal fissures being observed in 57% of teeth with chronic pulpitis. Unerupted permanent premolars are also affected in some cases, possibly as a result of apical vascular compromise resulting from the impaction caused by an obstructed eruption pathway. The location can be confined to a single pulp horn or multiple horns that may share communication with a common root pulp.[4,34]

Sectioning of teeth extracted because of pulpitis can reveal the presence of both vital and necrotic pulp in adjacent horns in the same tooth (**Fig. 12**). This fact,

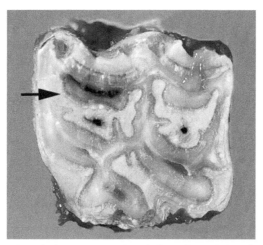

Fig. 12. This sectioned tooth shows 1 necrotic pulp horn (*arrow*), but the pulp horns on the remainder of the section appear to be vital.

combined with the upregulated ability of the dentinopulpar complex to produce secondary dentine, suggests that equine teeth can remain vital after pulpitis of individual pulps[4] in some cases.

Pulpitis results in reactive osteitis of the alveolar bone surrounding a diseased pulp with remodeling, expansion, lysis of the radicular endodontic dentine, lysis of the periodontium, and reactive sclerosis of the surrounding alveolar bone.[4] This process can result in localized bony swellings of the ventral mandible or maxilla with ipsilateral lymphadenitis, which can progress to the formation of a suppurating tract through the alveolar bone surrounding the diseased apex with discharging tracts exuding through the periodontium (rarely) (**Fig. 13**), ventral mandible, nasal cavity, maxillary bone, or into the rostral or caudal maxillary sinuses. These changes are shown on radiographs or computed tomograms.[34,36] Afflicted teeth also revealed fissures in occlusal secondary dentine in 57% of cases,[4] which are revealed well using dental endoscopy.[37]

Conservative treatments with antimicrobials for 1 to 4 weeks historically have been shown to result in amelioration of clinical signs temporarily, or permanently in a minority of cases, especially in young horses with wide apical foraminae.[35] This finding may indicate that the apical vascular is less prone to ischemic compromise in such teeth compared with those of older horses with narrower apical foraminae, which may be more vulnerable to vascular compromise.

Most chronically afflicted teeth traditionally and currently require extraction to eliminate the nidus of necrotic pulp and infection. Extraction techniques were described in the early literature and have altered little in fundamental principle. However, in recent years, refinements to case selection, improved sedative analgesic combinations, better instrumentation, and the widespread use of local analgesia have improved efficacy, precision, efficiency, and morbidity to the horse with fewer complications.[38]

It has been widely accepted that extraction of mature hypsodont teeth is a technically challenging invasive procedure and is a procedure that should only be performed by veterinary surgeons with appropriate expertise and training. The potential to cause irreversible iatrogenic damage with welfare effects after botched attempts is well recognized.

The use of better quality radiographic and tomographic images has enhanced the detection of diseased teeth and aided precise treatment planning.[36]

More recently, attempts to salvage the tooth after performing root canal ablation[39] or apicectomy[40] of the diseased root have been described, but thus far the success has not been widespread.

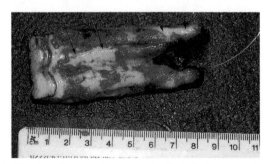

Fig. 13. An extracted tooth with a tract communicating via the periodontium to the apical foraminae (*arrows*), which can result in perioendodontic transmission of bacteria.

DENTAL EXTRACTION

In principle, dental extraction involves the separation of the periodontium and the removal of the tooth with minimal damage to the alveolus. This result is achieved most effectively by extraction per os along the normal eruption pathway.[38,41] Desensitizing the tooth using regional nerve blocks combined with subgingival infiltration reduces the morbidity to the patient and assists restraint, thereby allowing a precise, controlled procedure.[42] Nevertheless, periodontal separation remains challenging because of the poor access and, despite improving instrumentation, this remains primitive. Gingival elevation precedes periodontal separation, and is done using gingival elevators that expose the alveolar crest allowing access to the periodontium. Periodontal separation is achieved using periodontal elevators, molar separating forceps, and by stretching the periodontium gradually using repeated oscillation of molar forceps.

Permanent Premolar and Molar Extraction

Technique for oral extraction
The techniques described by O'Connor[43] (1942) and Guard[44] (1951) have been modified and are described in detail in more recent texts.[41] The recent advances in the techniques comprise the widespread use of local nerve blocks to provide effective analgesia, which enables a more controlled procedure that is less noxious for the horse. However, bilateral blockade of the inferior alveolar nerve should be approached with caution to avoid the horse self-mutilating its tongue following the bilateral desensitization of the lingual nerve branch with the mandibular nerve.[45] The evolution of better instrumentation has facilitated greater precision with dental extractions in recent years. Antibiotics are routinely given before surgery. A bright headlight is necessary for accurate instrument placement. The gag (speculum) is inserted and opened sufficiently wide to allow digital palpation to clearly identify the tooth to be removed. After visually and digitally identifying the tooth to be extracted, the gingiva on the buccal, palatal, or lingual aspects of the affected tooth are elevated from the tooth using a flat-bladed dental pick or small periodontal elevator. Specific instrumentation enables more effective separation of the periodontium before application of the molar separators than was previously possible (**Fig. 14**). The periodontium is strongest in the zone adjacent to the alveolar crest[5] and effective separation of this before attempting

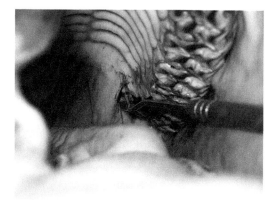

Fig. 14. The gingiva is elevated to the level of the alveolar crest before commencing a dental extraction.

extraction is crucial. Molar separators are placed rostral and then caudal to the affected tooth to loosen the rostral and caudal periodontal attachments. Aggressive use of the molar separators is unnecessary and also increases the risk of inadvertently loosening a healthy tooth, or fracturing the crown of the affected or adjacent teeth.

The molar extractors can then be placed on the tooth. Molar extractors come in different sizes and no single instrument is perfect for every tooth (good instrument-tooth contact is essential, and instruments with toothed or knurled jaws are preferable). The extractor handles are then fixed using the locking mechanism (or a rubber bandage or adhesive tape).

The extractors are oscillated with slow, low-amplitude movements in the horizontal plane only, down the center of the sagittal axis of the cheek tooth. A visual inspection during the first few oscillations should be performed to ensure that the extractor has maintained a grip on the tooth and that the tooth is moving slightly. When the periodontal attachments are loosened, a distinctive squelching sound can be heard, and the resistance to oscillation of the extractor decreases. In addition to disrupting the periodontal membrane, it has been suggested that this loosening contributes to stretching the alveolus, also facilitating extraction (Easley J, personal communication, 1998).

A dental fulcrum appropriate to the extractors is advanced to lie between the extractors and the cheek tooth rostral to the affected tooth. The mechanical advantage is maximized by advancing the fulcrum as far as possible along the row of cheek teeth, close to the jaws of the forceps. While keeping the molar extractors firmly gripped on the affected tooth, firm pressure is applied to the handles to lever the tooth over the fulcrum in an apical direction to extract it in a straight line parallel with its long axis. Once the tooth has been partially extracted (**Fig. 15**), it may be necessary to release the extractors and replace in a more apical position to extract the remaining part of the tooth. Once the tooth is partially extracted, it may be necessary to direct the clinical crown medially to allow extraction of the apical portion without obstruction from the opposing row of cheek teeth. Supernumerary maxillary distomolars (**Fig. 16**) can be extracted with care using the same technique.[46]

The alveolus should then be carefully digitally palpated for the presence of remaining dental fragments or alveolar bone fragments. If remnants remain, the alveolus is carefully curetted until the alveolus is smooth to digital palpation, and no dental fragments remain. Postextraction radiographs should be taken if the tooth fractures during extraction and dental fragments may remain.

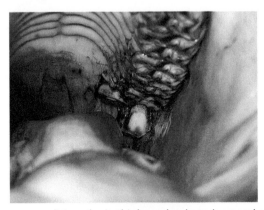

Fig. 15. The supernumerary distomolar in this horse has been loosened and, after complete periodontal separation, the tooth has been advanced from the alveolus using a fulcrum.

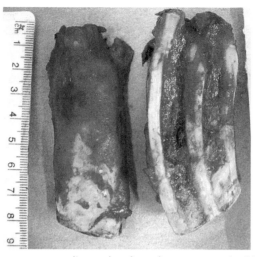

Fig. 16. These 2 supernumerary distomolars have been extracted with minimal alveolar trauma, resulting in uncomplicated healing.

The dental alveolus can be sealed using orthopedic polymethyl methacrylate bone cement or dental impression compound placed in the alveolar cavity. The alveolus should be cleaned and dried with gauze swabs before prosthesis placement (President putty, Henry Schein). Excessively long prostheses seem to result in delayed alveolar healing.

Aftercare
Minimal aftercare is necessary after oral extraction. However, nonsteroidal antiinflammatory drugs are suitable to provide analgesia for 24 to 72 hours. A soft or soaked diet can be fed for a few after surgery. Sinus lavage for several days may be necessary in cases with an associated sinusitis. A digital inspection of the alveolus 12 to 14 days after surgery for any remaining dental fragments is beneficial in cases in which the tooth was extracted in more than one fragment. There is significant mesial drift of the teeth distal to the alveolus vacated after dental extraction,[47,48] and this combined with the supereruption of the opposing tooth demands regular corrective dentistry annually or biannually after surgery.

OTHER METHODS FOR DENTAL EXTRACTION
Extraction of Fractured Teeth Under Endoscopic Guidance

Fractured teeth are challenging to extract using standard equipment because of the absence or friability of the clinical crown. An alternative technique recently described is to use the improved visibility provided by oral endoscopy to precisely elevate the periodontium using a range of specially developed periodontal elevators of varying sizes and shapes. The dental fragments are then extracted using specially designed low-profile fragment forceps.[49] This method is atraumatic and maintains the integrity of the dental alveolus, but requires a high level of sedation and analgesia, potentially expensive endoscopic equipment, and a range of specially designed dental elevators. However, the reduced incidence of complications compared with retrograde approaches justifies its use in selected cases.

Repulsion Techniques

Extraction along the eruption pathway is not possible in all cases, including those in which the clinical crown is fractured, affected by advanced caries, incompletely erupted or nonerupted, or when the crown fractures during attempted extraction leaving an apical fragment or fragments. Retrograde repulsion traditionally was widely practiced, although this method is destructive to surrounding alveolar bone, is inefficient at disrupting periodontium, and risks iatrogenic damage to related structures.[35] The increased awareness of the complications intrinsic to this technique has resulted in a decline in its popularity. Refinements of repulsion include the use of fluoroscopy to assist with punch positioning, and the use of smaller diameter Steinmann pins for repulsion of teeth that have undergone previous periodontal separation.[50–52] In addition to the improved precision afforded with real-time imaging, the use of a minimally invasive approach reduces the trauma to the dental alveolus (**Fig. 17**). The maintenance and sealing of the alveolus from the oral cavity is a crucial step in healing after dental repulsion and a minimally invasive approach that is sympathetic to the alveolus has much to recommend it. Furthermore, with the assistance of appropriate imaging, sedation, and local analgesia, less invasive repulsion techniques can be performed effectively in standing, conscious horses in selected cases.[52] However, after surgery, access to the alveolus for visual and digital inspection is limited and the narrow punches or Steinmann pins are not effective for separating intact periodontium. Such minimally invasive techniques are also useful to assist with the removal of root fragments, especially in cases in which an oral approach has been unsuccessful.

Buccotomy Techniques

Teeth that have not erupted or that are impacted are not amenable either to extraction per os or repulsion via an apical approach. For these, some form of transcortical approach is need, which usually involves an osteotomy of the buccal dental alveolar bone, and an incision through the soft tissues of the oral cavity to expose the clinical crown (buccotomy). These techniques have been used successfully for mandibular teeth 06 to 10 and maxillary teeth.[53,54] The removal of uninterrupted mandibular

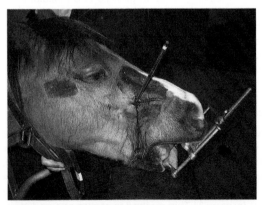

Fig. 17. Retrograde root fragment repulsion in a standing sedated horse with regional analgesia. This horse is undergoing minimally invasive root fragment removal, using a modified root fragment punch, which is positioned with radiographic guidance. This technique is applicable when the fragments are inaccessible per os. Careful restraint of the horse and precise technique are prerequisites to avoid iatrogenic damage and to succeed.

11s remains challenging and a modified vertical alveolar osteotomy has been used effectively. These buccotomy techniques that require precise surgical technique report a long-term success rate superior to repulsion (92%) but with more frequent complications (31%) than after extraction per os.[38] Incisional dehiscence is the most common complication and facial nerve dysfunction after trauma to the dorsal or ventral buccal nerves has also been reported.[53] The buccotomy/osteotomy techniques are performed with the horse anesthetized. A curvilinear incision is made over the apex of the afflicted tooth (or parallel with it for mandibular 11s). The soft tissues are carefully dissected, with cautious retraction of any nerves encountered, until the periosteum of the mandible or maxilla is encountered. Using Gelpi retraction forceps to retract the soft tissues, a longitudinal incision is made in the periosteum over the midline of the long axis of the tooth. Perpendicular incisions are made at each end and the periosteum is reflected using a periosteal elevator to expose the external lamina of the maxillary or mandibular cortex. After identifying the location of the mesial and distal borders of the afflicted tooth, an osteotomy is created using a sharp osteotome, bone burr, or oscillating saw. This osteotomy is extended coronally as far as the alveolar crest and an incision is made though the gingival mucoperiosteum at the level of the gingival reflection, into the oral cavity to reveal the clinical crown. The bony lamina is elevated and the buccal periodontium separated to reveal the buccal aspect of the reserve crown of the tooth (**Fig. 18**). The periodontal attachments of the mesial and distal reserve crown and the apex are separated using elevators, luxators, and gauges. Once the tooth is separated (apart from the inaccessible lingual/palatal periodontium), it is usually sectioned transversely and/or sagittally. Apical fragments can be extracted via the osteotomy and the coronal portion can usually be advanced out of the alveolus via the oral cavity. The alveolus is carefully palpated and any dental bone fragments are removed before irrigation. The apical alveolus is usually packed with a seton and the oral side sealed with polysiloxane putty. The soft tissues are apposed in 3 layers with the seton exiting a separate single-stab incision.

After surgery, the seton is removed after 48 hours. The oral polysiloxane implant sometimes becomes loose in the absence of a buccal alveolar wall and requires replacement. Soft, nonfibrous diets are fed for 48 hours and application of riding harness is avoided for 6 weeks. The cosmetic outcome is good even in cases that suffer incisional dehiscence.

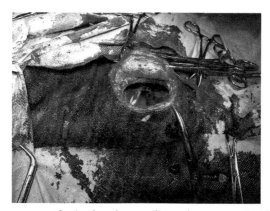

Fig. 18. This horse was anesthetized and a curvilinear buccotomy incision made through skin and soft tissues, avoiding branches of the facial nerve. The mandibular cortex and buccal alveolus have been removed to expose the reserve dental crown.

More recently a combination of the buccotomy approach and extraction per os has been described and instruments specific to this technique have been developed.[55,56] The minimally invasive transbuccal technique (MIT) facilitates a more direct approach to the periodontium, without destruction of the dental alveolus. Portals are created through the soft tissues including skin, musculature, and oral mucosa using a stab incision through the skin and the insertion of a trochar/cannula combination (**Fig. 19**). This technique allows the insertion of instruments through the cannula into the mouth to approach the cheek teeth occlusally rather than the inefficient oblique angle of approach restricted during an oral approach. The cannula accommodates a range of periodontal elevators that, when used thus, can be advanced apically to transect the periodontium more effectively than by using right-angled elevators per os. In addition, fractured fragments can be approached and, after drilling into the dental remnant via the cannula, a thread can be tapped and a threaded rod inserted into the dental fragment. Manipulation of the rod can facilitate further periodontal separation, allowing extraction of the tooth from the alveolus with an integral percussion device applied to the external end of the rod. Once free of the alveolus, the rod can be disengaged and the tooth withdrawn from the oral cavity. Small fragments within the alveolus can be removed using dedicated grasping forceps via the cannula. The stab incision in the skin is closed routinely after irrigation and the oral mucosa can be closed with absorbable monofilament material or can be allowed to heal spontaneously. This technique has shown particular promise for removal of fractured or carious maxillary 09s, which have a disappointing complication incidence using all other techniques.

Fractured Teeth

Removal of fractured teeth presents particular challenges. The presence of dental remnants prevents granulation of the alveolus and a fibrous, gingiva-covered, intact mucosa from healing and, as a consequence, food impaction in the alveolus, caries, and halitosis may ensue. Gradual fragmentation of dental remnants as caries progress will occur in subsequent years. However, many fractured teeth are asymptomatic and their removal can be technically challenging with the risk of morbidity causing clinical signs that are more obvious than the original dental remnant. Therefore each case should be evaluated thoroughly before embarking on attempted removal. This

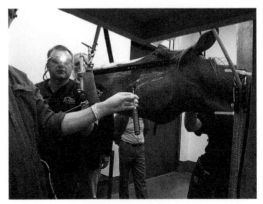

Fig. 19. A cannula has been carefully placed through the skin and buccal mucosa in this horse to enable periodontal separation and extraction using a minimally invasive transbuccal technique.

evaluation should include careful examination, radiography, and, in some cases, computed tomography. Calcium hydroxide can be administered to exposed pulp as a first aid measure in acute fractures and restorations can be performed in selected cases as described elsewhere in this issue, especially with incisors. For cheek teeth fractures, if there is an intact dental alveolus and the horse is clinically asymptomatic, there is an argument for a conservative approach. If there is penetration of the dental alveolus, then contamination from the buccal cavity bacteria in decaying food can ensue and removal of the fragments is necessary, especially if there are discharging cutaneous tracts or paranasal sinus involvement. The maxillary 09 is the most commonly fractured tooth and most fractures are pathologic. Slab fractures that do not involve the pulp may be treated conservatively, but many involve coalescing infundibulae or pulps and have advanced caries. If dental extraction is undertaken, then complete removal of all dental tissue and nonvital bone is essential before alveolar healing. Specialized instruments have been developed to assist with periodontal separation of fractured fragments and fragment removal (**Fig. 20**). Both orthograde approaches under endoscopic guidance using elevators and fine forceps and retrograde radiologically guided repulsion techniques must be considered. Extreme care should be taken to avoid additional iatrogenic damage to vital structures, especially when removing small retained root fragments. In some cases the fracture can be partially reduced and the fissure filled with bone cement to immobilize the fragments. Thereafter, extraction as if for an intact tooth can be possible (**Fig. 21**).

OCCLUSAL RESTORATION AND ENDODONTICS IN EQUINE TEETH

Dental extraction of a diseased tooth is considered a failure of salvage techniques, although it may be the most pragmatic solution to alleviate clinical signs. In other species, attempts to salvage the tooth are more extensively researched and tested. However, extrapolation of techniques that are effective in brachydonts to hypsodonts are rarely appropriate and there is limited understanding of the causes and development of equine pulp disease, although some bacteriology has been reported.[57] There are several significant challenges that remain before endodontic treatment of hypsodont teeth is routinely successful. Firstly, the continuous occlusal attrition and resulting exposed dentine on the occlusal surface renders it porous to microbes[1,2] and inevitably results in erosion of any occlusal restorative material. Secondly, the complex

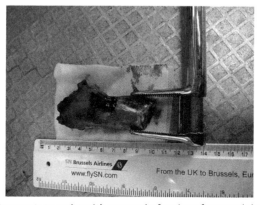

Fig. 20. Special instruments to assist with removal of carious fractured dental fragments can help avoid damage to the dental alveolus (Equine Blades Direct UK).

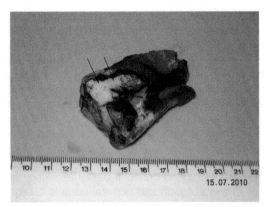

Fig. 21. This fractured tooth has been reduced and immobilized using polymethyl methacrylate (*arrow*) bone cement and subsequently extracted per os using extraction forceps.

and variable pulp anatomy of equine dentition makes endodontic debridement challenging.[1] Thirdly, the limited access to the pulp occlusally, and the moist environment, compromise many techniques that are successful in other species. Fourth, the desire to undertake dental treatment in the conscious horse results in movement, leading to compromise of the precision required for such technique to be successful.

Nevertheless there have been encouraging reports of the application of restorative techniques in carefully selected cases.[33] Materials used in equine dentistry are exported from other species and have yet to be systematically evaluated in equine teeth.[58]

Materials Used in Restorative Techniques

Cavity preparations

Cavity liners are used to protect the pulp, decrease dentinal sensitivity, and in some cases stimulate dentogenesis. The most popular is calcium hydroxide [$Ca(OH)_2$], which can be purchased in powder or paste form. Cavity bases provide structural support and protection for pulp and examples include zinc-oxide eugenol and zinc phosphate.[58]

The most popular direct-placement restorative material is glass ionomer. This material bonds chemically to dentine, although the bond is less secure than with resin composites. Their application is limited in hypsodont restorations because they are applicable to low stress, and require precise technique during handling and setting, which is less compatible with dental restorations in conscious horses.

Dental composites are the most commonly used materials. They are easy to apply, less technique sensitive, are practical, and bond well to equine dental material if prepared correctly. Products are either light-curing composites or self-curing flowable composites. The latter, although slightly reduced in quality of the seal because of their higher shrinkage during curing, are significantly more practical and hence the most popular.

Acute pulp exposure

Acute exposure of the pulp occurs as a result of dental fracture or during dental corrective procedures and is most commonly recognized involving incisors. Exposed pulp can be managed in most horses without the need for general anesthesia. Hemorrhage from traumatized exposed pulps should be recognized and, if the pulp exposure is the consequence of dental fracture, is an indication for radiography to determine the extent of the fracture. Removal of loose dental fragments is undertaken before careful debridement of the exposed contaminated dentine surrounding the exposed pulp using a high-speed burr. Hemostasis can be assisted with cotton buds or paper points soaked in adrenaline. Calcium hydroxide paste is placed in contact with exposed pulp, and resin containing calcium hydroxide preparations can be used as a second layer, although not in direct contact with the pulp. An alternative popular in human dentistry is to use mineral trioxide aggregate, which has the advantage of setting in a moist environment and facilitates dentogenesis.

Occlusal sealing of pulpar exposure associated with pulpitis
In horses with clinical signs of pulpitis, occlusal dental fissures are present in 57% of cases. The pulp anatomy is complex and vascular anastomoses and histology of diseased teeth suggests that local pulpitis is possible and that vital pulp can remain in such teeth.[1,59] The dentinal fissure is attributed to cessation of secondary dentine production occlusally to a pulp compromised by pulpitis and subsequent loss of odontoblast function. There are anecdotal reports that debridement of such exposed pulps followed by occlusal restoration can salvage the tooth, at least temporarily, delaying or avoiding the need for extraction in a proportion of cases,[60] although controlled detailed studies on its efficacy have yet to be completed. Careful debridement of the exposed pulps with a high-speed burr until apparently healthy dentine is exposed, followed by acid etching (**Fig. 22**), bonding, and setting with composite and glass ionomer has shown early promise, provided there is remaining vital pulp in the tooth.[40]

Endodontic root canal obturation
Root canal treatments in the horse remain in their infancy in terms of development. The incomplete understanding of the causes and development of pulpitis, the complex hypsodontic anatomy of the dentinopulpar complex, and instrument limitation remain obstacles to its widespread development. Endodontic treatments using a normograde (occlusal) approach[61] and a retrograde approach have been described with limited success.[62] Restoration of incisor teeth and using a normograde approach for root canal obturation in cheek teeth have been described, with good remission of clinical signs reported even after long-term follow-up, but such techniques have yet to become widespread and be validated after careful scientific scrutiny. Debridement of diseased pulp is essential and is achieved using a combination of high-speed burrs,

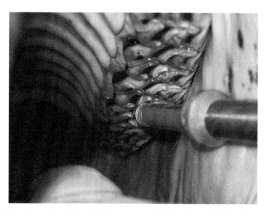

Fig. 22. Before occlusal restoration, this exposed dental pulp has been debrided and is being etched with phosphoric acid before application of flowable composite.

Hedstrøm files, and 2.5% sodium hypochlorite or 3% hydrogen peroxide. After irrigation with ethanol and drying, the obturated canals are filled using eugenol-free cements, composites, or gutta percha, before completing the occlusal seal. Root canal therapy using a retrograde approach is performed after a surgical approach to the dental apex, sectioning the diseased root (apicectomy) using a fine burr, and subsequent debridement and sealing of the exposed pulp.[62] Such techniques have resulted in limited success with approximately 50% of teeth restored in this fashion subsequently requiring extraction.[40] The task of creating a sterile, dry environment around the exposed and sectioned dental apex remains a technical challenge.

SUMMARY

There have been significant advances in dental therapeutic techniques in recent years. These advances have led to an overdue review of some traditional techniques, the justification of which is being questioned (eg, asymptomatic wolf tooth extraction). In addition, the overzealous use of modern powered tools to perform routine rasping in inadequately restrained horses has been shown to be potentially harmful and the risks of iatrogenic damage when performing techniques such as diastema widening (odontoplasty) have been revealed. The need for good-quality imaging to facilitate precise interventional techniques is inescapable, and refinement of traditional extraction techniques and the use of better analgesia and restraint have greatly reduced patient morbidity. The absolute requirement for specialized training and instrumentation to perfume equine dental techniques safely and effectively is now realized with an expansion of further education toward this goal. The development of restorative techniques remains embryonic in horses but the next decade promises great progress in this area.

REFERENCES

1. Windley Z, Weller R, Tremaine WH, et al. Two- and three-dimensional computed tomographic anatomy of the enamel, infundibulae and pulp of 126 equine cheek teeth. Part 1: findings in teeth without macroscopic occlusal or computed tomographic lesions. Equine Vet J 2009;41:433–44.
2. Marshall R, Shaw DJ, Dixon PM. A study of sub-occlusal secondary dentine thickness in overgrown equine cheek teeth. Vet J 2012;193:53–7.
3. van den Enden MS, Dixon PM. Prevalence of occlusal pulpar exposure in 110 equine cheek teeth with apical infections and idiopathic fractures. Vet J 2008; 178(3):364–71.
4. Casey MB, Tremaine WH. The prevalence of secondary dentinal lesions in cheek teeth from horses with clinical signs of pulpitis compared to controls. Equine Vet J 2010;42:30–6.
5. Warhonowicz M, Staszyk C, Rohn K, et al. The equine periodontium as a continuously remodeling system: morphometrical analysis of cell proliferation. Arch Oral Biol 2006;51:1141–9.
6. Cox A, Dixon PM, Smith S. Histopathological lesions associated with equine periodontal disease. Vet J 2012;194:386–91.
7. du Toit N, Burden FA, Kempson SA, et al. Pathological investigation of caries and occlusal pulpar exposure in donkey cheek teeth using computerised axial tomography with histological and ultrastructural examinations. Vet J 2008; 178(3):387–95.
8. Gere I, Dixon PM. Post mortem survey of peripheral dental caries in 510 Swedish horses. Equine Vet J 2010;42:310–5.

9. Ramzan PH, Palmer L. The incidence and distribution of peripheral caries in the cheek teeth of horses and its association with diastemata and gingival recession. Vet J 2011;190:90–3.
10. Huthmann S, Staszyk C, Jacob HG, et al. Biomechanical evaluation of the equine masticatory action: calculation of the masticatory forces occurring on the cheek tooth battery. J Biomech 2009;42:67–70.
11. Carmalt JL, Carmalt KP, Barber SM. The effect of occlusal equilibration on sport horse performance. J Vet Dent 2006;23:226–30.
12. Carmalt JL, Allen A. The relationship between cheek tooth occlusal morphology, apparent digestibility, and ingesta particle size reduction in horses. J Am Vet Med Assoc 2008;23:452–5.
13. Williams J. Effect of manual and motorized dental rasping instruments on thoroughbred's heart rate and behaviour. J Vet Behav 2012;7:149–56 [1558-7878].
14. Dacre IT, Shaw DJ, Dixon PM. Pathological studies of cheek teeth apical infections in the horse: 3. Quantitative measurements of dentine in apically infected cheek teeth. Vet J 2008;178:333–40.
15. Kilic S, Dixon PM, Kempson SA. A light microscopic and ultrastructural examination of calcified dental tissues of horses: 3. Dentine. Equine Vet J 1997;29: 206–12.
16. Allen M, Baker G, Freeman DE, et al. In vitro study of heat production during power reduction of equine mandibular teeth. J Am Vet Med Assoc 2004;224: 1128–32.
17. Wilson G. Temperature changes in dental pulp associated with use of power grinding equipment on equine teeth. Aust Vet J 2005;83:75–7.
18. O'Leary JM, Barnett TP, Parkin TD, et al. Pulpar temperature changes during mechanical reduction of equine cheek teeth: comparison of different motorised dental instruments, duration of treatments and use of water cooling. Equine Vet J 2013;45(3):355–60.
19. Tell A. The prevalence of oral ulceration in Swedish horses when ridden with bit and bridle and when unridden. Vet J 2008;178:405–10.
20. Walker H. Prevalence and some clinical characteristics of equine cheek teeth diastemata in 471 horses examined in a UK first-opinion equine practice (2008 to 2009). Vet Rec 2012;171:44.
21. Tremaine WH. Diastema and periodontal disease in the horse. Equine Vet Educ 2004;16:192–3.
22. Barakzai S. How to radiograph the erupted (clinical) crown of equine cheek teeth. Clin Tech Equine Pract 2005;4:171–4.
23. Dixon PM, Barakzai S, Collins N, et al. Treatment of equine cheek teeth by mechanical widening of diastemata in 60 horses (2000–2006). Equine Vet J 2008; 40:22–8.
24. Casey MB, Tremaine WH. Dental diastemata and periodontal disease secondary to axially rotated maxillary cheek teeth in three horses. Equine Vet Educ 2010;22:439–44.
25. Erridge ME, Cox AL, Dixon PM. A histological study of peripheral dental caries of equine cheek teeth. J Vet Dent 2012;29:150–6.
26. Simhofer H. The use of oral endoscopy for detection of cheek teeth abnormalities in 300 horses. Vet J 2008;178:396–404.
27. Ramzan PH. Cheek tooth malocclusions and periodontal disease. Equine Vet Educ 2010;22:445–50.
28. Lundström TS, Dahlén GG, Wattle OS. Caries in the infundibulum of the second upper premolar tooth in the horse. Acta Vet Scand 2007;49:102–7.

29. Fitzgibbon C. Anatomical studies of maxillary cheek teeth infundibula in clinically normal horses. Equine Vet J 2010;42:37–43.

30. Dixon PM. Equine idiopathic cheek teeth fractures: part 3: a hospital-based survey of 68 referred horses (1999–2005). Equine Vet J 2007;39:327–32.

31. Dacre I. Equine idiopathic cheek teeth fractures. Part 1: pathological studies on 35 fractured cheek teeth. Equine Vet J 2007;39:310–8.

32. Dacre I, Kempson S, Dixon PM. Pathological studies of cheek teeth apical infections in the horse: 5. Aetiopathological findings in 57 apically infected maxillary cheek teeth and histological and ultrastructural findings. Vet J 2008;178:352–63.

33. Pearce CJ. Equine cheek teeth infundibular restorations: long-term follow up results in 223 procedures in 92 horses. Proceedings of the 52nd Scientific congress of BEVA. Birmingham: Equine Veterinary Journal Limited; 2012. p. 103–7.

34. Windley Z, Weller R, Tremaine WH, et al. Two- and three-dimensional computed tomographic anatomy of the enamel, infundibulae and pulp of 126 equine cheek teeth. Part 2: findings in teeth with macroscopic occlusal or computed tomographic lesions. Equine Vet J 2009;41:441–7.

35. Dixon PM, Tremaine WH, Pickles K, et al. Equine dental disease part 4: a long-term study of 400 cases: apical infections of cheek teeth. Equine Vet J 2000;32:182–94.

36. Veraa S. Computed tomography of the upper cheek teeth in horses with infundibular changes and apical infection. Equine Vet J 2009;41:872–9.

37. Tremaine WH. Dental endoscopy in the horse. Clin Tech Equine Pract 2005;4:181–7.

38. Dixon PM, Dacre I, Dacre K, et al. Standing oral extraction of cheek teeth in 100 horses (1998–2003). Equine Vet J 2005;37:105–12.

39. Lundstrom T. Orthograde endodontic treatment of equine teeth with periapical disease: long-term follow up. Proceedings of 52nd BEVA congress. Birmingham: Equine Veterinary Journal Limited; 2012. p. 105–8.

40. Simhofer H, Stoian C, Zetner K. A long-term study of apicectomy and endodontic treatment of apically infected cheek teeth in 12 horses. Vet J 2008;178:411–8.

41. Tremaine WH, Schumacher J. Exodontia. In: Easley J, Dixon PM, Schumacher JS, editors. Equine dentistry. 3rd edition. Philadelphia: Elsevier; 2010. Chapter 20. p. 319–32.

42. Tremaine WH. Local analgesic techniques for the equine head. Equine Vet Educ 2007;19(9):495–503.

43. O'Connor. Operations. In: Dollar's veterinary surgery. 3rd edition. London: Bailliere Tindal and Cox; 1942. p. 250–61.

44. Guard WF. Equine operations in surgical principals and techniques. Columbus (OH): 1951. p. 78–89.

45. Caldwell FJ, Easley J. Self-inflicted lingual trauma secondary to inferior alveolar nerve block in 3 horses. Equine Vet Educ 2012;24:119–23.

46. Quinn G, Lane JG, Tremaine WH. Supernumerary cheek teeth (n = 24): clinical features, diagnosis, treatment and outcome in 15 horses. Equine Vet J 2005;37:505–9.

47. Vlaminck L. Radiographic evaluation of tooth drift after cheek tooth extraction and insertion of an intra-alveolar prosthesis in ponies. Vet J 2008;175:249–58.

48. Townsend NB. Evaluation of the long-term oral consequences of equine exodontia in 50 horses. Vet J 2008;178:419–24.

49. Ramzan PH, Dallas RS, Palmer L. Extraction of fractured cheek teeth under oral endoscopic guidance in standing horses. Vet Surg 2011;40:586–9.

50. Marzok M. Surgical repulsion of maxillary check teeth using C-arm fluoroscopy in horses. San Antonio: Online J Vet Res 2009;13:1–18.
51. Coomer R, Fowke G, McKane S. Repulsion of maxillary and mandibular cheek teeth in standing horses. Vet Surg 2011;40:590–5.
52. O'Neill H, Boussaw B, Bladon BM, et al. Extraction of cheek teeth using a lateral buccotomy approach in 114 horses (1999–2009). Equine Vet J 2011;43:348–53.
53. Tremaine WH, McCluskie L. Removal of 11 incompletely erupted, impacted cheek teeth in 10 horses using a dental alveolar transcortical osteotomy and buccotomy approach. Vet Surg 2012;39:884–90.
54. Vogt K. Lehrbuch der Zahnheilkunde. Germany: Schattauer; 2011. p. 209–13.
55. Stoll M. How to perform a buccal approach for different dental procedures. Proc of Am Assoc Eq Prtns. 64. 2007. p. 507–11.
56. Bienert A, Bartmann CP, Verspohl J, et al. Bacteriological findings for endodontical and apical molar dental diseases in the horse. Dtsch Tierarztl Wochenschr 2003;110(9):358–61 [in German].
57. Steenkamp G, Olivier-Carstens A, van Heerden WF, et al. In vitro comparison of three materials as apical sealants of equine premolar and molar teeth. Equine Vet J 2005;37:133–6.
58. Galloway S, Galloway M. Dental materials. In: Easley KJ, Dixon PM, Schumacher JS, editors. Equine dentistry. 3rd edition. Philadelphia: Elsevier; 2010. p. 345–65.
59. Casey MB, Pearson GR, Perkins JD, et al. Gross CT and histopathological findings in mandibular cheek teeth extracted from horses with clinical signs of pulpitis. Proceedings of the 50th BEVA Congress. Liverpool: Equine Veterinary Journal Limited; 2011. p. 179.
60. Schramme MC, Boswell JC, Robinson J, et al. Endodontic therapy for periapical infection of cheek teeth in 19 horses. In: Proceedings Am Assoc. Eq. Prtnrs. 46. 2000. p. 113–6.
61. Lungstrom T. Orthograde endodontic treatment of equine teeth with periapical disease: long-term follow-up. Proceedings of the 52nd Congress of the British Equine Veterinary Association. Birmingham: Equine Veterinary Journal Limited; 2012. p. 105–17.
62. Carmalt J, Barber S. Periapical curettage: an alternative surgical approach to infected mandibular cheek teeth in horses. Vet Surg 2004;33(3):267–71.

New Ways to Diagnose and Treat Equine Dental-Related Sinus Disease

Jeremiah T. Easley, DVM[a],*, David E. Freeman, MVB, PhD[b]

KEYWORDS

- Dental • Sinus • Equine • Disease • Surgery

KEY POINTS

- Equine dental disease is becoming increasingly important in veterinary medicine.
- Most secondary sinus disorders are related to dental disease.
- Diagnosis and treatment of dental-related sinus disease is challenging with a high risk of complications.
- In-depth understanding of anatomic structures and diagnostic and therapeutic options is vital to successful outcomes in dental-related sinus disorders.

INTRODUCTION

Advances in the diagnosis and treatment of dental-related sinus disease over the past 10 to 15 years are the result of a better understanding of primary dental disease and the role of equine cheek teeth and paranasal sinus anatomy in treatment. This has been accomplished by detailed cadaveric studies and advanced three-dimensional imaging. From a surgeon's perspective, a thorough understanding of anatomy is the cornerstone of an accurate diagnosis and successful treatment. Diagnostic imaging modalities (radiography, scintigraphy, computed tomography, and magnetic resonance imaging) are discussed in depth in other articles in this issue. This article focuses on the use of endoscopy and surgical techniques of the paranasal sinuses to evaluate, diagnose, and treat dental-related sinus disease.

DENTAL AND PARANASAL SINUS ANATOMY

Accurate diagnosis and treatment of dental-related sinus diseases in horses is challenging because of the complicated anatomy and difficulty of access to the oral cavity

[a] Surgical Research Laboratory, Department of Clinical Sciences, Colorado State University, 300 West Drake Street, Fort Collins, CO 80523, USA; [b] College of Veterinary Medicine, Department of Clinical Sciences, University of Florida, PO Box 100136, 2015 Southwest 16th Avenue, Gainesville, FL 32608–0136, USA
* Corresponding author.
E-mail address: jeremiah.easley@colostate.edu

Vet Clin Equine 29 (2013) 467–485
http://dx.doi.org/10.1016/j.cveq.2013.04.003
0749-0739/13/$ – see front matter Published by Elsevier Inc.

vetequine.theclinics.com

and the paranasal sinuses. Most maxillary sinuses in young horses younger than 5 years of age are filled with the tooth roots of the caudal four cheek teeth (fourth premolar and first, second, and third molars or 108–111 and 208–211). The apical portion of the hypsodont tooth develops a root for several years after eruption. These teeth change position in the sinuses as the skull grows and the deciduous teeth are shed and permanent teeth develop. In the mature horse, the fourth premolar and first molar alveoli lie within the rostral maxillary sinus (RMS), whereas the second and third molar alveoli lie within the caudal maxillary sinus. Cheek teeth reserve crowns become shorter as the horse ages, filling less of the rostral and caudal maxillary sinus (CMS) while at the same time the maxillary sinus enlarges. After 5 to 9 years of age, the roots of the fourth premolar no longer communicate with the RMS and instead, the reserve crown, roots, and alveolar structures of the fourth premolar form the rostral wall of the maxillary sinus.[1] The anatomic difference between young (<5 years) and older horses (>6 years) shows that maxillary trephination and sinusotomy, although diagnostically beneficial, are not without risk to the dental apices. An accurate understanding of anatomic variations between ages of horses can help rule out sinus disease secondary to disorders affecting the dental apices.

Most dental-related sinus disease is a result of infection within dental apices either primary in origin or secondary to other dental abnormalities, including trauma, idiopathic dental fractures, supernumerary cheek teeth, dental overgrowths, and diastemata.[2] Equine mandibular cheek teeth have two roots, except for the third molar, which has three; the maxillary cheek teeth have three roots, two of which are buccal and a larger, more complex palatal root.[3] In the maxillary arcade, there are 9 to 12 dental roots on each side that have the potential to become damaged or diseased from infection or surgery leading to secondary sinusitis.

The equine paranasal sinuses are complex and consist of seven pairs: (1) frontal, (2) dorsal conchal, (3) CMS, (4) RMS, (5) ventral conchal sinus (VCS), (6) ethmoidal sinus, and (7) sphenoplalatine sinus (**Fig. 1**). The frontal and dorsal conchal sinus is often referred to as one sinus, the conchofrontal sinus (CFS). The CFS, CMS, ethmoidal, and sphenopalatine sinuses communicate, and the RMS and VCS communicate with each other. Delicate scrolls of bone known as conchae (or turbinates) are attached laterally in the nasal cavity and contain the conchal sinuses. The right and left CFS are separated by a complete septum so there is no communication between them. A bony septum divides the maxillary sinus into rostral and caudal compartments. The septum traverses obliquely across the fourth and fifth cheek teeth (109, 110, and 209, 210) and the ventral conchal bulla (VCB) forms the dorsal aspect of this septum (**Fig. 2**). The infraorbital canal is the separation between the RMS and VCS. These two sinuses communicate, but drainage from the VCS must occur over the infraorbital canal by the conchomaxillary opening and into the RMS before drainage by the nasomaxillary opening (NMO) of the RMS. This indirect drainage along with numerous diverticulae of the VCS predisposes it to develop accumulations of inspissated pus and chronic infection.[4,5] This anatomic variation becomes important when treating difficult cases of chronic sinusitis.[5]

The NMO is the common exit of separate ostia draining the RMS and CMS, respectively (see **Fig. 1**). The CFS, ethmoidal, and sphenopalatine sinuses all drain into the CMS before exiting the CMS sinonasal ostia and similar drainage occurs from VCS into RMS before exiting the RMS sinonasal ostia.[6] There is a large opening in the caudomedial aspect of the CMS opening into the sphenopalatine sinus, a small medial opening into the middle conchal sinus and a large dorsally located opening into the frontal sinus, termed the frontomaxillary opening. Because of thin dorsal and lateral walls of the sphenopalatine sinus and a close relationship with the brain, optic

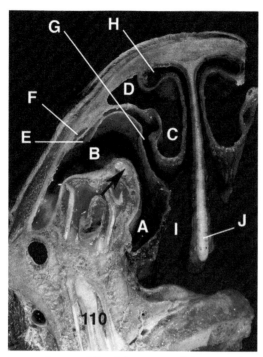

Fig. 1. Cadaveric transverse image of the right paranasal sinuses and nasal passage through the second maxillary molar (110) as viewed from the front. A, ventral conchal sinus; B, rostral maxillary sinus; C, dorsal conchal sinus; D, frontal sinus; E, opening of rostral maxillary sinus to the middle meatus; F, nasolacrimal duct; G, middle meatus; H, dorsal meatus; I, ventral meatus; J, nasal septum. *Black arrow* points to the infraorbital canal. (*Adapted from* Freeman DE. Sinus disease. Vet Clin North Am Equine Pract 2003;19:209–43; with permission.)

chiasma, pituitary gland, olfactory bulb, cranial nerves II (optic), III (oculomotor), IV (abducens), V (trigeminal), and VI (trochlear), and major blood vessels, disease within this sinus can lead to clinical signs referable to these structures, such as blindness or trigeminal dysfunction.[4,7,8] The NMO, located in the middle meatus, drains mucus secretions from the sinuses by mucociliary clearance toward the pharynx where it is eventually swallowed (see **Fig. 1**). The paranasal sinuses are lined with respiratory mucous membrane primarily composed of pseudostratified columnar epithelium and goblet cells. Any inflammation within the sinonasal mucosa can disrupt mucociliary clearance and narrow drainage pathways, leading to excessive sinus secretions and nasal discharge.[4] The blood supply to the paranasal sinuses is extensive and consists of blood flow from the ethmoidal artery (frontal sinus), branches of the sphenopalatine artery (maxillary sinus), and anastamosis of the internal and external ethmoidal arteries to form the aterial ethmoidal rete (ethmoidal sinus).[9]

The infraorbital canal and nasolacrimal duct are closely related to the paranasal sinuses (see **Fig. 1**). It is important to understand the anatomic location of both structures and realize that disease within the dental apices and sinuses can involve the infraorbital canal or nasolacrimal duct.[10,11] The nasolacrimal apparatus includes the lacrimal canaliculi, lacrimal sac, and the nasolacrimal duct. The duct functions as a passage for drainage of tears from the medial canthus of the eye. It courses rostrally from the lacrimal sac beneath the lacrimal, zygomatic, and maxillary bones within the

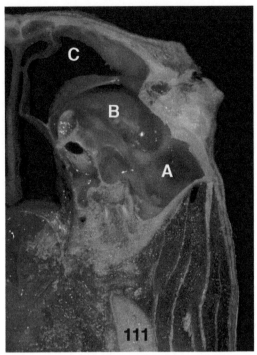

Fig. 2. Cadaveric transverse cross-sectional image of the right paranasal sinuses and nasal passage through the third maxillary molar (111) as viewed from the back. A, caudal maxillary sinus; B, ventral conchal bulla; C, conchofrontal sinus.

boney lacrimal canal and exits at the level of the conchal crest.[10,12] Whereas the nasolacrimal duct courses along the peripheral edge of the paranasal sinuses, the infraorbital canal courses within the paranasal sinus cavities. It is a thin-boned cylindrical structure containing the infraorbital nerve and separates the RMS from the VCS (see **Fig. 1**). In young horses it is located immediately dorsal to the dental apices.

CLINICAL DIAGNOSIS OF DENTAL-RELATED SINUS DISEASE

Sinusitis can be primary in origin or secondary to dental disease, mycotic infections, oromaxillary fistula formation, sinus cysts, sinus neoplasia, progressive ethmoid hematomas, or trauma. Primary sinusitis is a bacterial infection that develops without any apparent predisposing cause, such as the aforementioned diseases.[4,13]

Dental-related sinus disease is the most common cause of secondary sinusitis and arises from bacteria spreading from one or more infected dental apices on any of the caudal four maxillary cheek teeth (08, 09, 10, and 11) through the alveolar bone. The fourth premolar is a less likely cause of secondary sinusitis in horses older than 5 years of age.[1] Unilateral nasal discharge is the most common clinical sign in dental-related sinus disease (**Fig. 3**). Bilateral nasal discharge is uncommon with unilateral sinusitis, because the nasal septum prevents access of drainage to the contralateral nasal passage. Bilateral discharge is more common with diseases of the guttural pouches, lungs, and pharynx. If secondary sinusitis is caused by dental infection, the discharge is typically malodorous because of anaerobic bacterial infection. Malodorous nasal discharge can help to differentiate dental disease from other causes of secondary sinusitis in certain cases.

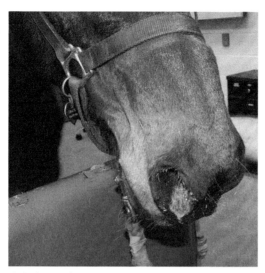

Fig. 3. Purulent nasal discharge from the right nostril in a horse with a periapical infection.

Severe secondary sinusitis of dental origin can cause facial distortion and even impinge on the medial walls of the conchae, pushing the conchae into the nasal passage and even displacing the nasal septum. In such cases, the resulting nasal occlusion can force some of the sinus drainage around the nasal septum and out the contralateral nostril. Although possible in cases of apical infection, distortion of boney structures and even exopthalmos is more common in cases of sinus neoplasia or cysts. The close anatomic location of the nasolacrimal duct can lead to epiphora because of compression or even erosion through the osseous wall.[10]

Space-occupying material within the sinus compartments can be diagnosed with the use of percussion with some reliability. Neoplasia of dental origin or inspissated pus cannot be differentiated from other space-occupying material by percussion alone without additional diagnostic tools. To percuss the sinuses, pointedly tap the overlying bones with the fingertips. With the horse's mouth open, the percussive sound can be heard more easily. After percussion of the affected side, the corresponding normal sinus should be percussed for comparison. If space-occupying material is present within the sinuses, the percussive sound is duller compared with the normal compartment. Along with percussion, a detailed oral examination, preferably with the aid of a dental mirror or oral endoscopic camera, should be performed before continuing with any imaging or diagnostic surgery. Blood count and blood chemistry can be performed, but changes in peripheral blood as a result of paranasal sinus disease are uncommon.

Ancillary diagnostic techniques for the evaluation of the sinus compartments and apices of the maxillary cheek teeth are extensive and include a detailed physical and oral examination, nasal endoscopy, sinoscopy, radiography, scintigraphy, computed tomography, magnetic resonance imaging, and microbiologic and histologic examinations in some cases.

Dixon and colleagues[14] reviewed the diagnostic findings of more than 200 cases with paranasal sinus disease. Twenty percent of cases were diagnosed with dental disease (**Tables 1** and **2**). Eighty-seven percent of the cases with dental-related paranasal sinus disease had exudate in the sinonasal ostium, 15% had a sinonasal fistula, and 28% had an open VCB diagnosed by nasal endoscopy or sinoscopy.

Table 1
Endoscopic, sinoscopic, and radiographic findings in 40 cases of primary dental-related sinus disease

Type of Sinus Disease Present	Dental N = 40
Exudate at sinonasal ostium	33 (87%)
Sinonasal fistula	6 (15%)
Sinoscopy performed	29 (73%)
Open VCB sinoscopically	11 (28%)
Radiography performed	40 (100%)
Intrasinus fluid lines	16 (40%)
Intrasinus radio-opacity	22 (55%)
Radiographic apical changes	34 (85%)
Radiographic sinus wall bone changes	1 (3%)

Abbreviation: VCB, ventral conchal bulla.
Data from Dixon PM, Parkin TD, Collins N, et al. Equine paranasal sinus disease: a long-term study of 200 cases (1997–2009): ancillary diagnostic findings and involvement of the various sinus compartments. Equine Vet J 2012;44:272–6.

Forty-percent of cases had an intrasinus fluid line, 55% with intrasinus radio-opacity, 85% with apical changes, and 3% with bone changes. All these changes were diagnosed by radiography.[14] Contrary to expectations, radiographic changes of the dental apices were not specific to dental sinusitis. Twenty-nine percent of chronic primary sinusitis cases and 16% of subacute primary simusitis cases also had radiographic changes to dental apices.[14]

Nasal Endoscopy

Endoscopy of the nasal cavity can be very helpful in the diagnosis of dental-related paranasal sinus disease. A flexible endoscope is passed through the ventral meatus to evaluate the nasal septum, the ethmoturbinates, ventral, middle, and dorsal meati.

Table 2
Proportions of individual sinus compartments affected in primary dental-related sinus disease

Type of Sinus Disease	Dental N = 40
CFS	12 (30%)
CMS	29 (73%)
RMS	31 (78%)
VCS	30 (75%)
SPS/ES	2 (5%)
CFS inspissated pus	1 (3%)
CMS inspissated pus	8 (20%)
RMS inspissated pus	6 (15%)
VCS inspissated pus	8 (20%)
SPS/ES inspissated pus	2 (5%)

Abbreviations: CFS, conchofrontal sinus; CMS, caudal maxillary sinus; ES, ethnmoidal sinus; RMS, rostral maxillary sinus; SPS, sphenopalatine sinus; VCS, ventral conchal sinus.
Data from Dixon PM, Parkin TD, Collins N, et al. Equine paranasal sinus disease: a long-term study of 200 cases (1997–2009): ancillary diagnostic findings and involvement of the various sinus compartments. Equine Vet J 2012;44:272–6.

The NMO or ostia is the shared unilateral exit for drainage of fluid (pus, blood, and so forth) from the CMS and RMS into the middle meatus and cannot be seen with the endoscope.[6] The most common clinical sign noted on nasal endoscopy in cases of dental-related sinus disease is pus from the NMO draining into the middle meatus and then into the ventral meatus (**Fig. 4**). In cases of large space-occupying lesions (neoplasia, granulomas, sinus cysts), the turbinates overlying the ventral and dorsal conchal sinus can be distorted, eroded (**Fig. 5**), or displaced axially preventing passage of the endoscope to the caudal most aspect of the nasal cavity. Portions of soft tissue masses can also be seen protruding through the NMO.

Recently, two studies have been published discussing nasal endoscopic access to the paranasal sinuses for improved diagnosis and treatment. Morello and Parente[15] describe the technique of laser vaporization of the dorsal turbinate to access and evaluate the paranasal sinuses. The procedure uses a flexible endoscope and a diode laser with a contact probe and a custom built laser introducer rod. Under endoscopic guidance, a site on the caudomedial aspect of the turbinate overlying the dorsal conchal sinus is identified and a stoma is created by contact laser vaporization. After stoma creation for passage of a flexible endoscope, the CFS and CMS, including the apical aspects of the alveoli of the caudal cheek teeth, could be evaluated. This study concluded that the stoma lasts at least 5 weeks and can be used as a successful alternative to more invasive sinusotomy techniques, with fewer complications and improved cosmetic results. Such an approach might also be useful in the treatment of sinusitis cases with poor or absent ventral drainage. The stoma location would be guided by other diagnostic or treatment goals. However, in cases of dental apical infection or inspissated pus within the VCS, a sinoscopy performed directly over the diseased apices or through the frontal sinus is likely to be more diagnostic and easier to perform.

Bell and colleagues[6] described the use of an endoscope-guided balloon sinuplasty through the NMO. Sinusitis can cause obstruction of drainage from the paranasal sinus system by narrowing of the NMO from inflammation of the sinus mucosa and accumulation of purulent material within the sinuses. Under endoscopic guidance, a balloon

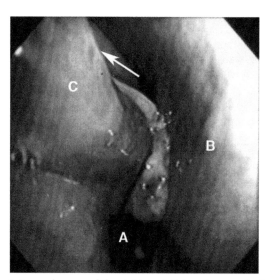

Fig. 4. An endoscopic image by way of the right nostril showing purulent drainage from the middle meatus (*arrow*). A, ventral meatus; B, nasal septum; C, medial wall of the ventral conchal sinus.

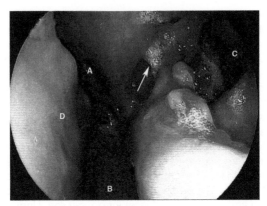

Fig. 5. An endoscopic image by way of the left nostril showing erosion through the medial wall of the ventral conchal sinus. A, ethomoid turbinates; B, pharynx; C, ventral conchal sinus; D, nasal septum. *Arrow* points to middle meatus toward nasomaxillary opening.

catheter was passed into the NMO and inflated to 6 atm for 30 seconds, three times, thereby dilating the NMO and improving drainage rates from the CMS. In most cases, surgical fenestration of the dorsal turbinate and NMO during flap sinusotomy is used to improve drainage. Improved drainage by fenestration along with antibiotic administration and lavage was shown to have an 84% success in cases of primary sinusitis.[16] The authors have successfully treated or improved paranasal sinusitis with fenestration, but do not have experience with the balloon dilation technique. This technique dilates the "natural" drainage opening without requiring fenestration of normal turbinate tissue. The technique is less invasive and has a decreased complication rate, is less expensive, and reestablishes drainage by the natural drainage angle compared with the surgical fenestration technique. Although this technique is not described as a diagnostic tool, there is potential for dilation of the NMO to allow passage of a narrow flexible endoscope into the CMS and CFS for evaluation in cases of sinus disease. Drainage through an enlarged natural orifice is preferred to creation of a second drainage opening by fenestration, because the latter alters passage of mucus in human patients and does not does not actually improve drainage time.[17]

Sinoscopy

Sinoscopy can be performed as a diagnostic aid following skull radiography and nasal endoscopy, or used as a treatment option for lavage of the sinus compartments. It can aid in the diagnosis of sinus-related diseases including primary sinusitis, dental-related sinusitis, sinus cysts, and progressive ethmoid hematomas.[13] With standing sedation and local anesthesia, a small trephine hole can be placed in the conchofrontal or rostral or CMS compartment for direct evaluation by a rigid or flexible endoscope. Traditionally, the following portals have been used: for the CMS, 2 cm rostral and 2 cm ventral to the medial canthus of the eye; for the RMS, 50% of the distance from the rostral end of the facial crest to the level of the medial canthus and 1 cm ventral to a line joining the infraorbital foramen and the medial canthus; and the frontal sinus, 60% of the distance from midline toward the medial canthus and 0.5 cm caudal to the medial canthus (**Fig. 6**).[8,18] More recently, Barakzai and colleagues[1] described an approach to the maxillary sinus located 40% of the distance from the rostral end of the facial crest to the level of the medial canthus of the eye, and 1 cm ventral to a line

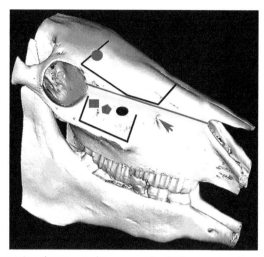

Fig. 6. A three-dimensional computed tomography (CT) reconstruction of the equine skull illustrating trephine and sinus bone flap locations. Red circle, trephine location for frontal sinus; red square, trephine location for caudal maxillary sinus; red pentagon, caudal trephine location for rostral maxillary sinus; black circle, rostral trephine location for rostral maxillary sinus[1]; red straight line, location of nasolacrimal duct; red arrow, infraorbital foramen; blue connected lines, approach to sinuses through a maxillary bone flap; black connected lines, approach to the sinuses through a frontonasal sinus flap.

joining the infraorbital foramen and medial canthus (see **Fig. 6**). The traditional approach described by Ruggles and colleagues[18] allowed for inadvertent trephination of the CMS in 33% of cadavers compared with 98% accuracy using the approach described by Barakzai and colleagues.[1] However, a more rostral approach carries a greater risk of encountering or damaging a tooth root, and it is advised that this approach be used with the assistance of radiographic guidance in horses less than or equal to 5 years of age.[1]

Sinoscopy carries great value in aiding diagnosis and providing for an opportunity to treat through a minimally invasive surgical approach. Sinoscopy provides a direct view of numerous sinus compartments. However, the ability to evaluate and diagnose the entire extent of sinus disease is limited in comparison with three-dimensional imaging, such as computed tomographic and magnetic resonance imaging. Sinoscopy also enables sample collection for histologic examination and microbial culture.[19] One study claims 69% resolution of paranasal sinus disease after sinoscopy and lavage.[19] Dental-related sinus disease can affect a single sinus or all sinus compartments. However, disease of the dental apices directly affects the RMS, CMS, or VCS. Recently, Perkins and colleagues[20] compared sinoscopic approaches to develop a reliable technique for sinoscopic examination of the ventral conchal and RMS of horses. Using 40 equine cadaver heads, six different sinoscopic approaches were evaluated for their ability to provide endoscopic access to the VCS and RMS. Success in examining the VCS and RMS with each approach are outlined in **Table 3**. This study showed that trephination of the CFS along with fenestration of the VCB (frontal VCB approach) provided adequate access to the rostral and caudal aspects of the RMS and VCS for diagnosis and therapy. It is recommended that a second trephine portal be made into the CMS if the VCB cannot be adequately observed through the frontal VCB approach alone.[20] Examination of the VCS is very important in dental-related sinus

Table 3
Success rates for identification of intrasinus structures within the ventral conchal sinus and rostral maxillary sinus

Approach	Entire Ventral Conchal Sinus	Entire Rostral Maxillary Sinus
Frontal VCB	24 (60%)	29 (73%)
Caudal VCB	16 (40%)	16 (40%)
Light RMS	12 (30%)	26 (60%)
Rostral RMS	0 (0%)	16 (40%)
Caudal RMS	5 (13%)	11 (28%)
Combined VCB	29 (73%)	35 (88%)

Data from Perkins JD, Windley Z, Dixon PM, et al. Sinoscopic treatment of rostral maxillary and ventral conchal sinusitis in 60 horses. Vet Surg 2009;38:613–9.

disease because it is the frequent site of accumulation of inspissated exudate, which is difficult to remove and treat successfully.[21,22] Perkins and colleagues[20] performed a follow-up study using the CFS trephination approach coupled with fenestration of the VCB (frontal VCB approach) to evaluate treatment of RMS and VCS sinusitis in 60 horses. The CFS approach with fenestration of the VCB provided adequate observation of the RMS and VCS in 88% of horses. This approach was diagnostically useful in 82% of horses with primary sinusitis and allowed for observations of neoplasia, sinus cysts, and progressive ethmoid hematomas. However, other diagnostic modalities were typically required for confirmation of diagnosis of dental-related sinusitis. Of the 60 cases treated in this study by CFS trephination, with fenestration of the VCB and sinoscopic lavage, 43% had complete resolution of sinusitis. Fifteen (25%) of the 60 horses had apical infections resulting in secondary sinusitis, and sinoscopy was helpful for diagnosis in only 20% and for treatment in 0% of these horses. Sinoscopic lavage as a sole treatment of dental-related sinus disease is never successful without removing the primary cause of the disease (dental extraction, repair of fistula, and so forth). However, sinoscopy can be a very useful minimally invasive adjunct therapy to tooth removal or fistula repair in dental-related sinus disease. It can be performed with very little morbidity to the patient and should be considered as a first-line treatment option before sinusotomy.

From the authors' experience, sinoscopy is very helpful as a diagnostic tool, but has limited value for treatment. When evaluating the sinus compartments for abnormalities or foreign objects (**Fig. 7**), sinoscopy is an excellent choice because there is minimal bleeding to obstruct the view. The authors have found sinoscopy especially helpful in cases where a secondary sinusitis is caused by foreign material, such as feed or devitalized, necrotic tissue localized to a specific area of the sinuses (see **Fig. 7**). A pair of endoscopic grasping forceps or Ferris-Smith rongeurs can help tremendously with removal of small foreign objects. In the case of dental-related sinus disease, inspissated pus can commonly be involved. The authors have found this to be especially true in older horses with chronic sinusitis that have been treated with long-term systemic antibiotics without complete resolution. Inspissated pus in the paranasal sinuses and most commonly the VCS is difficult to completely remove and resolve. Perkins and colleagues[20] describe the successful removal and resolution of inspissated pus in 44% of cases with primary sinusitis after endoscopic fenestration of the VCB, followed by endoscope-guided removal of inspissated exudate, and sinus lavage, with or without systemic antibiotics. However, the authors have found a large

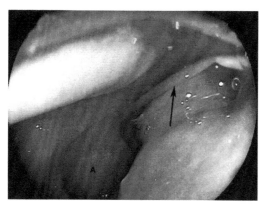

Fig. 7. A sinoscopic image through a right-sided frontal trephination in a horse with a large orosinus fistula after tooth repulsion of the first right maxillary molar (210). A, ventral conchal bulla. *Arrow* points to hay in the caudal maxillary sinus.

standing frontonasal sinus flap is likely to provide quicker resolution of clinical signs. A large frontonasal sinus flap improves access to all sinus compartments to allow aggressive removal of all inspissated exudate, fenestration of the VCB, and creation of a new nasosinus osteum for increased sinus drainage. Contrary to common belief, a large frontonasal sinus flap provides superior access to all sinus compartments, including RMS and CMS for treatment, compared with a maxillary sinus flap.

TREATMENT OF DENTAL-RELATED SINUSITIS

Dental-related sinusitis is typically the result of another disease, most commonly infection of dental apices. However, oromaxillary fistulas can also lead to secondary sinusitis as a result of severe periodontal disease or tooth removal with incomplete healing of the alveolar socket. In both scenarios, the sinus compartments are grossly contaminated with multiple bacterial organisms and even feed material. To resolve the secondary sinusitis, the initial disease must be resolved. In the case of dental apical infections, the diseased tooth must be removed by oral extraction, lateral buccotomy, tooth repulsion, or a minimally invasive extraction method through a buccal approach.[23–26] Endodontic therapy has been reported, but outcomes have been disappointing with long-term success rates ranging from 44% to 81%.[24] Carmalt and Barber[27] describe an alternative surgical approach to infected mandibular cheek teeth by periapical curettage. To the authors' knowledge, this technique has not been described in maxillary teeth through a sinus approach. However, the apical curettage method in mandibular teeth typically only spares the tooth and clears up signs of dental-related osteitis for the short term. The tooth needs to be removed eventually. Overall, complete removal of the diseased tooth is the preferred first step in resolving dental-related sinus disease.

Tooth Repulsion

To fit with the context of this article on sinus disease, only tooth repulsion is discussed. After the entire tooth is removed by any extraction method, it is important to evaluate the health of the alveolar socket. Tooth repulsion creates a communication from the RMS or CMS to the oral cavity and carries an increased complication rate when compared with oral extraction or lateral buccotomy. Tooth repulsion in older horses is especially at risk to form oromaxillary fistulas because the socket is shallow and difficult to protect with packing, so that healing does not proceed rapidly. Tooth repulsion has a 32% to 70% rate of serious complications including infection of a second tooth, bone sequestration, chronic sinusitis, draining tracts, retained dental packing, feed impaction of the alveolus or sinus, suture line dehiscence, or sloughed skin flaps.[2,16,25] Many surgeons have the common misconception that tooth repulsion is a quicker technique than extraction for tooth removal. This is true of the time required to remove the tooth, but does not account for any of the complications mentioned previously. The time and money required dealing with those complications far outweigh the initial decrease in surgical time compared with an oral extraction or lateral buccotomy approach. Therefore, a maxillary or frontonasal approach should be reserved strictly for teeth that have no exposed crown beyond the buccal surface and cannot be removed by any other method. However, Coomer and colleagues[28] reported repulsion of mandibular and maxillary teeth in 18 standing, sedated horses. Oral extraction was attempted in all cases in this study before repulsion. This study nicely describes the appropriate technique and emphasizes the importance of loosening the tooth beforehand by an oral approach and use of radiography to facilitate instrument positioning. Loosening of the affected tooth requires far less effort than extraction and reduces the risk of damage to surrounding alveolar structures during the repelling process. Twenty cheek teeth were successfully removed in 18 horses with 13 horses (72%) having involvement of teeth within the maxillary arcade. The median number of intraoperative radiographs was six. In the authors' opinion intraoperative radiographs are imperative to allow accurate placement of the punch, thereby reducing trauma to surrounding alveolar structures or apices of unaffected teeth. Maintaining correct placement of the dental punch on the appropriate tooth root after each impact is difficult. The third to sixth cheek teeth have considerable caudal curvature in horses younger than 8 years of age and radiographic assessment of the location of the dental punch with regards to the apex of the tooth is vital to proper repulsion along the normal eruption pathway of the tooth. Of the horses with maxillary involvement undergoing standing tooth repulsion, 6 of 10 horses had recurrent sinusitis requiring follow-up medical or surgical treatment.[28] Complications after standing repulsion were comparatively minor in contrast to repulsion under general anesthesia and were related to ongoing infection from the site rather than iatrogenic collateral trauma. The decreased complication rate with standing repulsion emphasizes the importance of prior loosening of the periodontal attachments before attempting repulsion standing or under general anesthesia. The authors do not recommend performing tooth repulsion in the standing horse if the tooth cannot be loosened beforehand. Prior oral loosening of teeth may not be required for repulsion under general anesthesia, but should be performed if possible to minimize complications as a result of trauma to surrounding structures.

The authors realize that tooth repulsion may be inevitable when the tooth has fractured and crown exposure is reduced or if the apical portion of tooth root has undergone chronic remodeling. Therefore, repulsion should be reserved for appropriate clinical cases and owners should be informed of the complications that can result from this technique.

Surgery of the Paranasal Sinuses

Sinus trephination is discussed in detail elsewhere in this issue as a surgical technique for diagnosis and treatment of sinusitis in the horse. It is minimally invasive compared with the larger bone flaps. However, a frontonasal or maxillary bone flap improves access to all paranasal sinus compartments, which can facilitate treatment of secondary sinusitis. Sinusotomy by a bone flap is not commonly performed for apical tooth infections that cause secondary sinusitis. However, removal of sinus-related tumors, foreign bodies, or inspissated pus, or repair of oroantral fistulas often requires a large frontonasal or maxillary bone flap.

Frontonasal flap

In the authors' opinion, the frontonasal flap approach is the ideal approach to the paranasal sinuses. It provides access to the conchofrontal and CMS and, by additional steps, the rostral maxillary and VCS.[29] The size of the flap can vary and depends on the lesion requiring the flap. This approach to the paranasal sinuses can be used for removal of the fourth, fifth, and sixth cheek teeth, large-volume lavage, and removal of inspissated pus, and removal of large soft tissue and dental-related tumors. This procedure can be performed under standing sedation or general anesthesia and the choice should be based on patient safety and surgeon comfort.

The uncut or hinged, medial edge of the frontonasal bone flap is the dorsal midline. The rostral and caudal edges are at right angles to the dorsal midline. The caudal edge is midway between the supraorbital foramen and the medial canthus, and the lateral edge starts 2 to 2.5 cm medial to the medial canthus of the eye, then runs dorsal to a line from the medial canthus to the nasoincisive notch. The point at which the nasal bones become parallel is the location of the rostral edge. The rostral edge should end before this point to avoid entering the nasal cavity, or severe hemorrhage and a permanent nasal blemish can result. This creates a flap of approximately 10 cm from caudal to cranial (see **Fig. 6**).[8,29] It is important to make the flap as large as possible without involving the nasolacrimal duct. A good way to locate the nasolacrimal duct is to draw a line from the medial canthus of the eye to the nasoincisive notch (see **Fig. 6**).

An incision through the skin and periosteum is made larger than the proposed bone flap to overlap the bone incision by 5 mm of the overlying soft tissues. The corners of the incision are curved. The periosteum is minimally elevated toward the proposed bone cut exposing a 3- to 5-mm wide strip of bone. It is important to preserve as much soft tissue attachment as possible to the bone flap to prevent bone necrosis. The blood supply to the skin and periosteum in the frontal region primarily comes from a branch of the maxillary artery called the rostral deep temporal artery. It emerges from the alar canal through the temporal foramen, and ascends in the rostral part of the temporal fossa to supply blood to the temporalis muscle and gives off branches to the frontal region.[30,31] The caudal incision disrupts branches of the rostral deep temporal artery because they extend from caudal to rostral, making preservation of soft tissue attachments vital to the underlying bone health.

After the bone flap is cut along its edges, an osteotome is inserted progressively under the cut edges around the flap to test the completeness of the bone cuts. An osteotome is then inserted along the inner surface of the flap at its rostromedial end to cut any trabecular attachments and to partly separate the underside of the flap from the reflection of the dorsal nasal concha. Two osteotomes are inserted under the lateral edge of the flap and close to its underside to start to pry it into an open position. After the lateral edge is open sufficiently, the surgeon places the index finger of each hand under the lateral edge and pries the flap upward. Downward pressure from the thumbs on the dorsal midline as the flap is pried upward forces the flap to fracture on this medial edge and also allows the surgeon to sense that the flap is free enough to fracture during this step. If excessive resistance to fracture is encountered, then additional cuts to the underside are required.

Standing flap

A maxillary nerve block can be used for a frontonasal bone flap in the standing position, although this might not anesthetize the entire surgical region and is not required.[21,30] However, local anesthesia of the incision site and sinus mucosa is important. The authors perform a line block along the rostral, caudal, and lateral edges of the sinus flap with 20 to 35 mL of either 2% lidocaine or 2% mepivicaine. After the three-sided skin incision is made, a 2- to 3-mm diameter Steinman pin is used to create a small hole in the upper axial corner to accommodate a 14-gauge needle so that another 35 mL of lidocaine or mepivicaine can be infused into the paranasal sinuses. Depending on the lesion, local anesthesia may or may not drain from the corresponding nostril. Along with local anesthesia, the authors recommend a detomidine constant-rate infusion (CRI) with or without the addition of butorphanol. The CRI protocol is as follows: (1) administer an intravenous bolus of detomidine, 0.02 µg/kg, and butorphanol, 0.02 mg/kg; (2) followed by a CRI of 0.02 mg/kg/h detomidine and 0.024 mg/kg/h butorphanol. For a 450-kg horse, add 15 mg of butorphanol and 12.5 mg of detomidine to a 500-mL bag of sterile saline and infuse at a rate of one drop per second (using a 10 drops per milliliter drip set) depending on the sedation level of the horse. The solution typically lasts approximately 90 minutes. A CRI provides a consistent level of sedation for the entirety of the surgery, minimizes movement from the patient, and is financially comparable with using multiple intravenous injections. The CRI can be placed in a fluid pump for increased accuracy of drug delivery, although a carefully monitored drip set provides excellent sedation and analgesia.

The decision to perform a frontonasal sinus flap in the standing position versus under general anesthesia should be based on patient safety and surgeon comfort and preference. Surgeons that continue to perform sinus surgery with the horse under general anesthesia are either unfamiliar or uncomfortable with standing surgical procedures, or have not attempted a sinus flap in the standing position. The standing position provides numerous advantages in most cases. Aside from the obvious risks and increased costs of general anesthesia, blood loss from hemorrhage seems to be far greater in the anesthetized patient. Positioning of the patient's head under general anesthesia at a point lower than or level with the heart combines with a high rate of intravenous fluid delivery to create thickened, edematous sinus mucosa that bleeds excessively on incision (**Fig. 8**).

Increased hemorrhage leads to excessive blood loss, which increases the need for a blood transfusion, which is not without its own risks. To decrease the need for transfusion, the surgeon must work quickly and hastily, which could result in surgical errors. As with any surgery, bleeding also obscures the view requiring most sinus surgery under general anesthesia to be performed more by "feel" than by sight. In the standing horse, bleeding of incised sinus mucosa is minimal and with the help of gravity, is removed from the surgical field, which improves the view of the lesion (ie, inspissated pus, tooth roots, tumors). The ability to actually see the lesion is a great advantage and aids in surgical accuracy and helps to ensure complete removal of the lesion. Although sinus packing is required after cases under general anesthesia to control hemorrhage, standing procedures rarely require any packing. Packing is left for 48 to 72 hours after surgery and then must be removed. A blood-soaked packing can lead to increased infection rate, and when removed can lead to severe hemorrhage. Usually, the patient is left on systemic antibiotics until or shortly after the packing is removed, which increases hospitalization time, risk of antibiotic-induced diarrhea, and overall cost. Although standing sinus surgery is considered a contaminated surgery because of inability to adhere to aseptic technique, the authors typically treat with only 24 hours of antibiotic therapy.

Although the authors prefer performing sinus surgery in the standing position, there are cases when general anesthesia may be required. Highly vascularized tumors

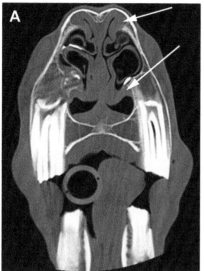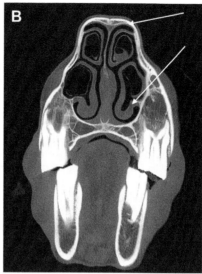

Fig. 8. (*A*) Transverse CT image at the level of the third premolar performed under general anesthesia. (*B*) Transverse CT image at the level of the third premolar performed in the standing position. *Arrows* point to the thickened sinus mucosa that occurs during anesthesia in dorsal recumbency during CT imaging. Note the difference in mucosal thickness between images *A* and *B*.

should be reserved for removal under general anesthesia to improve patient and surgeon safety. Also, it is not recommended in uncooperative patients. In summary, standing sinus surgery can result in decreased risk to the patient and minimize cost to the owner in most scenarios.

Maxillary flap technique

For diseases involving the RMS and premolar teeth, the maxillary sinus flap may be most useful. However, the maxillary sinus flap is smaller and allows only minimal access to the RMS or CMS. The large reserve crowns in horses younger than 5 years of age fill most of the RMS and a maxillary sinus flap may only provide access to the tooth roots. This is obviously ideal for tooth repulsion, but not if access to other paranasal sinus compartments is needed. This flap can be performed successfully in the standing horse. The surgical technique is similar to the frontonasal bone flap. Location and size of the flap may vary depending on the reason for surgery. The caudal margin is a vertical line 1 to 2 cm in front of the medial canthus to the dorsal aspect of the facial crest, the ventral margin is a line 0.5 cm above and parallel to the facial crest, and the rostral margin is a vertical line extending dorsally from the rostral aspect of the facial crest. The bone is fractured along the dorsal margin, which is immediately ventral to a line drawn from the medial canthus of the eye to the infraorbital foramen, to stay below the nasolacrimal duct (see **Fig. 6**). From the authors' experience, there is limited use of this flap alone, except for the very rostral aspect of the CMS. It can be helpful in conjunction with a frontonasal sinus flap if improved access to the RMS or VCS is required. Dental-related tumors, such as compound odontomas that fill the entire paranasal sinuses, are very difficult to access through a single frontonasal or maxillary bone flap. However, successful removal can be accomplished with the use of both flaps simultaneously. Boutros and Koenig[32] describe the use of a combined frontal and maxillary sinus approach for repulsion of a third maxillary molar (211) with a fractured crown. A large maxillary flap was created combined with a 2.5-cm trephination hole in the frontal sinus. The dental punch was placed through the frontal trephine hole and guided and held in placed on the root of the third molar through the maxillary bone flap. The combined maxillary and frontal sinus approaches provide excellent exposure for sinus debridement and tooth repulsion in such cases and facilitated a complete alveolar seal.

Two facial muscles, the levator labii superoris and levator nasolabialis, have been transposed to prevent or repair orosinus fistulas.[33,34] Both techniques require the creation of a maxillary bone flap or trephine hole. Transposition of the levator labii superioris muscle is theoretically more appropriate for repairing larger orosinus fistulas. In the authors' limited experience with either technique, the levator labii superioris transposition is slightly easier to perform. Large, chronic orosinus fistulas are extremely frustrating and difficult to successfully repair. Successful repair requires persistence on the part of clinician and an owner that is completely committed financially. The use of either technique should be considered after other less invasive treatment options have been exhausted.

Bilateral sinus disease is uncommon in horses. There are limited indications for surgical access to the right and left paranasal sinuses. In a study involving 277 horses with sinonasal disease, only 9% of cases had bilateral nasal discharge, and only 3% of those cases had disease with bilateral sinus involvement.[13,16] None of those horses had bilateral dental-related sinus disease. In a more recent report on 200 horses with diseases of the paranasal sinuses, nine horses had bilateral sinus disease.[14] Bilateral dental-related sinus disease may result from tumors of dental origin, most likely compound odontomas. The authors have experience with two unrelated American Miniature horses with a bilateral mucocele. It is not uncommon for American Miniature horses to have slight deformation of frontal bones, small sinus cavities, disproportionately large teeth for their skull size, and a high curvature of the tooth roots. In these two cases, this combination of anatomic variations possibly resulted in distortion of sinuses and bilateral obstruction of the sinus ostium. If surgery is

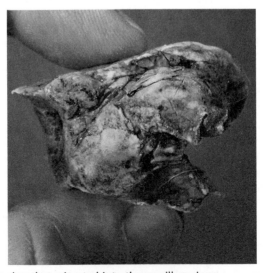

Fig. 9. An alveolar plug that migrated into the maxillary sinus.

required for a bilateral disease, each side can be approached through bone flaps as staged procedures, approximately 3 weeks apart. Alternatively, a single flap approach can be used to access both frontonasal sinuses simultaneously.[29,30]

Although dental-related sinus disease may not require a sinusotomy approach to remove the primary cause, sinusotomy is often necessary for complete resolution of the resulting sinusitis. Tremaine and Dixon[16] showed that 40.7% of cases that had dental repulsion required a sinusotomy to remove residual bony or dental sequestra, or to improve nasomaxillary drainage for complete resolution of clinical signs. Four of 54 cases of tooth repulsion developed an oromaxillary fistula and two had dental wax plugs become displaced into the sinuses (**Fig. 9**). In a more recent study by Dixon and colleagues,[35] 51% of horses with dental-related sinus disease were treated with a maxillary sinus flap and 5% were treated with a frontonasal sinus flap. Eight horses were diagnosed with dental-related oromaxillary fistulas; 38% of those horses were treated with a maxillary flap and 25% were treated with a frontonasal flap. A maxillary sinusotomy was the preferred sinus approach in this study, although reasons were not provided for the preference.

SUMMARY

Dental-related sinus disease can be challenging diagnostically and therapeutically, often resulting in high financial burdens on the owner and long-term morbidity for the horse. An accurate diagnosis is paramount to the successful treatment and overall positive outcome for the horse. Thorough understanding of sinus and dental anatomy is the first step, followed by use of the numerous diagnostic and advanced imaging modalities described throughout this article. Dental-related sinus diseases are never considered true emergencies and are rarely life threatening to the horse. Because of this, invasive therapy should never be performed without a confident understanding of the disease and the potential complications of surgical intervention. Seeking guidance through surgery and radiology specialists is highly recommended in challenging cases.

REFERENCES

1. Barakzai SZ, Kane-Smyth J, Lowles J, et al. Trephination of the equine rostral maxillary sinus: efficacy and safety of to trephine sites. Vet Surg 2008;37:278–82.
2. Dixon PM, Tremaine WH, Pickles K, et al. Equine dental disease. Part 4: a long-term study of 400 cases: apical infections of cheek teeth. Equine Vet J 2000;32:182–94.
3. Lane JG. The management of sinus disorders of horses. Part 1. Equine Vet Educ 1993;5:5–9.
4. O'Leary JM, Dixon PM. A review of equine paranasal sinusitis. Aetiopathogenesis, clinical signs and ancillary diagnostic techniques. Equine Vet Educ 2011;23:148–59.
5. Perkins JD, Windley Z, Dixon PM, et al. Sinoscopic treatment of rostral maxillary and ventral conchal sinusitis in 60 horses. Vet Surg 2009;38:613–9.
6. Bell C, Tatarniuk D, Carmalt J. Endoscope-guided balloon sinuplasty of the equine nasomaxillary opening. Vet Surg 2009;38:791–7.
7. McCann JL, Dixon PM, Mayhew JG. Clinical anatomy of the equine sphenopalatine sinus. Equine Vet J 2004;36:466–72.
8. Freeman DE. Sinus disease. Vet Clin North Am Equine Pract 2003;19:209–43.
9. Bell BT, Baker GJ, Abbott LC, et al. The macroscopic vascular anatomy of the equine ethmoidal area. Anat Histol Embryol 1995;24:39–45.

10. Cleary OB, Easley JT, Henrikson MDL, et al. Purulent dacryocystitis (nasolacrimal duct drainage) secondary to periapical tooth root infection in a donkey. Equine Vet Educ 2011;23:553–8.
11. Ramzan PH, Payne RJ. Periapical dental infection with nasolacrimal involvement in a horse. Vet Rec 2005;156:184–5.
12. Latimer CA, Wyman M, Diesem C, et al. Radiographic and gross anatomy of the nasolacrimal duct of the horse. Am J Vet Res 1984;45:451–8.
13. Tremaine WH, Dixon PM. A long-term study of 277 cases of equine sinonasal disease. Part 1: details of horses, historical, clinical and ancillary diagnostic findings. Equine Vet J 2001;33:274–82.
14. Dixon PM, Parkin TD, Collins N, et al. Equine paranasal sinus disease: a long-term study of 200 cases (1997-2009): ancillary diagnostic findings and involvement of the various sinus compartments. Equine Vet J 2012;44:267–71.
15. Morello SL, Parente EJ. Laser vaporization of the dorsal turbinate as an alternative method of accessing and evaluating the paranasal sinuses. Vet Surg 2010;39:891–9.
16. Tremaine WH, Dixon PM. A long-term study of 277 cases of equine sinonasal disease. Part 2: treatments and results of treatments. Equine Vet J 2001;33:283–9.
17. Wagenmann M, Naclerio RM. Anatomic and physiologic considerations in sinusitis. J Allergy Clin Immunol 1992;90:419–23.
18. Ruggles AJ, Ross MW, Freeman DE. Endoscopic examination of normal paranasal sinuses in horses. Vet Surg 1991;20:418–23.
19. Ruggles AJ, Ross MW, Freeman DE. Endoscopic examination and treatment of paranasal sinus disease in 16 horses. Vet Surg 1993;22:508–14.
20. Perkins JD, Bennett C, Windley Z, et al. Comparison of sinoscopic techniques for examining the rostral maxillary and ventral conchal sinuses of horses. Vet Surg 2009;38:607–12.
21. Schumacher J, Dutton DM, Murphy DJ, et al. Paranasal sinus surgery through a frontonasal flap in sedated standing horses. Vet Surg 2000;29:173–7.
22. Schumacher J, Honnas C, Smith B. Paranasal sinusitis complicated by inspissated exudate in the ventral conchal sinus. Vet Surg 1987;16:373–7.
23. Dixon PM, Dacre I, Dacre K, et al. Standing oral extraction of cheek teeth in 100 horses (1998-2003). Equine Vet J 2005;37:105–12.
24. Baker GJ. Endodontic therapy. In: Baker GJ, Easley KJ, editors. Equine dentistry. 1st edition. London: WB Saunders; 1999. p. 250–9.
25. Prichard MA, Hackett RP, Erb HN. Long-term outcome of tooth repulsion in horses: a retrospective study of 61 cases. Vet Surg 1992;21:145–9.
26. Stohl M. How to perform a buccal approach for different dental procedures. In: Proceedings of the Annual Convention of the AAEP, vol. 53. Lexington (KY): AAEP; 2007. p. 507–11.
27. Carmalt JL, Barber SM. Periapical curettage: an alternative surgical approach to infected mandibular cheek teeth in horses. Vet Surg 2004;33:267–71.
28. Coomer RP, Fowke GS, Mckane S. Repulsion of maxillary and mandibular cheek teeth in standing horses. Vet Surg 2011;40:590–5.
29. Freeman DE, Orsini PG, Ross MW, et al. A large frontonasal bone flap for sinus surgery in the horse. Vet Surg 1990;19:122–30.
30. Easley JT, Freeman DE. A single caudally based frontonasal bone flap for treatment of bilateral mucocele in the paranasal sinuses of an American Miniature Horse. Vet Surg 2013. http://dx.doi.org/10.1111/j.1532-950X.2013.01093.x.
31. Hillmann DJ. Skull. In: Getty R, editor. Sisson and Grossman's the anatomy of the domestic animals. 5th edition. Philadelphia: WB Saunders Co; 1975. p. 318.

32. Boutros CP, Koenig JB. A combined frontal and maxillary sinus approach for repulsion of the third maxillary molar in a horse. Can Vet J 2001;42:286–8.
33. Brink P. Levator labii superioris muscle transposition to treat oromaxillary sinus fistula in three horses. Vet Surg 2006;35:596–600.
34. Orsini PG, Ross MW, Hamir AN. Levator nasolabialis muscle transposition to prevent an orosinus fistula after tooth extraction in horses. Vet Surg 1992;31:150–6.
35. Dixon PM, Parkin TD, Collins N, et al. Equine paranasal sinus disease: A long-term study of 200 cases (1997-2009): Treatment and long-term results of treatments. Equine Vet J 2012;44:272–6.

The Gold Standard of Dental Care
The Juvenile Horse

Cleet Griffin, DVM

KEYWORDS

- Juvenile horse • Craniofacial abnormality • Malocclusion • Facial swelling
- Dental eruption

KEY POINTS

- Postpartum evaluation of the foal's head and mouth are performed to detect craniofacial malformations and other congenital defects.
- Important abnormalities of foals include wry nose, cleft palate, overbite (parrot mouth), and underbite (monkey mouth, sow mouth).
- Tumors and cysts such as equine juvenile ossifying fibroma, paranasal sinus cysts, aneurysmal bone cyst, and epidermal inclusion cysts of the false nostril can be detected in young horses.
- In juvenile horses, primary dental care procedures include oral examination, management of sharp enamel points, management of deciduous teeth, and management of wolf teeth.

EXAMINATION OF FOALS

During postpartum examination, an external evaluation of the foal's head is performed to evaluate for symmetry. The lips and gums of the incisive area are examined for abnormalities, and occlusion of the upper and lower jaw is evaluated simultaneously. Brief inspection of the palate, tongue, and oral soft tissues is performed by gently retracting the cheek and shining a bright light into the oral cavity. If indicated a more detailed oral examination can be performed using appropriate sedation and a small dental speculum designed for use on ponies. Radiography or computed tomography (CT) is useful to gain further information when craniofacial malformations are present.[1]

Wry nose (campylorhinus lateralis) is an uncommon congenital deformity of the nasal bones, premaxilla/maxilla, hard palate, and nasal septum that causes lateral deviation of the nose, respiratory stridor, and improper dental occlusion[2–5]; additional deformities of the limbs, head, and neck also can accompany the condition.[6] Inheritance has not been reported,[7] but results of 1 retrospective study[6] indicate that the deformity could be a result of improper uterine positioning and inability of the uterus

College of Veterinary Medicine and Biomedical Sciences, Texas A&M University, College Station, TX 77843-4475, USA
E-mail address: cgriffin@cvm.tamu.edu

to distend sufficiently during gestation to accommodate the growing fetus. A different potential cause has been proposed from a CT study of an affected foal. Three-dimensional reconstructions revealed fusion between the incisive bone and nasal bone only on 1 side of the nose (on the short side). Continued growth and elongation on the opposite side push the premaxilla into a wry position.[8] Mildly affected foals do not require immediate treatment, and mild facial deformity may straighten significantly with growth.[6,7] It is speculated later in life that mildly affected foals may develop a diagonal plane of occlusion between the upper and lower incisor teeth to accommodate the deformity. Severely affected foals may need prompt intervention for survival, such as feeding by nasogastric tube.[9] Symptoms in moderately to severely affected foals may include:

- Dysphagia[10]
- Malocclusion of the incisors and cheek teeth
- Difficulty nursing or eating[9]
- Stridorous breathing and airflow obstruction caused by nasal septum deviation[11]
- Collapse of the nostril on the convex side of the deviation[11]
- Chronic, foul odor from the mouth caused by accumulation of feed material[12]

Surgical correction of wry nose, resulting in favorable cosmetic appearance and good dental occlusion, has been performed in foals and yearling age horses.[4,7,9,12,13] Surgical treatment can be accomplished in 1 or 2 stages and involves performing an osteotomy of the maxilla/premaxilla for realignment of the nose, stabilization of the realigned segment using bone plates or Steinman pins and a rib graft, and removal of the deformed portion of the nasal septum to improve airflow. Other methods of correction include using external fixators[4] and distraction osteogenesis principles[12] to successfully treat the condition. The prognosis of obtaining an athletic animal after surgery is poor except in mild cases.[11]

Cleft palate (palatoschisis) is an uncommon congenital anomaly, resulting from failure of the transverse palatal folds to fuse within the mouth.[14,15] Clefts potentially involve the external nares, lip, hard palate, and soft palate[16] but all cases reported in the veterinary literature involve isolated defects of the soft and hard palates[15,17–22] (there is a single case report of a foal affected with cleft of the lower lip, mandible, and tongue).[23] The inheritance or cause of cleft palate in foals is not known but is speculated to be multifactorial,[18,21] and numerous sources have suggested not to breed the affected animal.[10,14,16,19] Foals affected with cleft palate are noticed to drip milk from the nostrils after suckling (however, persistent dorsal displacement of the soft palate may also cause milk to drip from the nose).[11] Impaired suckling ability and dysphagia in foals with cleft palate can often result in failure of passive transfer, aspiration pneumonia, and chronic malnutrition.[14,16,17,21] The palatal defect can be usually diagnosed by oral examination with a bright light source, and endoscopy may provide more comprehensive evaluation of the cleft.[24]

Case reports of surgical repair of cleft palate in foals include using a mandibular symphysiotomy approach, followed by mucosal suturing techniques to close the palatal defect. The surgery is invasive, and postoperative complications occur frequently, including persistent nasal discharge, formation of oronasal fistula, dehiscence of the palate repair, dehiscence of the lower lip, and osteomyelitis of the mandible.[17,21,22] (A lip sparing technique can be used to alleviate the potential for dehiscence of the lip incision.)[25] More recently, there has been a case report of less invasive, successful correction of a cleft soft palate in a 1-year-old pony using a laryngeal tie-forward technique.[20] Alternatively, a transoral approach using laparoscopic principals to repair defects in the palate may become possible in foals.[10]

Overbite (Parrot Mouth) and Overjet

Overbite and overjet of the incisor teeth are classified as class II malocclusions[26] and result from a relative difference in the length of the maxilla and mandible. This disparity can be the result of either mandibular brachygnathism or maxillary prognathism.[27] The term overjet is used to describe affected horses in which the maxillary incisors project horizontally beyond the labial edge of the occlusal surface of the lower incisors. A small degree of incisor overjet is a common finding and is not generally considered to be associated with significant clinical problems. The degree of incisor overjet that is observed in a horse can be influenced by the position of the horse's head and normal rostral-caudal movement of the mandible (ie, when the horse's poll is extended, the mandible retracts caudally; and when the poll is flexed, the mandible normally protrudes in a rostral direction).

With more severe disparity in jaw length, the upper incisors could project beyond the labial side of the lowers to such an extent that the occlusal surface of the upper incisors deviates ventrally, dropping below the occlusal surface of the lower incisors, creating an overbite (parrot mouth). The lower incisor teeth become trapped behind the palatal side of the uppers, limiting rostral growth and movement of the mandible.[28] Over time, the lower unopposed incisors continue to erupt and may come into contact with and traumatize the mucosa of the hard palate.[29] With overbite and overjet, the maxillary cheek teeth tend to be positioned more rostrally relative to their mandibular counterparts, resulting in focal dental elongations (hooks) of the rostral aspect of the maxillary arcade and the caudal aspect mandibular arcade.[29] Overjet and overbite have also been associated with the presence of exaggerated transverse ridges of the cheek teeth, which further limit mobility of the mandible.[28] Parrot mouth is generally considered to be heritable, and the defect may develop in foals during the first few months of life that were known to be normal at birth (**Fig. 1**).[30]

In young horses with overjet, regular occlusal adjustment is performed to reduce dental elongations and exaggerated transverse ridges of the cheek teeth. In foals, this procedure is believed to help achieve correction of the condition by reducing dental interlock, increasing mandibular mobility, and eliminating restriction to mandibular growth.[27] Caretakers can also be instructed to feed affected foals and weanlings at ground level to promote protrusion of the mandible.

Orthodontic techniques involving application of tension band wires to retard maxillary growth, with or without application of an acrylic bite plane to the upper incisor

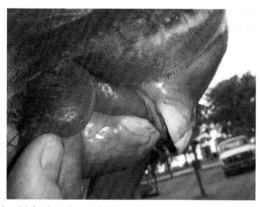

Fig. 1. Three-month-old foal with overbite.

teeth, have been reported in the management of overjet and overbite in foals.[8,27,29,30] Tension band wires extending from the maxillary premolars to the incisors can be surgically placed in the mouth to slow growth and correct the condition,[30] but when used without an acrylic bite plane, it is believed that the tension wires pull the premaxilla more ventrally and potentially exacerbate the condition.[27,31] An acrylic bite plane is affixed to upper incisors and extends in a palatal direction, providing the lower incisor teeth with an opposing occlusal surface. Over time, this plane alleviates ventral deviation of the upper incisors, allows less restricted motion, and permits maximal growth of the mandible (**Fig. 2**).[27]

Mandibular osteodistraction, a surgical technique used to treat mandibular shortness in humans, has been used to successfully manage overbite in horses.[31,32] Under general anesthesia, a complete osteotomy of both mandibles is performed rostral to the second premolars. Depending on the technique, an external fixator or a ratchet device implant is attached to the mandibles. Lengthening of the mandible can be achieved by application of distraction forces across the osteotomy site. Once the occlusal abnormality is corrected and appropriate healing of the bone and soft tissue has occurred, the appliance is removed.

Underbite (Sow Mouth, Monkey Mouth)

When the maxilla is shorter than the mandible, the mandibular incisors may protrude past the maxillary incisor teeth to a variable degree, resulting in either an underjet or an underbite. These conditions are classified as class III malocclusions[26] and are most commonly noted in miniature horse breeds. With underbite, unopposed upper incisors continue to erupt over time and may damage the mucosa behind the lower incisors. Focal elongations develop on the rostral portion of the lower cheek teeth quadrants and the caudal portion of the upper cheek teeth quadrants. These elongations may be severe in some cases, resulting in painful trauma and inflammation of the opposite soft tissue and bone. Regular occlusal adjustment and similar orthodontic and surgical principals used in the management of overbite can be used to manage underjet/underbite.[1]

Tumors and Cysts

Equine juvenile ossifying fibroma is a rapidly growing, fibro-osseous tumor of the head, which may be seen in very young horses (birth to 12 months of age).[33,34] These tumors have a predilection for the rostral part of the mandible[35] but can occur at other locations, such as the paranasal sinuses and nasal cavity, resulting in abnormal

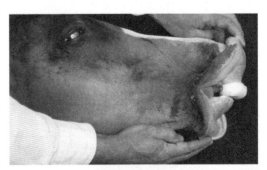

Fig. 2. Seven-month-old foal with overbite. An acrylic bite plane has been affixed to the upper incisors to provide an opposing occlusal surface for the lower incisor teeth.

respiratory noise.[36-39] Radiographically, the tumor can appear as a dense, bony mass[36,40] and may involve lytic changes of the roots of associated teeth.[35] Successful reports in the management of equine juvenile ossifying fibroma include surgical resection,[36] systemic and local injections of cisplatin,[33] radiation therapy,[38,40] and rostral mandibulectomy.[35] Incomplete surgical resection is a key factor in local recurrence of the tumor.[35] Differential diagnoses for equine juvenile ossifying fibroma include osteoma, fibrous dysplasia, osteosarcoma, and fibrous osteodystrophy.[34]

Tooth formation and location rely on embryonic interactions between ectoderm of the first branchial arch and migration of neural crest-derived ectomesenchymal cells.[41,42] Heterotopic polydontia has been defined as an extra tooth situated separately from the dental arcades.[43] One example is an ear tooth, which develops within an epithelial-lined cyst near the base of the ear in young horses. When an ear tooth occurs, it develops from misplaced tooth germ of the first branchial arch that becomes abnormally located in the ear region.[43] Tooth structures contained within the cyst can be loosely attached or may be tightly adhered to underlying bone,[34,44] and the cystic enlargement contains a fistula that opens along the margin of the ear pinna.[44,45] Ectopic tooth cysts have also been reported to occur intracranially,[46] intranasally,[47] and within the paranasal sinuses.[48] Other terms in the veterinary literature used to describe an ear tooth include dentigerous cyst, aural fistula, and temporal teratoma.[44-49] These types of cysts are identifiable in young foals but may not be recognized until later in life and occasionally occur bilaterally.[1,43,44,50,51] Radiography can help confirm the diagnosis, but small ectopic teeth may not be evident.[44] CT or magnetic resonance imaging may allow more detailed assessment of the proximity of important structures before surgical removal.[50,51] Complete surgical removal is curative,[44] but reported complications include profuse hemorrhage, infection, incomplete removal of the cyst, damage to the ear, dehiscence, damage to auriculopalpebral nerves,[45] and death.[46]

Paranasal sinus cysts can develop in any of the paranasal sinuses and may extend into the nasal passages.[3,52] The cysts, which can affect horses of any age, are of uncertain cause and typically consist of epithelial-lined, fluid-filled cavities.[1,52] Clinical signs include facial swelling, sinus dullness on percussion, nasal discharge, and dyspnea.[1,3,52,53] As a sinus cyst enlarges, pressure causes distortion to the skull[54] and may affect the developing tooth buds of the permanent dentition.[1] Nasal endoscopy commonly reveals narrowing of the nasal passage, and in some instances, the cystic structure may be visualized within the nasal cavity.[3,52,53] Centesis of an affected sinus typically yields viscous fluid (clear to amber color) and cytology may reveal abundant erythrocytes and leukocytes.[52,53] Radiography and CT are useful for defining the severity and extent of the cystic lesions. Sinus endoscopy can be used to identify the cysts[53] but may be limited by distention and distortion of the sinus.[3] Definitive treatment of sinus cysts involves surgical removal of the cystic structures and lining via a sinus flap approach, combined with postoperative irrigation to remove debris and blood clots.[3,52-54] Postoperative improvement of nasal airway obstruction and facial deformity more likely occurs in the young, growing horse (**Fig. 3**).[1]

Mandibular aneurysmal bone cysts are rare but can occur in a young horse as an expansile swelling of the lower jaw.[55-59] There is a report[58] of dystocia in a mare delivering a foal affected with a large congenital mandibular aneurysmal bone cyst. Radiographically, an aneurysmal bone cyst appears as a complex, multiloculated structure with a thin rim of bone around the periphery.[56] Progressive destruction of bone and dental supporting structures may result in pain and pathologic fracture of the mandible.[56,59] Drainage and aggressive surgical curettage of uncomplicated aneurysmal bone cysts can be curative.[57] An epidermal inclusion cyst (atheroma) is a

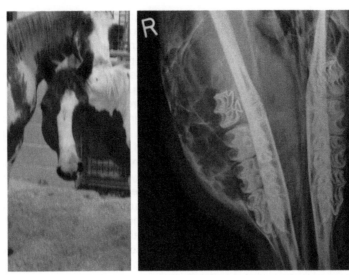

Fig. 3. Weanling with swelling of the right maxillofacial region. A dorsoventral radiograph revealed an expansile osteolytic lesion involving the right maxillary sinuses with distortion of the nasal septum. There also seems to be bone loss along the buccal alveolar margin of the right maxillary cheek teeth. The presence of a large sinus cyst was confirmed at surgery. (*Courtesy of* Carolyn Arnold, DVM, College Station, TX.)

spherical, epithelial-lined cyst that occurs between the skin and mucous membrane in the dorsolateral aspect of the nasal diverticulum (false nostril).[60,61] Keratinized and nonkeratinized squamous epithelial cells with keratin debris comprise the contents of the cyst.[62,63] These cysts vary between 3 cm and 5 cm in diameter, usually occur unilaterally, and rarely interfere with breathing.[61,62] Elimination of the cyst with good cosmetic result has been accomplished via surgical extirpation,[61] ventral drainage of the cyst and removal of the lining with a laryngeal burr,[60] and desiccation of the cyst by intralesional administration of formalin.[62]

YEARLING TO 5 YEARS OF AGE
Examination

For all dental cases, examination begins with visual evaluation of the head. The ear pinnae, orbits, globes, eyelids, facial bones, and nostrils are inspected for symmetry. Causes of facial asymmetry include:

- Craniofacial deformity
- Muscle atrophy
- Neurologic disease
- Bony depression of the skull
- Soft tissue enlargement
- Bony enlargement

Further diagnostic evaluation of facial asymmetry may be indicated in some instances. In horses between the ages of 1 year and 5 years, 24 permanent cheek teeth and 12 incisors erupt sequentially, causing the deciduous cheek teeth and incisors to shed. Objectives of an oral examination during this period include evaluation for appropriate dental eruption, assessment of occlusion, identification of sources of pain, and evaluation of the oral soft tissues (cheeks, tongue, lips, and palate) for problems such as bleeding, erosions, or tumors. The periodontal tissues and endodontic elements of the teeth should also be evaluated during oral examination. In order to visualize the gums and occlusal surface of the cheek teeth, a dental mirror or intraoral scope is necessary. When gingival recession or periodontal pocketing of feed is encountered, the area is irrigated to remove impacted plant material to better assess the gingiva and a periodontal probe is used to measure pocket depth. Normal depth of the gingival sulcus of the incisors is less than 3 mm, and for the cheek teeth, less than 5 mm.[64] On the occlusal surface of the crown, necrotic pulp exposure appears as an area of dark, discolored secondary dentin. Closer examination with a mirror or dental scope usually reveals feed material packed within the necrotic pulp, and probing with a dental explorer can confirm the finding. If the occlusal defect communicates with the apical part of the pulp canal, then periapical infection can result; however, it is possible in some instances that healthy pulp exists in an apical direction from an occlusal pulp defect.[65] Radiography is often warranted when periodontal disease or necrotic pulp exposure is identified to evaluate the tooth, surrounding bone, and periapical region.

Juvenile horses tend to tolerate oral examination well. Placement of a full mouth dental speculum and use of a bright light source are required to perform a thorough visual and tactile examination of the oral cavity. Some speculum bite plate designs may irritate the gum tissue on the lingual side of the mandibular incisors in juvenile horses because of short deciduous incisor crown length. Sedation protocols vary, but adequate sedation and analgesia for primary dental care procedures in juvenile horses can generally be obtained by intravenous (IV) administration of an α_2 agonist (eg, detomidine at 0.01–0.02 mg/kg IV). After sedation and rinsing the mouth, the head should be supported at an appropriate height. Caretakers should be instructed to eliminate access to hay and feed for 4 hours after sedation to eliminate potential problems with dysphagia, esophageal choke, aspiration, and so forth.

Management of Sharp Enamel Points

Problems that occur during performance, such as bit chewing, tail wringing, gaping the mouth, excessive head tossing, and ear pinning, have been associated with conditions causing oral pain.[66,67] Erosion of the cheek mucosa associated with sharp enamel points is more common in juvenile horses,[68] and erosion occurs with greater frequency in horses ridden with a bit and bridle compared with unridden horses.[69] The buccal space along the upper cheek teeth is extremely narrow in the caudal part of the mouth, making the cheeks in close apposition to sharp areas[70]; as a result, sharp enamel points can be easily palpated by placing the fingers on the outside of the cheeks along the buccal edge of the upper cheek teeth. If mild pressure is placed on the cheeks over sharp enamel points of the more caudally located cheek teeth, the horse generally begins to gape the mouth and toss the head. Sharp points on the lingual side of the lower cheek teeth can also irritate or cause erosions of the tongue.[70] Sharp elongations such as those on the mesial part of the upper first cheek teeth or on the distal aspect of the last lower molars may traumatize the mucosa and are associated with bitting problems and abnormal head carriage.[71] Sharp dental points require floating along the buccal side of the upper cheek teeth and the lingual side of the lower cheek teeth using hand instruments or motorized equipment. The horse's narrow oral opening, large tongue, and narrow buccal space create challenges for the veterinarian performing primary dental care procedures such as dental flotation. In juvenile horses, enamel points are often sharp, yet tend to be easily and quickly removed by dental flotation compared with mature horses. It is important to carefully palpate the upper and lower cheek teeth quadrants to verify that floating has successfully removed sharp points and hooks. When floating the teeth of juvenile horses, caution should be exercised not to damage the mucosa located over erupting caudal permanent cheek teeth. Juvenile horses should be reexamined for sharp enamel points every 6 to 9 months.

In horses, the cheek teeth normally have palpable transverse ridges located across the chewing surface. In some instances (eg, horses with overjet or overbite), 1 or more elongated long transverse ridges may occur.[28] It is generally believed that an excessively large transverse ridge may cause excessive wear or create a pathologic diastema.[28,72] When encountered, large transverse ridges can be reduced to a more normal length with a dental float, taking care not to eliminate normal transverse ridges.[28,72]

It is common practice to contour and round the mesial edge of the occlusal surface of the second premolars. This procedure is performed in an attempt to alleviate potential discomfort as the bit pulls or presses the buccal mucosa against the premolar teeth. When performed appropriately, gentle and conservative rounding of the sharp point that occurs at the mesial aspect of the second premolar can be performed safely. The practice of aggressively contouring the clinical crown and occlusal surface (ie, bit seating) is inappropriate and may result in iatrogenic tooth damage and pain.

Management of Wolf Teeth

Wolf teeth (Triadan 05) are rudimentary first premolars that erupt just mesial to the second premolar teeth (**Fig. 4**). Most wolf teeth cause no problems for the horse and are often shed during eruption of the permanent second premolars (Triadan 06). However, in some instances, wolf teeth are blamed for causing discomfort when the mucosa of the cheek presses against the sharp point of the tooth. Loose, displaced, enlarged, or fractured wolf teeth have also been implicated as being potentially problematic for the bitted horse.[8] If present, mandibular wolf teeth should be suspected as a source of discomfort in horses showing bitting problems. Unerupted wolf teeth (known as blind or impacted wolf teeth) are believed to cause pain when the gingiva is compressed against the underlying tooth. If it is determined that wolf tooth extraction is indicated, the procedure can be performed in standing, sedated horses and is facilitated by the use of a dental speculum and local anesthesia. After sedation, a bleb of local anesthetic is deposited near the lateral aspect of the rugae of the palate at the level of

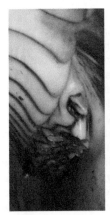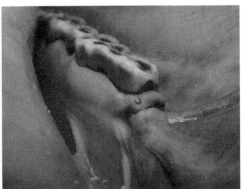

Fig. 4. Examples of erupted wolf teeth: an upper left wolf tooth (Triadan 205, *left*) and left mandibular wolf tooth (Triadan 305).

the wolf tooth, and in the mucogingival fold on the buccal aspect of the wolf tooth. The gingival tissue is elevated around the circumference of the tooth, and using a straight elevator, the tooth is loosened, then grasped for removal with forceps. Aftercare is usually minimal, although tetanus prophylaxis is advised after extractions. Upper wolf tooth extraction sites are left open for healing and epithelialization. Lower wolf tooth extraction sites can become contaminated with feed material; as a result, daily irrigation of lower extraction sites is recommended until granulation tissue has filled the alveolus. Horses may resume training 24 hours after wolf tooth extraction.

Management of Deciduous Teeth

Deciduous incisors may fail to shed as the permanent incisor erupts.[73] When the deciduous incisor does not shed properly, the permanent incisor is displaced lingually, resulting in malocclusion of the permanent incisor arcade (**Fig. 5**). In most cases, the retained deciduous incisor and root remnant can be removed in a standing patient after administration of a sedative analgesic (eg, detomidine 0.01–0.02 mg/kg IV, or xylazine 0.25–0.50 mg/kg IV) and infiltration of a local anesthetic or nerve block (eg, a mental foramen nerve block for lower teeth or infraorbital foramen nerve block for upper teeth). A small elevator loosens the attachments of the tooth for removal. If the deciduous incisor tooth fractures during removal, the gingiva needs to be incised over the labial aspect of the root to expose and remove the root spicule. Radiography can be used to assist with surgical planning and confirm complete removal of all deciduous remnants. After removal of the retained deciduous incisor, the displaced permanent incisor tooth should gradually drift into proper alignment. Aftercare is minimal, but tetanus prophylaxis is indicated after tooth extractions in horses.[74]

As a juvenile horse matures, the crowns of the deciduous premolars wear thin, and the roots resorb as the underlying permanent teeth erupt. A thin portion of the deciduous crown with slender, sharp root spicules remains. As the permanent tooth continues to erupt into the mouth, a small gap develops between the erupting permanent tooth and the deciduous premolar. Necrosis of the soft tissue attachments associated with the deciduous premolar occurs as feed material and bacteria become trapped in this space. As a result, variable degrees of gingivitis and halitosis are associated with eruption of permanent premolars in juvenile horses. Deciduous premolars that are loose,

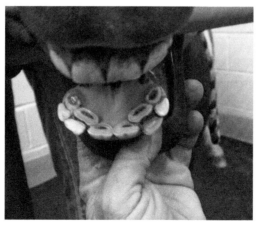

Fig. 5. Retained deciduous incisors in a juvenile age horse (incisors 702, 703, 802, 803 retained).

fractured, or that fail to shed properly may cause discomfort or irritatation.[28,75] Failure of a deciduous premolar to shed may be caused by abnormality or previous trauma to the underlying permanent tooth. Because the crown of the deciduous premolars closely resembles the crown of the permanent tooth, it may be difficult to determine whether the deciduous premolar tooth has been appropriately shed or not. When investigating inappropriate retention of deciduous premolar teeth, an open-mouth, lateral oblique radiograph can be helpful to evaluate the deciduous tooth, permanent tooth, alveolar bone, and adjacent teeth. A deciduous premolar can usually be identified on a radiograph as a short, thin tooth situated over the underlying permanent premolar (**Figs. 6** and **7**).

Deciduous premolar teeth can be safely extracted when a line of demarcation is visible between the deciduous premolar and the erupting permanent tooth. The thin deciduous premolar can be grasped with 4-prong forceps and rolled toward midline. Premature removal of deciduous premolars may damage blood supply to the developing infundibula of the permanent tooth, resulting in cemental hypoplasia, predisposing the tooth to infundibular decay and fracture. An index of suspicion for the presence of fractured deciduous premolar remnants should exist when performing primary dental care of juvenile horses. These small remnants may cause a substantial amount of mucosal and gingival irritation and have been suspected to interfere with eruption of permanent teeth. When identified, deciduous premolar remnants should be elevated and removed.

Facial and Mandibular Swelling

Eruption cysts are firm, bony enlargements, which can be observed in juvenile horses on the ventral aspect of the mandible and on the dorsolateral aspect of the maxilla (**Fig. 8**).[76] These swellings are associated with the apices of erupting permanent premolar teeth in 3-year-old and 4-year-old horses. On radiographic examination, the enlargements normally appear as a smooth-bordered, periapical lucency with sclerotic margins (**Fig. 9**).[77] The facial and mandibular enlargements normally associated with eruption cysts tend to regress in subsequent years.[28,78,79] In some instances, an eruption cyst may occur from overcrowding and vertical impaction of the erupting permanent tooth because of excessive angulation of adjacent teeth.[80,81] If dental impaction is suspected, a thorough oral examination and radiographic examination should be performed. With normal growth of the young horse, the impacted tooth may gain room to erupt as the jaws elongate; however, it is also possible that the impacted tooth could undergo ankylosis to the mandible and fail to erupt.[80]

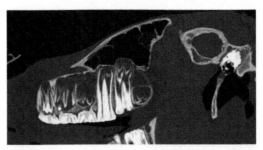

Fig. 6. Normal 2-year-old horse. Sagittal CT section of the left maxilla (*rostral direction is to the left*). Individual developing permanent premolars can be visualized above each deciduous premolar. The first molar is erupted, the second molar appears to be erupting, and the developing third molar is visible.

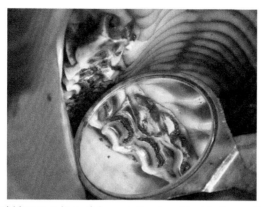

Fig. 7. Three-year-old horse. A line of demarcation is evident between the erupting permanent premolar (106) and worn deciduous premolar (506).

Blood-borne infection of the pulp and periapical tissues can occur in young horses, resulting in an excessively large, warm, painful eruption cyst or swelling of the maxilla or the mandible (which may be accompanied by a draining skin tract).[8] If an enlarged eruption cyst is encountered, a thorough oral examination should be performed to detect fractured teeth, retained deciduous premolars, deep periodontal problems, or necrotic pulp exposure. Radiographic examination is also warranted to assess for evidence of periapical disease and to evaluate the dental and bone structures associated with the swelling. If a skin tract is present, placing a malleable wire probe into the tract and obtaining an oblique lateral radiograph can be helpful to identify an infected cheek tooth.[82] If periapical infection associated with an enlarged eruption cyst is identified, then extraction of the affected tooth should be considered. However,

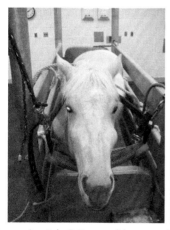

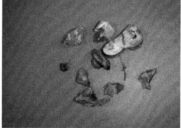

Fig. 8. Approximately 3.5-year-old mare with firm, nonpainful swellings involving the left and right maxilla. Oral examination of the same horse showed retained remnants of maxillary deciduous premolars (bilaterally, small retained remnants of deciduous fourth premolar teeth were wedged tightly in the interproximal space between the erupting upper permanent fourth premolar and first molar). These retained deciduous teeth fragments were removed along with multiple retained portions of deciduous mandibular premolars (*right*).

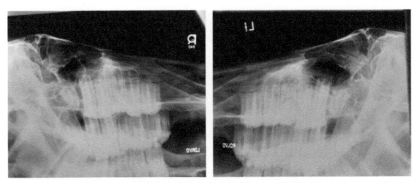

Fig. 9. Dorsal oblique extraoral radiographs of the right maxilla (*left*) and left maxilla (*right*) of same horse as in **Fig. 8**. Radiographic findings included periapical lucency of the third and fourth premolars bilaterally with sclerosis of adjacent maxillary bone (presumed maxillary eruption cysts).

in some instances, it is reasonable in juvenile horses to initiate conservative medical therapy for periapical infection with a 2-week to 4-week course of systemic antibiotics.[8,81] Extraction of the affected tooth can be attempted later, if after a reasonable duration of antibiotic therapy, the periapical infection fails to resolve or reoccurs.

Causes of a firm swelling of the maxilla or mandible also include tumors of dental origin. These types of tumors are rare and include ameloblastoma, ameloblastic odontoma, ameloblastic carcinoma, odontoma, complex odontoma, compound odontoma, and cementoma.[28,56,83–88] An ameloblastoma consists of odontogenic epithelium and may occur at any age.[56] These slowly progressive tumors cause an expansive swelling of the jaw and may result in destruction of bone and adjacent structures.[43] Ameloblastomas are nonmetastatic, invasive, and have a cystic radiographic appearance, with a spherical or multilocular shape; wide surgical excision may result in cure of ameloblastoma if performed early.[56] Odontomas are tumorlike malformations of fully differentiated dental tissues, which may occur on the maxilla or mandible.[56,84,85] These tumors result in bony distortion and swelling within the jaw of young horses and can be classified as a compound odontoma or complex odontoma, depending on the histologic organization of the dental tissues.[43,56,85,88] Compound odontoma and complex odontoma have been reported to appear radiographically as a well-marginated, osseouslike mass involving the mandible or maxilla.[84,85] Removal of affected tissues is the treatment of horses with odontoma, and prognosis is good with complete excision.[56,84,85,88]

Injuries

Juvenile horses commonly sustain trauma to the incisive region of the premaxilla or mandible, resulting in fractures of bone and avulsion and fractures of teeth, as well as damage to the gums and developing permanent tooth buds. Radiography is warranted to provide information about the injury in relation to the teeth and to help formulate a treatment plan. Additional diagnostic imaging in the form of CT provides excellent information in regard to management of craniofacial fractures.[32] In some horses, maxillary or mandibular fractures that are unilateral and stable can be managed conservatively (**Fig. 10**).

Clinical signs associated with injuries to the incisive area may be minimal. Fractures in this area should be irrigated and any food material, clotted blood, bone fragments,

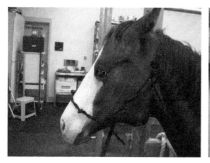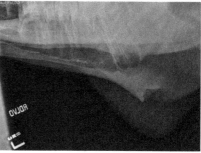

Fig. 10. Two-year-old horse with swelling and draining tract involving the left mandible. No significant clinical abnormalities were detected on oral examination; a small amount of thin, purulent material was encountered on probing of the skin tract. A ventral oblique radiograph of the left mandible of the same horse showed soft tissue swelling and a smoothly marginated and irregularly shaped concave defect of the ventral part of the mandibular ramus. No abnormalities of the dental structures are identified. The defect was presumably caused by previous fracture and was managed with conservative treatment.

and detached teeth should be carefully removed.[89] Care is taken with debridement to avoid damage to underlying permanent tooth structures. Avulsed incisor teeth and fractures of the incisive bone, mandibular symphysis, and premaxilla can be stabilized with cerclage wire fixation using standing sedation and nerve block or under general anesthesia.[8,32,89,90] When a fracture of the clinical crown of an incisor tooth and exposed vital pulp is encountered, an intraoral radiograph is recommended to evaluate the affected tooth, alveolar bone, and pulp canal. Tetanus prophylaxis and systemic antibiotic therapy are also recommended.[8] The idea with any interventional procedures involving fractured incisor teeth is to create an environment that allows the pulp to heal:

- When attempting first-aid treatment of pulp exposure, debris and fragments are removed from the exposed area with a needle[8] and irrigated thoroughly with sterile saline solution.
- A calcium hydroxide liner (Ultra-Blend plus, Ultradent Products, South Jordan, UT) can be applied and light-cured to seal the occlusal end of the pulp canal to eliminate oral contamination of the pulp and promote formation of reparative dentin by odontoblast cells residing in the pulp.[8]
- Flowable composite restorative material (StarFill 2B, Danville Materials, San Ramon, CA) is applied to fill the remaining pulp cavity after acid etching and application of a bonding agent (Adper Single Bond Plus Adhesive Kit, 3M, St Paul, MN).[8]
- For these procedures, the horse should be sedated and provided with local anesthesia by local anesthetic infiltration along the mucogingival junction or by performing a nerve block.
- In some young horses, with fractured incisor teeth and pulp exposure, the formation of reparative dentin and healing of affected tissues occurs without endodontic or restorative treatment.[73]

Mandibular fractures are an important differential diagnosis in horses with dysphagia and excessive swelling of the jaw.[5,90] Fractures through the interdental space of the mandible may be bilateral and unstable, resulting in difficulty eating or nursing, slobbering, and misalignment of the upper and lower incisors.[90] Techniques for stabilization of mandibular fractures through the interdental space include tension band wiring, u-bar placement, intraoral acrylic splinting, screws, and external fixators.[5,32,90] Fractures involving the body of the mandible are usually unilateral and therefore stabilized to some degree by the opposite intact mandible.[90] Mandibular body fractures have been repaired with bone plating or external fixator.[5,32,90] Some maxillary or mandibular fractures may involve 1 or more cheek teeth, and damage to developing permanent cheek tooth buds potentially results in abnormalities of the dentition later in life.[1,5] If an oral fracture component or avulsed teeth are present, halitosis develops after the injury; if present, any loose, avulsed fragments of cheek teeth should be removed in these instances.

Trauma to the head also potentially results in soft tissue injury to the skin, lips, and cheeks. Fresh, minimally contaminated head lacerations are good candidates for primary closure with standing sedation and local anesthesia. Routine wound care techniques are indicated for skin injuries that are left to heal by second intention. Full-thickness lacerations to the lips, if left untreated, may result in feed or saliva drooling from the mouth because of inadequate buccal seal.[91]

SUMMARY

During postpartum examination, the head and mouth of the foal are examined to detect congenital abnormalities. As foals mature, primary dental care involves oral examination to monitor normal dental eruption, floating sharp enamel points, removal of inappropriately retained deciduous teeth, and evaluation of facial and mandibular swellings.

REFERENCES

1. Easley JA. Review of equine dentistry: the first year of life. In: American Association of Equine Practitioners. Focus on the first year of life. July 27–29, 2008. Austin (TX). p. 155–68.
2. Baker GJ. Gastrointestinal disease. In: Reed S, Bayly W, editors. Equine internal medicine. Philadelphia: WB Saunders; 1998. p. 602–8.
3. Gaughan EM, DeBowes RM. Congenital diseases of the equine head. Vet Clin North Am Equine Pract 1993;9(1):93–110.
4. Cousty M, Haudiquet P, Geffroy O. Use of an external fixator to correct a wry nose in a yearling. Equine Vet Educ 2010;22(9):458–61.
5. Blackford JT, Blackford LW. Surgical treatment of selected musculoskeletal disorders of the head. In: Auer J, editor. Equine surgery. Philadelphia: WB Saunders; 1992. p. 1075–92.
6. Vandeplassche M, Simoens P, Bouters R, et al. Aetiology and pathogenesis of congenital torticollis and head scoliosis in the equine foetus. Equine Vet J 1984;16(5):419–24.
7. Schumacher J, Brink P, Easley J, et al. Surgical correction of wry nose in four horses. Vet Surg 2008;37(2):142–8.
8. Dixon P, Gerard M. Oral cavity and salivary glands. In: Auer J, Stick J, editors. Equine surgery. 4th edition. St Louis (MO): Elsevier; 2012. p. 339–67.
9. McKellar GM, Collins AP. The surgical correction of a deviated anterior maxilla in a horse. Aust Vet J 1993;70(3):112–4.
10. Cruz A. Congenital problems of foals. In: McKinnon A, Squires E, Vaala W, et al, editors. Equine reproduction. 2nd edition. West Sussex (United Kingdom): Wiley-Blackwell; 2011. p. 663–72.

11. Parente E. Congenital abnormalities of the respiratory system. In: McKinnon A, Squires E, Vaala W, et al, editors. Equine reproduction. 2nd edition. West Sussex (United Kingdom): Wiley-Blackwell; 2011. p. 609–14.

12. Puchol JL, Herrán R, Durall I, et al. Use of distraction osteogenesis for the correction of deviated nasal septum and premaxilla in a horse. J Am Vet Med Assoc 2004;224(7):1147–50, 1112.

13. Valdez H, McMullan WC, Hobson HP, et al. Surgical correction of deviated nasal septum and premaxilla in a colt. J Am Vet Med Assoc 1978;173(8):1001–4.

14. Tulleners E, Schumacher J, Johnston J, et al. Pharynx. In: Auer J, editor. Equine surgery. Philadelphia: WB Saunders; 1992. p. 453–9.

15. Jones RS, Maisels DO, Geus JJ, et al. Surgical repair of cleft palate in the horse. Equine Vet J 1975;7(2):86–90.

16. Chan C, Munroe G. Congenital abnormalities of the mouth and associated structures. In: Robinson N, editor. Current therapy in equine medicine. 4th edition. Philadelphia: WB Saunders; 1997. p. 144–6.

17. Kirkham LE, Vasey JR. Surgical cleft soft palate repair in a foal. Aust Vet J 2002;80(3):143–6.

18. Stickle R, Goble D, Braden T. Surgical repair of cleft palate in a foal. Vet Med 1973;68(2):159–62.

19. Mason TA, Speirs VC, Maclean AA, et al. Surgical repair of cleft palate in the horse. Vet Rec 1977;100(1):6–8.

20. Charman R. Correction of pharyngeal and soft palate dysfunction associated with a cleft palate in a miniature pony using a laryngeal tie-forward. Australian Veterinarian 2011;30(3):63.

21. Keeling N, Moll D. Use of mucosal graft to augment cleft palate repair in a foal. Equine Pract 1995;17:34–9.

22. Bowman KF, Tate LP, Evans LH, et al. Complications of cleft palate repair in large animals. J Am Vet Med Assoc 1982;180(6):652–7.

23. Aksoy O, Kilic E, Kacar C, et al. Congenital glossocheilognathoschisis and persistent frenula linguae in a foal: a case report. J Equine Vet Sci 2007;27(6):277–80.

24. Ducharme NG. Pharynx. In: Equine surgery. 4th edition. Elsevier; 2012. p. 569–91.

25. Grossman BS, Brinkman JF, Grant B. A new approach for intra-oral surgery in the horse. J Equine Vet Sci 1981;1(3):107–9.

26. Wiggs R, Lobprise H. Basics of orthodontics. In: Veterinary dentistry, principles and practice. 1st edition. Philadelphia: Lippincott; 1997. p. 438–41.

27. Klugh D. Acrylic bite plane for treatment of malocclusion in a young horse. J Vet Dent 2004;21(2):84–7.

28. Dixon PM, Dacre I. A review of equine dental disorders. Vet J 2005;169(2):165–87.

29. Easley J. Equine orthodontics. In: American Association of Equine Practitioners. Focus on dentistry. 2006.

30. Gift LJ, DeBowes RM, Clem MF, et al. Brachygnathia in horses: 20 cases (1979-1989). J Am Vet Med Assoc 1992;200(5):715–9.

31. Verwilghen D, Van Galen G, Vanderheyden L, et al. Mandibular osteodistraction for correction of deep bite class II malocclusion in a horse. Vet Surg 2008;37(6):571–9.

32. Auer JA. Craniomaxillofacial disorders. In: Equine surgery. 4th edition. Elsevier; 2012. p. 1456–82.

33. Pellmann R, Jaugstetter RJ. Equines juveniles ossifizierendes mandibuläres Fibrom bei einem Vollblutfohlen behandelt mit Cisplatin. Pferdeheilkunde 2002;18:467–70 [in German].
34. Thompson K. Tumors and Tumor-Like Lesions of Bones. In: Maxie MG, editor. Jubb Kennedy & Palmer's Pathology of Domestic Animals (fifth edition), Vol. 1. Edinburgh: Elsevier Saunders; 2007. p. 110–30.
35. Morse CC, Saik JE, Richardson DW, et al. Equine juvenile mandibular ossifying fibroma. Vet Pathol 1988;25(6):415–21.
36. Trostle SS, Rantanen N, Anderson M, et al. Juvenile mandibular ossifying fibroma in a 12-week-old foal. Equine Vet J 2005;17:284–6.
37. Puff C, Ohnesorge B, Wagels R, et al. An unusual mucinous osteoma with features of an ossifying fibroma in the nasal cavity of a horse. J Comp Pathol 2006; 135(1):52–5.
38. Orsini JA, Baird DK, Ruggles AJ. Radiotherapy of a recurrent ossifying fibroma in the paranasal sinuses of a horse. J Am Vet Med Assoc 2004;224(9):1483–6.
39. Cilliers I, Williams J, Carstens A, et al. Three cases of osteoma and an osseous fibroma of the paranasal sinuses of horses in South Africa. J S Afr Vet Assoc 2008;79(4):185–93.
40. Robbins SC, Arighi M, Ottewell G. The use of megavoltage radiation to treat juvenile mandibular ossifying fibroma in a horse. Can Vet J 1996;37(11):683–4.
41. Cobourne M, Mitsiadis T. Neural crest cells and patterning of the mammalian dentition. J Exp Zool B Mol Dev Evol 2006;260:251–60.
42. Cobourne MT, Sharpe PT. Tooth and jaw: molecular mechanisms of patterning in the first branchial arch. Arch Oral Biol 2003;48(1):1–14.
43. Brown I, Baker C, Barker I. Oral Cavity. In: Maxie MG, editor. Jubb Kennedy & Palmer's Pathology of Domestic Animals (fifth edition), Vol. 2. Edinburgh: Elsevier Saunders; 2007. p. 3–32.
44. Fessler J. Heterotopic polydontia in horses: nine cases (1969-1986). J Am Vet Med Assoc 1988;192(4):535–8.
45. Rashmir-Raven A, DeBowes R, Cash W, et al. Dentigerous cysts. Compendium on Continuing Education for the Practicing Veterinarian 1990;12(8):1120–6.
46. Hunt R, Allen D, Mueller E. Intracranial trauma associated with extraction of a temporal ear tooth (dentigerous cyst) in a horse. Cornell Vet 1991;81(2):103–8.
47. de Mira MC, Ragle CA, Gablehouse KB, et al. Endoscopic removal of a molariform supernumerary intranasal tooth (heterotopic polyodontia) in a horse. J Am Vet Med Assoc 2007;231(9):9–12.
48. McClure SR, Schumacher J, Morris EL. Dentigerous cyst in the ventral conchal sinus of a horse. Vet Radiol Ultrasound 1993;34(5):334–5.
49. Gardner DG. Dentigerous cysts in animals. Oral Surg Oral Med Oral Pathol 1993;75(3):348–52.
50. Easley JT, Franklin RP, Adams A. Surgical excision of a dentigerous cyst containing two dental structures. Equine Vet Educ 2010;22(6):275–8.
51. Smith LC, Zedler ST, Gestier S, et al. Bilateral dentigerous cysts (heterotopic polyodontia) in a yearling Standardbred colt. Equine Vet Educ 2012;24(11): 573–8.
52. Waguespack RW, Taintor J. Paranasal sinus disease in horses. Compend Contin Educ Vet 2011;33(2):E1–12.
53. Woodford N, Lane J. Long-term retrospective study of 52 horses with sinusal cysts. Equine Vet J 2006;38(3):198–202.
54. Lane J, Longstaffe JA, Gibbs C. Equine paranasal sinus cysts: a report of 15 cases. Equine Vet J 1987;19(6):537–44.

55. Bryant U, Fallon L, Lee M, et al. Congenital aneurysmal bone cyst in a foal. J Equine Vet Sci 2012;32(6):320–3.
56. Knottenbelt D, Kelly D. Oral and dental tumors. In: Easley J, Dixon P, Schumacher J, editors. Equine dentistry. 3rd edition. London: Elsevier; 2010. p. 149–81.
57. Stenberg T, Dowling B, Dart AJ. Mandibular bone cysts in two horses. Aust Vet J 2004;82(7):417–8.
58. Lamb C, Schelling S. Congenital aneurysmal bone cyst in the mandible of a foal. Equine Vet J 1989;21(2):130–2.
59. Purdy C. Mandibular aneurysmal bone cyst in a foal. Equine Pract 2012;7(1):22–4.
60. Schumacher J, Moll H, Schumacher J, et al. A simple method to remove an epidermal inclusion cyst from the false nostril of horses. Equine Pract 1997;19(1):17–20.
61. Nickels F, Tulleners E. Nasal passages. In: Equine surgery. Philadelphia: WB Saunders; 1992. p. 433–46.
62. Frankeny RL. Intralesional administration of formalin for treatment of epidermal inclusion cysts in five horses. J Am Vet Med Assoc 2003;223(2):221–2.
63. Tremaine WH, Clarke CJ, Dixon PM. Histopathological findings in equine sino-nasal disorders. Equine Vet J 1999;31(4):296–303.
64. Gieche J. Oral examination of equidae. In: American Association of Equine Practitioners 360. Basic dentistry. 2012. p. 22–42.
65. Van den Enden MS, Dixon PM. Prevalence of occlusal pulpar exposure in 110 equine cheek teeth with apical infections and idiopathic fractures. Vet J 2008;178(3):364–71.
66. Scrutchfield L, Schumacher J. Examination of the oral cavity and routine dental care. Vet Clin North Am 1993;9(1):123–31.
67. Bennet D. An overview of bits and bitting. In: American Association of Equine Practitioners. Focus on dental procedures. 2006. p. 181–95.
68. Allen T. Incidence and severity of abrasions of the buccal mucosa adjacent to the cheek teeth in 199 horses. In: American Association of Equine Practitioners. 2004. p. 31–6.
69. Tell A, Engvell A, Lundstrum T, et al. The prevalence of oral ulceration in Swedish horses when ridden with a bit and bridle and when unridden. Vet J 2008;178(3):405–10.
70. Orsini P. Oral cavity. In: Auer J, editor. Equine surgery. Philadelphia: WB Saunders; 1992. p. 218–305.
71. Dixon P, Tremaine W, Pickles K. Equine dental disease part 2: a long term study of 400 cases: disorders of development and eruption and variations in position of the cheek teeth. Equine Vet J 1993;31(6):519–28.
72. Johnson TJ, Porter CM. Dental overgrowths and acquired displacement of cheek teeth. In: American Association of Equine Practitioners. Focus on dental procedures. 2006.
73. Dixon P, Tremaine W, Pickles K, et al. Equine dental disease part 1: a long-term study of 400 cases: disorders of incisor, canine, and first premolar teeth. Equine Vet J 1999;31(5):369–77.
74. Tremaine WH, Lane J. Exodontia. In: Easley J, Baker G, editors. Equine dentistry. 2nd edition. Philadelphia: WB Saunders; 2005. p. 267–94.
75. Stubbs RC. Dentistry of equine cheek teeth. In: American Association of Equine Practitioners. 2004. p. 1–6.
76. Griffin C. Routine dentistry in juvenile performance horses. Comp Equine 2009;402–15.

77. Gerard M, Wotman K, Komaromy A. Infections of the head and ocular structures in the horse. Vet Clin North Am Equine Pract 2006;22:591–631.

78. Dixon P. Dental anatomy. In: Baker G, Easley KJ, editors. Equine dentistry. 2nd edition. Philadelphia: WB Saunders; 1993. p. 3–28.

79. Dacre I. Equine dental pathology. In: Baker G, Easley J, editors. Equine dentistry. 2nd edition. Philadelphia: WB Saunders; 2005. p. 91–109.

80. Dixon P. Disorders of development and eruption of the teeth and developmental craniofacial abnormalities. In: Easley J, Dixon P, Schumacher J, editors. Equine dentistry. 3rd edition. London: Elsevier; 2010. p. 99–113.

81. Dixon P, Tremaine W, Pickles K, et al. Equine dental disease part 4: a long-term study of 400 cases: apical infections of cheek teeth. Equine Vet J 2000;32(3): 182–94.

82. Tremaine WH. Oral extraction of equine cheek teeth. Equine Vet Educ 2004; 16(3):151–8.

83. Dillehay DL, Schoeb TR. Veterinary pathology online. Vet Pathol 1986;23:341–2.

84. Brounts SH, Hawkins JF, Lescun TB, et al. Surgical management of compound odontoma in two horses. J Am Vet Med Assoc 2004;225(9):1423–7.

85. Snyder C, Dubielzig RR, Gengler W, et al. Surgical treatment of a rostral mandibular complex odontoma in a 3-year-old horse. Equine Vet Educ 2008;20(12): 647–51.

86. Kreutzer R, Wohlsein P, Staszyk C, et al. Dental benign cementomas in three horses. Vet Pathol 2007;44(4):533–6.

87. Tremaine WH. Oral cavity neoplasia. In: American Association Equine Practitioners. Focus on dentistry. 2006.

88. Hackett ES, Baxter GM. Odontogenic tumours in the horse. Equine Vet Educ 2008;20(12):652–4.

89. Wilson D, Kramer J, Constantinescu G, et al. Manual of equine field surgery. St Louis (MO): Saunders Elsevier; 2006. p. 122–6.

90. Schneider R. Mandibular fractures. In: White N, Moore J, editors. Current practice of equine surgery. Philadelphia: Lippincott; 1990. p. 589–95.

91. Stashak T, Theoret C. Equine wound management. 2nd edition. Ames (IA): Wiley-Blackwell; 2008. p. 273–332.

The Gold Standard of Dental Care for the Adult Performance Horse

David L. Foster, VMD

KEYWORDS

- Performance horse • Wolf teeth • EOTRH

KEY POINTS

- Although uncommon, mandibular wolf teeth, if present and contacted by the bit, will likely cause biting problems in a horse of any age.
- Removal of the wolf teeth in performance horses is widely accepted.
- Due to the age of emergence and the shedding of the deciduous teeth, the formation of hooks usually does not become a major concern in the performance horse before the age of 5 years.
- Equine odontoclastic tooth resorption and hypercementosis plays a minor role in the mature performance horse.
- In the adult performance horse primary dental problems are less common than in younger performance horses.
- Many adult performance horses that are presented for a suspected dental problem actually suffer from a problem elsewhere.

DEFINITIONS

On contact. A horse is ridden or driven on contact when the rider or driver offers resistance to the horse's mouth via the reins or lines. The horse responds to this pressure by engaging the bit and a dynamic interplay between horse and rider or driver is established. This contact is an essential element of many styles of riding (eg, dressage, hunter seat, flat racing, jumping) and all elements of driving. In its simplest interpretation, one might confuse this action with the desire of the rider or driver to slow the horse. This is not the intent of the rider, who will simultaneously be pushing the horse forward with his or her legs and weight. The driver achieves a similar effect by urging the horse forward into the bit with the whip and the lines, as needed. The horse's natural inclination to go forward is moderated by the rider or driver by establishing the appropriate degree of bit contact or collection. Riding or driving a horse on contact

Department of Surgery, University of Pennsylvania School of Veterinary Medicine, New Bolton Center, Kennett Square, PA 19348, USA
E-mail address: davidlfostervmd@cs.com

Vet Clin Equine 29 (2013) 505–519
http://dx.doi.org/10.1016/j.cveq.2013.04.012
0749-0739/13/$ – see front matter © 2013 Elsevier Inc. All rights reserved.

actually enhances the horse's ability to achieve a balanced, efficient gait. This is distinct from an attempt to slow the horse down.

Puller, rusher. A horse that, when driven or ridden, requires far more force on the lines or reins to rate than an average horse does on contact. To keep the horse at the desired speed, one has to pull harder on the reins than would be required of a horse that is not a puller.

Line (lines). The reins used on a driving horse.

On a line. Commonly used in standardbred racing, this refers to the degree to which the driver must resist (pull against) the horse's preferred direction of motion to keep the horse traveling in a straight line. For example, a horse being driven is constantly drifting to the left. To keep the horse traveling in a straight line, the right line must be pulled harder than the left line. This horse is said to be "on the right line."

Lugging in or out, or drifting in or out. This is the preference of the horse, when being exercised, to drift to the inside or outside of the course (or jump). For the rider to keep the horse on a straight course, the opposite rein must be under more tension. For example, a thoroughbred that lugs in while traveling on a counterclockwise course tends to want to turn toward the inside rail while at speed. To correct this, the rider must pull harder on the right rein than the left rein to prevent the horse from moving toward the rail. The terms on the line (right or left) and lugging or drifting (in or out) describe the same phenomenon from different perspectives: man versus horse.

Tongue-tie. This is a device applied to the tongue of racehorses to entrap and stabilize the tongue to the mandible. Typically made of flexible material (cotton felt or nylon stocking), it is about 45 cm long and 3 cm wide. It is applied by loosely tying a simple overhand knot, inserting the tongue with the knot on the dorsum of the tongue, then tightening the ends and tying the free ends snugly around the mandible. The tongue-tie prevents dorsal displacement of the tongue over the bit and can limit the horse's ability to retract the tongue distally within the oral cavity. In the young horse, the tongue-tie additionally functions to maintain proper position of the bit in the young horse's mouth.

PRIMARY ODONTOGENIC PROBLEMS OF THE MATURE PERFORMANCE HORSE
Wolf Teeth

The wolf teeth rarely present a problem in a mature performance horse. If they were present and caused biting issues, they would have been removed earlier in the horse's career. There are a few exceptions to this. Consider the horse that was not put into training until later in life. The first premolars may have never been addressed. Another relatively common situation is with a horse that switched careers. A thoroughbred racehorse may perform unaffected by the presence of unerupted (blind) wolf teeth while racing, but the introduction of a double bridle, as for an advancing dressage horse, may cause problems with the same wolf teeth. A western pleasure horse that switches careers to an English hunter offers a similar possibility, changing from being ridden off contact to on contact. Any change in bit or bridle that causes problems in the horse's performance demands a thorough visual and digital examination of the mouth for the presence of wolf teeth or their fragments. Be sure to examine carefully the maxilla and the mandible. Although uncommon, mandibular wolf teeth, if present and contacted by the bit, will likely cause biting problems in a horse of any age.

Removal of the wolf teeth in performance horses is widely accepted. Visual inspection alone is not sufficient to confirm that the wolf teeth have been removed. Digital palpation will often reveal unerupted or fractured wolf teeth (**Fig. 1**). These may or

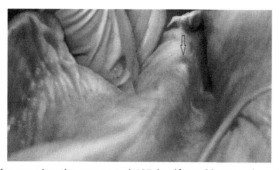

Fig. 1. (*Arrow*) The covering the unerupted 405 (wolf tooth) operculum. (*Courtesy of* Jack Easley, DVM, Shelbyville, KY.)

may not cause the horse discomfort. On the normal horse, one can apply thumb pressure on the area mesial to the 06s with all one's strength and elicit little or no reaction from a normal, unsedated patient. If the horse consistently responds to this pressure, suspect a problem. Any reddening or evidence of a draining tract associated with a first premolar should be regarded as highly suspicious. Radiographs of the area may prove valuable in these cases.

Hooks on 106 or 206 and 311 or 411

Because of the age of emergence and the shedding of the deciduous teeth, the formation of hooks usually does not become a major concern in the performance horse before the age of 5 years. The permanent 06s do not come into occlusal contact until the middle of the second year, and the third molars until the third year. If we assume an eruption rate of about 2 to 3 mm per annum,[1,2] the fastest a 1.0 cm hook can form is about 3 years from occlusion. This explains why hooks alone rarely become large enough to cause performance issues in the young performance horse. This is not always true in the older athlete.

There is a lack of evidence-based information regarding the effect of hooks on the performance of the mature (or young) performance horse. However, one condition affects the performance of many older competing horses. 106/206 hooks, when present and of sufficient length, will affect the horse that is ridden or driven on contact (**Fig. 2**).

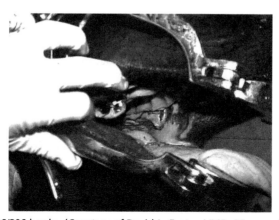

Fig. 2. Mesial 106/206 hooks. (*Courtesy of* David L. Foster, VMD, Morganville, NJ.)

The clinical presentation of these horses is consistent. When asked to engage the bit, the horse raises her or his head, shakes it from side to side, and then drops it. The horse assumes contact only to repeat this behavior until contact with the bit is released by the rider. Several other conditions can produce similar behavior, including headshaking syndrome, poorly fitting tack, and a horse that has not been sufficiently trained to accept the bit. It is on oral examination that the offending 106 or 206 hooks are recognized and the examiner's suspicion should be directed to these hooks until their involvement in the behavior is proven otherwise. One additional insight into this condition concerns the type of bit used. Often, at the first signs of this behavior, the horse owner or trainer will exchange the horse's regular bit for one of a larger diameter. It is commonly assumed that a bit that has larger diameter cannons is better accepted by horses that are experiencing biting issues. In this case, the larger diameter bit exacerbates the horse's discomfort and actually makes the condition worse; whereas a narrow diameter bit will often improve the behavior temporarily (until the hook becomes larger).

Reduction of the identified hooks will often ameliorate the symptoms immediately. Care should be taken to be judicious with the amount of dental tissue removed when reducing these hooks. One must strive to keep the protective dentin-filled pulp chambers intact. Staging these reductions for large hooks (greater than 1 cm) over 2-month intervals may be indicated. By suggesting a smaller diameter bit and a staged reduction of the hooks, a happy medium can be achieved. The reduction of the hook can be staged and the horse will immediately perform better.

The development of 311 or 411 overgrowths are also delayed in the aging horse because of the progressive eruption of the molars.[3] It has been suggested that these hooks or overgrowths will restrict the rostral or caudal mobility of the mandible. Although physical manipulation of a horse's atlas or axis joint normally produces rostrocaudal motion of the mandible, these extremes of flexion and extension are not common (or desirable) during the normal performance of most competitive horses. This may explain why 311 or 411 overgrowths impart a smaller impact on the performance than do the 106 or 206 hooks seem to do.

Overbite, Overjet, Underjet, and Wry Bite

Overbite, overjet, underjet, and wry bite, and their treatments, are common and well described.[4,5] It is unlikely that a young horse with severe wry bite (one that would impact the breathing) could be chosen as a performance horse. Many horses with slight maxillary deviations compete successfully. Often this deviation is overlooked while the horse is young. As the horse ages, the development of an uneven (tilted) incisor bite will indicate a slight wry bite. It is the author's experience that a horse with a wry bite that does not affect his breathing is unaffected in the performance arena.

As horses with overjet conformations mature, they develop partial overbites to varying degrees. These conditions do not seem to affect the athletic performance of the affected horses, despite an assumed interference with the rostrocaudal motion of the mandible.[4] One must keep in mind that horses with overjet conformation may have similar incongruity of the cheek teeth. This conformation will result in the eventual formation of hooks (overgrowths) of the involved teeth. Underjet conformation is uncommon in performance breeds. In the author's experience, affected horses have minimal expression of the condition and it plays no noticeable role in the horse's ability to perform.

Equine Odontoclastic Tooth Resorption and Hypercementosis

Equine odontoclastic tooth resorption and hypercementosis (EOTRH) plays a minor role in the mature performance horse (ages 5–15 years). Clinical expression of this condition is rarely reported in horses younger than 15 years.[6,7] However, there is a small but significant population of aged competition horses that continue to perform well after 15 years of age. Dressage, roping, combined training, and competitive trail horses come to mind. The cause of this condition is unknown at present. The author has treated several of these horses with 1 to 2 week courses of systemic antibiotics and oral flushes (dilute chlorhexidine) to reduce the periodontal disease before an important competition. The water additive, Healthy Mouth (Healthy Mouth LLC) has proven useful in reducing periodontal disease in some of these cases. These treatments are intended to offer transient relief of the symptoms of EOTRH and are not intended to be curative. If the incisors are removed en bloc, be aware that the horse will extend his tongue out of the mouth. This tongue lolling is severely penalized in dressage tests, essentially rendering the horse uncompetitive.

Infundibular Caries

The development of infundibular caries occurs within the 5 to 15 year age group. There has been some contention regarding their pathogenesis and treatment. The author is not aware of any study of the specific effects of this condition in the aging performance horse and can only speak from personal experience. Although the caries develop and advance over time, no appreciable effects are noted on the performance of these horses. If, however, the tooth fractures or an endodontic infection should develop, appropriate treatment should be pursued.

SECONDARY ORAL PROBLEMS

This topic may seem to be out of place in this article, but nothing could be further from the truth! Often, I am called to examine a performance horse that comes back from performing with a bit covered with blood and/or a report that the horse displays control issues while training. The owner or trainer calls me to address what is assumed a dental problem.

The problem cannot by solved with dental care because the cause of the horse's behavior was not due to a primary oral or dental problem. In these cases, the issue is the result of the rider or driver trying to control a noncompliant horse. The problem might be an inappropriate bit or ill-fitting tack. Often the reason for the horse's unacceptable behavior can be found elsewhere in the horse. The oral issues are only a manifestation of the rider or driver's attempt to control the horse. On occasion, human error can create a response in the horse that mimics a dental problem.

Human dentistry has put significant effort into exploring the diagnosis and management of nonodontogenic tooth and oral pain.[8–11] This is driven by a simple fact: patient pain and discomfort suffered is real. That its cause cannot be shown to be of dental origin presents the human dentist with a conundrum: how can one best serve the needs of the patient? "It is critical to keep in mind that whereas patients (humans or the caretakers of an equine patient) will provide information about the perceived site of pain, it is the clinician's examination that will reveal the true source of their pain… If after completing the subjective examination all items on the differential are outside the clinician's scope of practice, then the clinician should continue the examination until he or she has a firm idea of the possible diagnosis so that a proper referral can be made. In addition, it is paramount that all odontogenic sources have been ruled out and that this information is communicated to the health care provider to which the patient is referred."[11]

I am not suggesting that these horses sense a referred oral pain and this causes the undesirable behavior. In the case of the performance horse, a nonoral issue seems to the caretaker to be an oral problem. I find it fascinating that, although the human non-odontogenic pain and the dentist's paradigm are fundamentally different than that of the horse and veterinary dentist, the resolution of the situations is similar.

I have been frustrated, attracted, and mystified by these cases for years. As a veterinarian, I believe I have a deeper insight into these horses than non veterinary equindental care providers. Having taken an oath to help all horses, I am compelled to give the trainer or owner of a given horse my best service. Many horses fail to succeed because their trainers and veterinarians do not recognize these symptoms. Merely to examine, float, and hope fails to fulfill the mission of a veterinarian. "An unthinking dentist is a bad dentist. Perfect technique misapplied is at least as unconscionable as sloppy work."[12] I am convinced that dental care alone will not cure these horses of their problems. Although it is not my role to address the nondental problems of horses, I make every effort to support and direct the caretakers of these horses toward a resolution of the horse's primary nondental issues. This is also a terrific argument for having veterinarians perform all equine dental care.

Pullers

A puller is a horse that consistently increases the tension on the reins or lines while being exercised. This apparent desire of the horse to gain speed requires that the rider or driver resist the acceleration of the horse by pulling back on the lines or reins. Pullers are not bolting as if from a threatening situation. Pulling is a purposeful, elective action taken by the horse. Most pullers will pull at almost any gait excepting, in some cases, the walk. It is the author's belief that pullers exhibit this behavior as a means to ease the pain of a chronic condition that the horse experiences while training or competing. I suspect that pulling is an evasive action learned by the horse to relieve or diminish a painful, repetitive, or perhaps a self-inflicted injury such as lameness or some sort of gait interference. In the author's experience, it is rare, to find pullers under the age of 4 years. A horse is not a quick learner; it takes years to discover and reinforce this behavior. However, once the horse has committed to pulling, little can be done to stop it unless the underlying pain or interference is ameliorated.

I believe that pulling is a trade-off behavior wherein the horse endures pain in his mouth (caused by bit pressure) to reduce a greater pain somewhere else in his body. They do this by committing their center of gravity forward, thus pulling of the reins or lines. The rider or driver then pulls backward, balancing the horse. The driver perceives the horse as accelerating and pulls back on the lines to rate the horse. This dynamic balance is constantly modified by both the horse and rider or driver. Essentially, the horse trains the man to resist his forward acceleration; thus allowing the horse to shift his center of gravity forward and off his hind end while the rider or driver offers the balancing caudal resistance. The driver or rider (a quick learner) on sensing the horse is running away with him or her, willingly resists the horse's efforts by pulling back on the reins or lines with effort. I have driven a few of these horses (as slowly as possible) and can assure the reader that it is an unforgettable and unpleasant experience. The excessive force that is applied to the lines or reins is translated to the bit–mouth interface. The damage to the oral cavity created by pullers is chronic and significant. Through the bit, the pulling horse and rider or driver apply pressure onto the gingival tissue mesial to 306 and 406.

Driven horses produce greater pulling forces than horses that are ridden. These forces include the greater mass of the driver, the physics of the driver's position, the fixed stirrups, the strength of the modern race bike, and the use of handholds (ie, adjustable loops that capture the wrists and allow the driver to pull on the lines with force exceeding his ability to hold the lines with hand strength alone). These all contribute to the great amount of force that the driver can exert on the pulling horse. Typically, the older standardbred horse races weekly and jogs (ie, exercises) many miles between races. Ironically, the reason standardbred horses pull harder than horses ridden astride is that the sulky driver is equipped to pull back on the lines harder than a rider is. Without the driver's mass, the fixed platform to resist the horses' pull, and no hand holds, the rider is limited to taking hold of the reins (grip strength and endurance alone), lifting his body from the saddle and into a sitting or standing position, and shifting his weight rearward, away from the horses head. The rider's weight is balanced through the legs and feet into the stirrups and is maintained by tension on the reins of the horse. This is awkward to describe, yet is a feat of dexterity performed daily by thousands of exercise riders! The harder the horse pulls, the farther back the rider adjusts his or her center of gravity and thus delivers greater rein pressure to the bit.

On oral examination, the trauma to the pulling horse's mouth is readily identified if the examination is performed within a day or two of competition or hard training. There are large, usually bilateral (1 cm or greater) erosions in the gingiva immediately mesial to 306 and 406. They bleed freely if palpated and are very painful to the horse if any pressure is applied. Bilateral buccal erosions caused by the bit forcing the soft tissue into contact with the second premolars often accompany these lesions. If the examination is performed more than 4 or 5 days after racing or training, care must be taken not to overlook the chronic appearance this condition assumes. The superficial gingiva and mucosa will heal quickly. The healing tissue is often somewhat excessive and creates a fold of tissue that lies against the mesial border of the mandibular 06s. However, there is a persistent sign of this condition. Digital palpation will reveal that the normal attachments of the gingiva to the mesial aspect of 306 and 406 are essentially nonexistent. A periodontal probing of the area will reveal there is a deep periodontal pocket that usually can be probed to the mandibular bone. In some long-standing pullers, the mandibular bone can also be traumatized and recede from the reserve crown. The rostral aspect of 306 and 406 will appear to have super erupted because of the excessive exposed crown. This finding is may be mistaken as ramping of 306 and 406. However, examination of the occlusal surface of the associated arcade will reveal no supereruption of the second premolars. No ramp formation is present. Bits of food material are commonly trapped within these periodontal pockets. Eventually, if the horse is not exercised (or does not wear a bit), the area will re-epithelialize and the gingiva will appear to grow down to the ventral aspect of the pockets. It is rare for the gingiva to reconnect spontaneously to the mesial aspects of the 06s.

Treatment of these pre-306 or pre-406 pressure lesions is straightforward. I recommend oral flush of dilute chlorhexidine solution and application of OraGel TM to the lesions three times a day. Care must be taken to avoid any possibility of violating any drug-treatment restrictions when working on any competition horse! I refrain from dispensing any oral medication to a horse in regular competition that might test positive. In the author's opinion, it is not worth the risk of a positive test! If an oral medication that has the potential to test positive is dispensed, I will only dispense the medication to the trainer of record, who has a stake in assuring my treatment instructions are followed to the letter. Key to getting these lesions to heal is to restrict use of the bit. Changing the bit offers little or no promise to altering this condition. Trainers, out of frustration may try severe bits (eg, twisted wire, wrapping the bit with fence wire, etc).

This results in more injury to the horse's mouth. The great forces directed on the periodontal tissues by the bit cause the oral lesions in this condition. The horse behaves on the track as if it is unresponsive to this pain. I discourage the wrapping of the bit with latex or some other product because it only aggravates the soft tissue damage. Latex and damaged plastic-coated bits become more abrasive and increase the damage done to the soft tissue. A highly polished metal bit that exposes no sharp edge to the interdental space creates the least trauma.

I commonly suggest to trainers that they consult their regular barn veterinarian and have the horse evaluated for a possible lameness (particularly hind end) or interference problem. I may personally contact the barn veterinarian and discuss the case. If I have an indication that the problem is a shoeing problem, I will advise the trainer and try to discuss the issue with the farrier. If the problem was easy to solve, the issue would have been addressed and I would have not been called! If possible, have the trainer tow, pony, or swim the patient between races. This will allow some healing of the gingiva.

I often recognize this condition in standardbred racehorses. Just about any stable with 15 to 20 mature racehorses has at least one puller. I have also recognized this condition in thoroughbred horses, steeplechase horses, show jumpers, polo ponies, combined training horses, and occasionally in dressage horses. The range of occurrence of this condition is likely greater than that mentioned because of the limits of my experience within my practice. I assume that any horse ridden or driven under rein or line contact might be vulnerable to pulling. Pulling is a common problem in many older racing horses. It is not a primary dental problem, but is often a reason that I am asked to examine and treat a horse. These cases are examples of oral lesions that are not the primary issue, but are the secondary result of another primary condition.

Horses on the Line, Lugging, or Drifting

Horses that drift to the left or right while at a performance gait require rider or driver correction to remain on the desired course. This correction is achieved by resisting (pulling) on the rein or line on the side opposite to the direction the horse is drifting. Although this condition occurs commonly in young and older performance horses, it often occurs for different reasons. The force required to keep the horse on course can be significant. Again, the standardbred driver has a mechanical advantage over a rider.

Several primary dental conditions might cause a horse to want to avoid bit contact unilaterally. Wolf teeth (05s), fractured premolar caps, and ill-fitting or damaged bits are easily identified in the performance horse and they will cause the horse to avoid bit contact on the affected side. With a young horse, avoiding the discomfort of bit contact on the affected side will cause it to drift toward the unaffected side. This will result in the horse appearing to move away from the oral pain associated with the condition. These conditions are the primary dental issues that cause the horse to try to avoid bit contact.

In the older performance horse, bearing in/out or being on one line usually occurs for different reasons. In these horses, I believe the primary reason for drifting out is pain experienced elsewhere. I consider most horses that demonstrate a preference to drift consistently to one side or the other as unilateral pullers. These horses have developed this habit in the response to consistent and predictable pain while exercising. Again, they rely on the predicable response of the rider or driver to pull on the appropriate rein or line to maintain directional control of the horse. Horses with arthritis, suspensory desmitis, tendon injuries, incomplete fractures, sesamoiditis, shoeing imbalance, conformation faults (causing interference), and so forth are prime candidates for being on a line. All the dental care in the world will not resolve this behavior. Sometimes the cause may be very subtle.

"These changes that alter a horse's way of going even to a minor degree are what I have in mind when I say that shoeing and balancing is a science of inches and ounces.

A horse that is missing his hind shins by a sixteenth of an inch is just as good as one that is missing by the proverbial mile. Often times, a very slight change, one whose effect is measures in tiny fractions of inches, may be absolutely all that you need."[13]

"Many times the cause (of a horse being on one line) is acute lameness and you have a major problem on your hands. But more often than not the cause is something less drastic, something a trainer can control. Perhaps the teeth need attention, the bit is too severe, the noseband too tight, or the shadow roll too high. Maybe your horse is going crooked simply from habit of perhaps he is just a little lame and shows it going into the turns and nowhere else."[14]

The oral consequences of a horse being on one line can also be significant. To keep the horse on course, the rein or line opposite to the horse's direction of drift has to be pulled on by the driver or rider. Most racing horses wear some sort of snaffle bit.[15] When one side of the bit is pulled with the determination of the rider or driver to keep the horse on course, several things happen. First, the bit has the tendency to slide through the oral cavity and the cannon emerges from the corner of the horse's mouth that is being restrained. This can place excessive pressure on the side of the tight rein to the buccal tissue associated with the commissure of the lips, forcing them against the buccal aspect of the maxillary second premolars. However, consider the situation in which the horse, while being restrained by a tight rein, bends its head and neck toward the tight rein. In this situation, the cheek piece of the bit can be elevated off the buccal tissue and little buccal injury may occur. With the bit pulled through the mouth, buccal pressure can be applied by the cheek-piece of the bit on the opposite side of the resistance! The result of this is that, on examination, the horse exhibits buccal trauma on the side opposite to the rein being pulled. In other words, one cannot reliably determine which side a horse is on the line by oral examination of the buccal tissue alone. Despite careful reduction of the 06s in this area (bit seat), the pressure placed on this tissue will cause contusions, if not small lacerations, in this tissue. In addition, premandibular erosions and denuding of the mesial aspect of the 306 or 406 commonly occur (similar to a puller-caused lesion) (**Fig. 3**). One lesion that may be easily missed can be found by lifting the tongue and examining the sublingual, medial aspect of the mandible about 3 to 4 cm rostral to the 06 on the rein pressure side (**Fig. 4**). The joint of a broken (hinged) snaffle bit engages the mandible at this point and can produce painful injuries. Note that all aforementioned

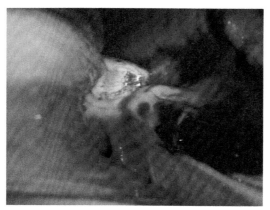

Fig. 3. Soft tissue trauma mesial to 306 due to bit pressure. (*Courtesy of* David L. Foster, VMD, Morganville, NJ.)

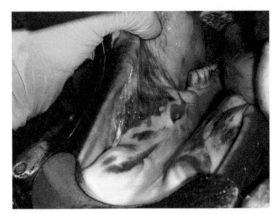

Fig. 4. Bar injury showing bone. (*Courtesy of* Jack Easley, DVM, Shelbyville, KY.)

injuries occur as the result of the horse being on the line as opposed to causing the horse to be on the line. This essential distinction must be expressed to the trainer or owner.

Basically, primary oral treatment for these lesions is the same for pullers. Conservative treatments work well with these soft tissues. The denuding of the gingiva mesial to 306 and 406 will heal, but the periodontal damage remains largely untreatable. I must admit that more aggressive treatment (eg, debridement, packing, root planning) of this condition seems futile as long as the horse remains on the line and continues to traumatize the area. The larger question of how one might get the horse off the line and alleviate the cause of the oral lesions is another matter. There are myriad bits, burrs, head poles, line burrs, bridles, and so forth that have been devised to counteract a horse's efforts to drift. Equestrians apply them with varying success. Nevertheless, they represent, in the author's opinion, an attempt to address the symptom of the horse's problem. They are not the solution to the problem itself.

Headshaking

I will mention this subject only for completeness on the subject. There is much new and ongoing research on this subject. Headshaking in younger horses due to dental problems and other training issues is common. In older horses, I find that headshaking due to a primary dental problem is not as common. They usually have very normal dentition yet demonstrate the headshaking behavior. One exception to this is the presence of 106 or 206 hooks.

IATROGENIC INJURIES TO THE OLDER PERFORMANCE HORSE
Bit Seat Reduction

Overzealous removal of dental material in the formation of the so-called bit seat is a common finding in the performance horse community. Because standards for this procedure are lacking, one must rely on experience and the data that have been reported in the literature for guidance in this controversial area. Aggressive removal of the mesial aspects of all the 06s can result in violations of the rostral (#6) pulp horns of these teeth. This is not good practice. While examining a mature performance horse, I will often probe the dentin covering these pulp horns to evaluate a potential pulp exposure. Often an incomplete closure of the pulp horn is found in a horse with an aggressively performed bit seat reduction.

If an open pulp canal is discovered on examination, I will ask the trainer or owner if there have been any signs of a biting problem. I ask them about the history of the horse's dental care, point out the defect, and suggest we keep an eye on it. If I suspect there might be significant endodontic disease, I recommend a radiographic examination and proceed accordingly from there.

Although pulp exposures should be avoided, I believe there is a solid basis for performing some reduction of the buccal aspect of 106 or 206, the lingual aspects of 306 or 406, and judicial smoothing of the rostral border of all the 06s. My confidence in this matter comes from the examination of hundreds of thoroughbred and standardbred horses, combined training horses, and dressage horses following competition. I believe that a properly performed bit seat reduction can improve the performance of these horses by reducing trauma to the horse's mouth. I cannot speak for those equine competitors that perform off bit contact.

Canine Teeth

Pulp exposure of the canines due to overreduction of the canine crown is also a common finding in the mature male performance horse. There is no place for cutting or nipping the canine teeth in modern equine dentistry. Although I do remove the sharp enamel edge of these teeth with a diamond-coated S float, I see no advantage to removing more than 1 to 2 mm of the crown. This is just enough softening of the edge to prevent lacerations to the tongue while applying a tongue-tie and to the handler's hand while inserting the bit.

My clinical experiences with horses that have had endodontic disease after canine pulp exposure are rare but memorable. Most of these horses violently resisted bit contact on the affected side, showed radiographic signs of apical disease in the affected tooth, and improved dramatically after extraction of the tooth. Every canine tooth pulp exposure should be evaluated for vital pulp therapy and treated appropriately.

Tongue-Tie

Oral injuries to the mature racehorse caused by the tongue-tie are common. This should come as no surprise considering the popularity of the tongue-tie among trainers and the nearly universal dislike of the tongue-tie among racehorses! While applying the tongue-tie, the tongue should be handled as gently as possible. Severe avulsion injuries to the tongue and hyoid bones are some of the results of attempting to apply a tongue-tie using brute force. Lacerations of the tongue by the canine teeth and bit are also possible. Tying the tongue so tightly that it becomes cyanotic during the horse's performance may induce muscle and nerve injury. Keep in mind that the trainer of the horse may or may not have been present while this device is applied. A diplomatic inquiry into the chain of events that led to a tongue injury makes good sense.

Mandibular Periostitis

This condition has been reported in the literature[16–18] as a cause for the horse to resist bit contact while performing. Excessive pressure placed on the interdental mandible can cause a periosteal reaction. Future pressure applied to this reactive tissue can lead to headshaking or other signs of the horse to resist bit contact. Physical examination will often reveal thickened, sensitive areas on the mandible that correspond to the location of bit contact and the previous injury. A surgical procedure can be performed to remove the affected tissue and alleviate the horse's pain.[4]

Operator Error

The range of talent within the world of competition horses is great. This applies to the horses, their riders, drivers, and trainers. Operator error occurs when a horse's unacceptable behavior is caused or exacerbated by a lack of skill of the person controlling them. The horse is not the primary problem in these situations and this possibility should not be ignored. A heavy-handed rider or driver can cause oral trauma to a normal horse. There are times in the heat of competition when even a skilled rider or driver may need to apply excessive force to the bit to avoid disaster.

It is difficult to offer guidance to the reader on this delicate matter. Diplomatic discussion of the issue with the concerned parties offers the possibility of a positive resolution to the problems. To keep the discussion positive, I often suggest that a client seek the advice of a professional in their chosen equine venue. There is a long learning curve for the amateur and professional horseperson. They are not all destined to become experts and ride their horses in the Olympics or race in the Breeder's Cup.

ALL THE REST
Trauma

All horses are vulnerable to physical injury. The performance horse is at greater risk because of the nature of their work. Oral injuries due to falls, collisions, kicks, starting gates, polo mallets, and trailer accidents all contribute to these risks (**Fig. 5**). Stall injuries such as incisor avulsions and electric shock are also possible. A seasoned, mature competition horse may be less likely to incur these injuries than an inexperienced youngster. All the teeth present in the mature performance horse are permanent teeth. There are times when one is confronted with a decision whether or not to attempt to salvage an injured incisor tooth. Although one could argue that the loss of such a tooth will not affect the performance of a patient, one might consider the impact of this loss on the future oral health in the horse's retirement.

HISTORY, ORAL EXAMINATION, AND DIAGNOSTIC NERVE BLOCKS

When called to examine a mature performance horse for what is believed to be a dental problem, it is beneficial to obtain a complete history of the problem before examining the horse.

When taking the history, questions and descriptions should include the following:

1. Have the problem described by the rider or driver of the horse, if possible. He or she will give vital information that might not be known by a trainer, groom, or owner. What is the rider or driver's skill level? Could the operator be causing the problem?
2. How long has the problem been noticed? How long have they had the horse in their care?
3. How consistent is the problem? Does it occur only when the horse is bitted? Does it occur when the horse is lightly exercising, lunging, towed, led in hand, or only at speed? Does the problem go away if the horse is not wearing a bit? Has the horse ever been fitted with a bitless bridle? Did this make a difference in the expression of the behavior?
4. Has the tack, bit, or rider or driver been changed lately? Did this coincide with the development of the behavior?
5. Can the behavior be demonstrated at the time of your examination?
6. Has the horse experienced lameness?
7. Have there been changes in the horse's shoeing?

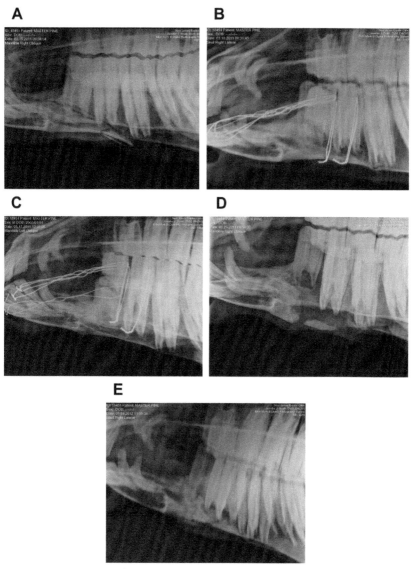

Fig. 5. "Master Pine" STB gelding, 2003. Fractured mandible. (*A*) Original injury, March 15, 2011. (*B*) Postoperative, March 17, 2011. (C) May 17, 2011. (*D*) Removal of 306, June 23, 2011. (*E*) January 4, 2012. (*Courtesy of* Jennifer J. Smith, DVM, DAVCS.)

8. When was the last time the horse performed? Describe that performance.
9. Does the horse demonstrate the behavior only while doing a specific function, such as turning to the right at high speed, when being rated or pulled up, or (much worse) when going the right way (counter clockwise in North America) on the racetrack? Is the problem worse in a turn versus on the straight portion of the course?
10. Does the horse improve or get worse on different surfaces? For example, is it better on the training track but worse at the racetrack?

11. If permitted, examine the horse's tack. Is this the tack the horse performs in or just the training bridle? Does the horse perform with any special equipment (eg, head pole, Murphy blind, shadow roll, blinkers)?
12. Has the horse had any significant treatments lately? For example, joint injections, dental care, and so forth. If treatments have occurred, do they coincide with the appearance of the dental problem? Did they improve the suspected dental problem?
13. Has the horse's eating habits changed? Is it selective in its diet?
14. What does the rider or driver think the problem is?

The Physical Examination

The physical examination should be conducted as follows:

1. Begin with a general visual assessment and carefully examine and palpate the horses head, poll, mandible, and lips.
2. If the legs are bandaged, ask why and whether there are any significant physical problems. If there is an indication of lameness contributing to the problem, ask to have the leg wraps removed.
3. Examine the horse for evidence of interference injury such as superficial trauma to the legs. Ask if the horse performs in bandages or protective boots. Does the horse show signs of interference after performing? Although protective boots will spare the horse from lacerations to the skin, the horse will often continue altering its gait while wearing the protective boots.
4. Check for basic function of the cranial nerves and vision.
5. Gently attempt to grasp the tongue with a gloved hand and note the horse's response. Is the tongue tone within normal limits? Does the tongue show signs of trauma?
6. Perform a casual oral examination with a headlamp, but without a speculum, looking and feeling for any abnormal tissue and or pain. Carefully palpate and visually examine the interdental spaces, the buccal tissue, and (if possible) the hard palate.
7. Then sedate the horse and apply an oral speculum to perform a more complete oral examination.
8. A thorough oral examination is conducted.

Diagnostic Nerve Blocks

Performing diagnostic nerve blocks on the tissues of the oral cavity of a horse and then asking a rider or driver to test the results on the performance horse should give the practitioner cause for concern. Will blocking the tissue cause the rider or driver to have less control of the horse? Will this cause a dangerous situation? Caution has led me to the following conclusions:

1. Blocking the oral tissues and sending the horse out to perform is a procedure that I reserve as a diagnostic test of last resort.
2. I personally advise the rider or driver of the potential risks he or she may be exposed to. If the rider or driver is not a seasoned veteran of the sport, I will not proceed.
3. I pick a time and location for the test so that other horses and people are not at risk. I try to choose an enclosed or fenced area to perform.
4. I try to limit my use of anesthetic to local infusion and avoid regional nerve blocks if possible.

Having followed these guidelines, I am relieved to say that I have never experienced a case of a "runaway" horse. We should more thoroughly explore this area!

REFERENCES

1. Dyce KM, Sack WO, Wensig CJ. Textbook of veterinary anatomy. 19897. Philadelphia: WB Saunders; p. 473–7.
2. Baker GJ. Oral examination and diagnosis: management of oral diseases. In: Harvey CE, editor. Veterinary dentistry. Philadelphia: WB Saunders; p. 217–28.
3. Dixon P. In: Easley J, et al, editors. Equine dentistry. 3rd edition. Elsevier; 2011. p. 100.
4. Dixon P. In: Easley J, et al, editors. Equine dentistry. 3rd edition. Elsevier; 2011. p. 99–100.
5. DeLorey MS. A retrospective evaluation of 204 diagonal incisor malocclusion corrections in the horse. J Vet Dent 2007;24(3):145–9.
6. Staszyk C, et al. Equine odontoclastic tooth resorption and hypercementosis. Vet J 2008;178:372–9.
7. Rice MK. Prevalence of incisor and canine tooth resorption. In: Proceedings of the 26th Veterinary Dental Forum. 2012. p. 167.
8. Melis M, Lobo SL, Ceneviz C, et al. Atypical odontalgia: a review of the literature. Headache 2003;43:1060.
9. Marbach J, Raphael KG. Phantom tooth pain: a new look at an old dilemma. Pain Med 2000;1:68.
10. Lipton J, Ship JA, Larach-Robinson D. Estimated prevalence and distribution of reported orofacial pain in the United States. J Am Dent Assoc 1993;124:115.
11. Mattscheck S, Saw AS, Nixdorf R. In: Hargreaves KM, Cohen S, editors. Pathways of the pulp. 10th edition. Elselvier; 2011. p. 49–70, 62.
12. Jeffcoat M. In: Hargreaves KM, Cohen S, editors. Pathways of the pulp. 10th edition. Elselvier; 2011. p. 49.
13. Simpson JF Sr. In: Care and training of the trotter and pacer. U.S. Trotting Assoc; 1968. p. 335–6.
14. O'Brien JC. In: Care and training of the trotter and pacer. U.S. Trotting Assoc; 1968. p. 420.
15. Bennett DW. In: Easley J, et al, editors. Equine dentistry. 3rd edition. Elsevier; 2011. p. 30.
16. Johnson TJ. Surgical removal of mandibular periostitis (bone spurs) caused by bit damage. In Proceedings of the 48th Annual Meeting of the American Association of Equine Practitioners. 2002. p. 458–62.
17. Van Lancker S, Van Den Broeck W, Simoens P. Incidence and morphology of bone irregularities of the equine interdental spaces. Equine Vet Educ 2007;19: 103–6.
18. Bennett D. In: Easley J, editor. Equine dentistry. 3rd edition. Elsevier; 2011. p. 27–8.

The Gold Standard of Dental Care
The Geriatric Horse

Nicole du Toit, BVSc, MSc, CertEP, PhD, MRCVS[a],*,
Bayard A. Rucker, DVM[b]

KEYWORDS

- Dental disease • Geriatric • Equine

KEY POINTS

- The change in normal equine dental anatomy with age results in dental disease specific to the geriatric horse.
- The culmination of dental disease throughout the life of horses often results in advanced dental disease in older horses.
- The approach to treatment of specific dental disease conditions has to be adapted for older horses to compensate for the reduction in reserve crown and occlusal enamel.
- Ensuring oral comfort and maximizing masticatory ability are the mainstays of geriatric dental treatment.
- Older patients often require long-term management changes, such as dietary modification, to manage dental disease effectively.

INTRODUCTION

The natural ageing process of equine teeth contributes to the majority of dental disease observed in geriatric equids. Central to the ageing changes seen in equine teeth are that they are hypsodont and have a finite length.[1,2] Various factors, such as management and type of diet, may also contribute to the rate at which teeth are worn and may accelerate age-related changes. For example, if a horse has had a lot of dental treatment throughout its life, involving reduction of the occlusal surface, this reduction decreases the functional length of the teeth. Horses that have been fed a coarse forage-based diet with lots of silicates may increase the amount of wear on the teeth.

The decrease in enamel thickness and enamel infolding further apically in teeth means less enamel is exposed on the occlusal surface as the teeth wear down,[3] resulting in teeth that are not able to resist wear as effectively younger horses' teeth

The authors have nothing to disclose.
[a] Equine Veterinary Dentistry, PO Box 210, Tulbagh 6820, Western Cape, South Africa;
[b] Southwest Virginia Veterinary Services, 309 Overlook Drive, Lebanon, VA, USA
* Corresponding author.
E-mail address: equinevetdentist@gmail.com

and the rate of attrition increasing. As a result of the teeth narrowing apically, aged horses have less tooth surface area and less tooth angulation, and the compression forces in each cheek teeth row are unable to maintain close interdental contact between teeth, which may result in multiple diastemata developing along a cheek teeth row, termed *senile diastemata*.[4]

A recent detailed biomechanical study determined that in older horses, mandibular cheek teeth became more curved rostrocaudally but did not change their dental positions. In contrast, the maxillary cheek teeth did not become more curved but did have an increase in mesio-occlusal angle (ie, changed their dental position).[5] Because the mandibular cheek teeth become more curved and the maxillary cheek teeth don't, the occlusal contact between them changes. This alteration in occlusal contact may contribute to changes in wear pattern observed in geriatric horses. Incisors also decrease in length with age and the contact angle between the maxillary and mandibular incisors becomes more acute. If this change of angle is not equal on both upper and lower jaws, it may adversely affect the normal wearing of the occlusal surfaces and inhibit normal prehension.

The mainstay of dental treatment in older horses is aimed at ensuring oral comfort and maximizing masticatory ability. The short remaining reserve crown limits dental crown reduction treatment in geriatric horses, especially if prophylactic dental care has not been maintained throughout a horse's life. Trying to achieve major changes in the cheek teeth row occlusal profile is more detrimental than more conservative treatment to patients at an advanced age.

Geriatric horses often have the culmination of dental disease that accrued throughout their lives. Due to the ageing process, dental diseases, such as worn teeth, periodontal disease, and diastemata, are common in older horses.[6] A study in a large population of donkeys showed a significant increase in the prevalence of dental disease as the animals aged. In particular, there was a significant increase in dental disease in the 15-year-old to 20-year-old age range.[6]

Missing teeth are more common in older than younger horses because teeth lose their stability once the reserve crown has reached a certain minimum length. Also, it may be more likely that over the years of horses' lives, they have had to have a tooth extracted due to fractures or apical infections. Diastemata are common in geriatric horses and were shown present in 85% of donkeys with a median age of 31 years.[7] Diastemata and displaced teeth are often accompanied by significant periodontal disease, regarded as the most painful dental disease, which needs to be treated accordingly.[8,9] Furthermore, periodontal disease contributes to the further displacement of teeth and loss of teeth due to periodontal ligament damage.

Equine odontoclastic tooth resorption and hypercementosis (EOTRH) is a dental disease specific to incisors and canines. It is characterized by gingivitis of the incisors and the canines in the early stages.[10] This gingivitis needs to be differentiated from gingivitis secondary to senile incisor diastemata with food impaction, common in elderly horses. EOTRH is a progressive inflammatory reaction within the alveolus resulting in necrosis of alveolar cementum and periodontal ligament by odontoclastic cells and simultaneous production of reparative cementum by odontoblasts. As EOTRH advances, it usually separates to 2 distinct clinical forms, with some overlap. The more serious form has lysis invading the tooth enamel, dentin, and alveolar bone, leading to a weakened tooth subject to fracturing. Eventually small draining abscesses appear on the buccal mucosa corresponding to the incisor apices. With the hypercementosis form, excess cementum is layered around the tooth within the alveolus, causing significant enlargement of the reserve crown. Both forms cause multiple incisor displacement, moderate to severe gingival recession, and painful teeth in geriatric horses. Radiographic assessment provides definite diagnosis. All medical treatments advocated for EOTRH to date slow the progression of the disease but do not provide cure. Successful treatment is usually only achieved with incisor extraction (see article by Rawlison elsewhere in this issue).

DENTAL EXAMINATION OF GERIATRIC PATIENTS

When geriatric patients are presented with clinical signs or history suggesting a systemic illness, physical examination and laboratory tests are indicated before the dental examination. Older horses often have worn incisors, which have to be taken into consideration before applying a full-mouth speculum (**Fig. 1**). If the incisors are worn, padded speculum bars instead of bite plates rest more comfortably and securely in the interdental space. Often, older patients have lots of food accumulation due to displaced teeth, missing teeth, diastemata, or other wear abnormalities, resulting in inefficient mastication and food accumulation. Therefore, it is important to ensure that the mouth is sufficiently flushed out before attempting an examination. Before probing and examination, periodontal pockets and diastemata may require cleaning with small dental picks, scalers, or commercially available high-pressure low-volume dental spray units or sprayers made from air tool hoses, connectors, and sprayers from home improvement stores.

Dental mirrors and periodontal probes are also essential tools when examining the geriatric equine mouth. Lesions in the caudal mouth, such as mandibular diastemata, need to be visually assessed to determine the severity of the lesion. A periodontal probe is useful in determining the depth of gingival and periodontal pockets, which are more common in older than younger horses. Careful evaluation of the lip and buccal mucosa is important to detect any chronic ulcers or ulcers that are proportionately large and deep for the associated dental lesion, which may be indicative of other systemic diseases, such as pituitary pars intermedia dysfunction, which are more common in older horses.[11]

Radiography may be a useful ancillary diagnostic aid when examining older patients with dental disease and is essential to make a diagnosis of EOTRH or apical disease but may also be useful when assessing fractured teeth or diastemata. Radiographic assessment is indicated when formulating a treatment plan for displaced teeth, periodontal pocketing, and diastemata. Periodontal lesions may have significant apical involvement, which is not revealed by oral examination, probing, or tooth mobility.

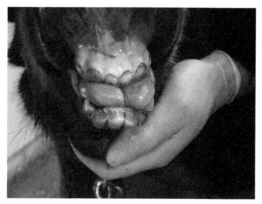

Fig. 1. Severely worn incisors in geriatric horses are common and may be due to normal age-related wearing of teeth or accelerated by vices, such as crib biting.

When assessing, in particular, the mandibular cheek teeth apices, the latero 35° to 45° ventral-dorsal oblique projection needs to be at the higher angle than the standard views to ensure that the apices are separated and visualized due to the shorter reserve crown. The open-mouthed oblique views are particularly useful for assessing problems associated with the cheek teeth crowns.[12]

TREATMENT OF SPECIFIC GERIATRIC DENTAL DISEASE CONDITIONS

Wave mouth is an uneven wear pattern of the occlusal surfaces with a proportion of teeth overgrown and/or worn within the same cheek teeth row. The opposing arcade usually has corresponding worn and/or overgrown teeth. Treatment of this condition is aimed at reducing the overgrown teeth. It is important to carefully float the overgrown teeth by only a few millimeters, because reduction of these teeth effectively takes them out of occlusion, reducing a horse's masticatory ability until the continued eruption of worn teeth effects occlusal contact again. During this interim period, owners may have to provide a dietary supplement to compensate for the decreased mastication. This treatment needs to be repeated approximately 3 months later. If a reasonably even occlusal surface has been achieved, treatment has to be repeated at 6-month intervals to ensure no further deterioration. In these older patients, it is rare that a complete even cheek teeth occlusal row is achieved, and these horses often maintain a mild wave mouth.

Smooth mouth is often characterized by smooth cupped-out teeth with sharp peripheral edges. These sharp edges should only be rasped if likely to cause cheek or tongue mucosal ulceration, because reducing them decreases the small amount of remaining enamel even further. Smooth mouth may affect only a portion of the cheek teeth rows and in these cases some functional masticatory ability is maintained. In cases of a complete smooth mouth of all 4 cheek teeth rows, dietary management is required to provide nutritional needs.

In some instances, smooth mouth may be characterized by the presence of worn teeth involving all the mandibular cheek teeth but not maxillary cheek teeth. As a consequence, the maxillary cheek teeth are often overgrown, which also may be seen in some cases of cheek teeth missing from an entire row (either mandible or maxillae). There is often some contact with the opposing gingiva, but it is important that the pressures exerted by the overgrown teeth on the soft tissues are not excessive. It is for this reason that the overgrown teeth in the opposing row be carefully reduced. Again, these patients have little or no masticatory ability and need dietary supplementation.

In some older patients, there may be multiple dental disorders, including worn teeth, displaced teeth, overgrown teeth, sharp points, and diastemata. These disorders are often referred to as broken mouth and are usually a result of a neglected mouth that has had minimal or no dental treatment in the past (**Fig. 2**). These horses have to be

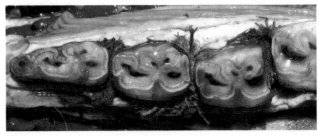

Fig. 2. A typical broken mouth with the presence of sharp points, overgrown teeth, worn teeth, diastemata, and periodontal disease.

evaluated on a case-by-case basis and the basic principles of geriatric dental care need to be applied.

The presence of displaced teeth is more common in geriatric than younger horses because teeth can displace secondary to periodontal disease or missing teeth, known as *acquired displacement*.[2,4] Some patients may have developed displaced teeth at a young age associated with the eruption process, termed *developmental displacements*.[4] Regardless of the initial cause of the displaced teeth, they are likely to progress and become exaggerated with old age for 2 reasons: the shorter reserve crown, which means less stability within the alveolar socket, and the development (or progression) of periodontal disease, which is more common in older than younger horses. If displacement is mild and there is no associated periodontal disease, the protruding edges may be floated lightly so that they are rounded, minimizing soft tissue lesions associated with abnormal pressure from these displaced teeth. Soft tissue lesions may also develop on the tongue with medial displacements, because they are often present on the buccal mucosa with lateral displacements. In cases of severely displaced teeth, there is often associated periodontal disease, which needs to be treated. Furthermore, floating of the protruding teeth is often not sufficient to alleviate discomfort. Thus, oral extractions of these severely displaced teeth are often indicated. Extraction of displaced teeth can be more difficult due to the abnormal angle of the teeth. In geriatric patients, however, the reduced reserve crown should facilitate extraction of these teeth.

The treatment of diastemata in geriatric patients is often more difficult than in younger patients for 2 reasons. First, there are often multiple diastemata present in older horses, and second, there are less compression forces on the cheek teeth row (**Fig. 3**). Treatment of multiple diastemata requires a compliant patient (ie, well sedated). If the diastemata are painful, the addition of dental nerve blocks facilitates examination, evaluation, and treatment.

Floating of opposing overgrowths and sharp points alleviates the impaction forces on the diastema. When diastemata are due to apical narrowing of the teeth (senile diastemata), treatment is aimed at alleviating the associated gingivitis and periodontal disease. Within the same cheek teeth row, there may be open and closed diastemata. Consequently, not all diastemata have secondary gingivitis or periodontal pockets.[13] Cleaning out and flushing of periodontal pockets and bridging with materials, such as polysiloxane, or composite, such as Structur 2 (VOCO, Cuxhaven, Germany), may be

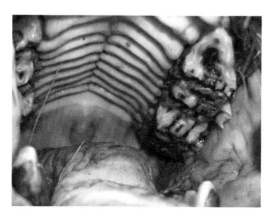

Fig. 3. Multiple senile diastemata with food impaction in a mandibular cheek teeth row. Note how the 310/11 and 309/10 diastemata are valve diastemata whereas the 308/09 diastema is an open diastema.

indicated for individual diastemata.[14] In selected cases, diastema burring may be beneficial. Ultimately, in geriatric patients, unlike in younger patients due to the lack of cheek teeth row compression forces, there is unlikely resolution of the diastemata. Other adjunct therapies, such as analgesia, antibiosis, regular oral rinsing with 0.12% chlorhexidine gluconate, and dietary management, may be required when treating diastemata.

EOTRH has been managed, with limited success, by application of corticosteroid cream, injection of corticosteroids submucosally, pulsed oral antibiotics (7–10 days per month), and nonsteroidal anti-inflammatory drugs. Daily application of 0.12% chlorhexidine gluconate until there is an obvious decrease in avoidance of percussion of the incisors, followed by application 3 times per week, is effective in controlling the pain.[15] Eventually, severely effected teeth require extraction and in some cases all the incisors require extraction at one time.

FEEDING MANAGEMENT

It has also been shown that older horses have decreased masticatory force as a result of a decrease in the curve of Spee,[5] which, along with the fact that the teeth are smoother, causes an even greater reduction in the masticatory ability. Ultimately, geriatric patients have difficulty maintaining their minimum daily energy intake. Not only is it important to consider the need to increase the digestible energy in the diet but also it is essential to ensure that the fiber component in the diet is sufficient for gastrointestinal health. Geriatric horses generally manage well on fresh pastures because the high moisture content and lower levels of acid detergent fiber allow for more efficient digestion despite minimal mastication. Diets composed of chopped forage may be beneficial in horses with reduced occlusal grinding ability. Certain types of chopped forage (eg, lucerne), however, may be contraindicated in cases of diastemata because the short hard fibers may lodge within the diastemata. Most major horse food brands produce pelleted forage, which is an ideal supplement in geriatric horses. In severe cases of smooth mouth or of patients having multiple missing teeth, fiber pellets can be soaked to aid ingestion. The addition of fat in the form of oil, instead of carbohydrates, to increase the caloric intake should also be considered. High levels of carbohydrates in the diet have been shown associated with an increased incidence of gastric ulceration.

Older horses, ponies, and donkeys with dental disease can continue to have a good quality of life with correct management. It is important for owners to understand that long-term management, consisting of regular veterinary treatment and dietary alteration, is required to maintain geriatric horses in good health.

REFERENCES

1. Dixon PM, Copeland AN. The radiological appearance of mandibular cheek teeth in ponies of different ages. Equine Vet Educ 1993;5:317–23.
2. Dixon PM. The gross, histological, and ultrastructural anatomy of equine teeth and their relationship to disease. In: Proceedings of the 48th American Association of Equine Practitioners Annual Convention. 2002. p. 421–37.
3. du Toit N, Kempson SA, Dixon PM. Donkey dental anatomy. Part 1: gross and computed axial tomography examination. Vet J 2008;176:338–44.
4. Dixon PM, Dacre I. A review of equine dental disorders. Vet J 2005;169:165–87.
5. Huthmann S, Gasse H, Jacob HG, et al. Biomechanical evaluation of equine masticatory action: position and curvature of equine cheek teeth and age-related changes. Anat Rec 2008;291:565–70.

6. du Toit N, Burden FA, Dixon PM. Clinical dental examinations of 357 donkeys in the UK: part 1-Prevalence of dental disorders. Equine Vet J 2009;41:390–4.

7. du Toit N, Gallagher J, Burden FA, et al. Post mortem survey of dental disorders in 349 donkeys from an aged population (2005-2006): part 2—epidemiological studies. Equine Vet J 2008;40:209–13.

8. Greene SK, Basile T. Recognition and treatment of equine periodontal disease. In: Proceedings of the 48th American Association of Equine Practitioners Annual Convention. 2002;48:463–6.

9. Dixon PM, Barakzai S, Collins N, et al. Treatment of equine cheek teeth by mechanical widening of diastemata in 60 horses (2000-2006). Equine Vet J 2008;40:22–8.

10. Stazyk C, Bienert A, Kreutzer R, et al. Equine odondoclastic tooth resorption and hypercementosis. Vet J 2008;178:372–9.

11. Dybdal N. Pituitary pars intermedia dysfunction (equine cushing's-like disease). In: Robinson NE, editor. Current therapy in equine medicine. Philadelphia: WB Saunders; 1997. p. 499–501.

12. Barakzai S. Dental Imaging. In: Easley J, Dixon PM, Schumacher J, editors. Equine dentistry. 3rd edition. Edinburgh: Saunders Elsevier; 2010. p. 199–230.

13. Walker H, Chinn E, Holmes S, et al. A study of the prevalence and some clinical characteristics of equine cheek teeth diastema in 471 horses examined in a UK first opinion practice (2008 – 2009). Vet Rec 2012;171:44.

14. Pearce C. Periodontal Disease Lecture WebLeC from Ledston Education Centre West Yorkshire (UK): Ledston Equine Clinic; 2012.

15. Rucker BA. Clinical observation. Lebanon, Virginia: South West Virginia Veterinary Services.

Index

Note: Page numbers of article titles are in **boldface** type.

Vet Clin Equine 29 (2013) 529–540
http://dx.doi.org/10.1016/S0749-0739(13)00045-X
0749-0739/13/$ – see front matter © 2013 Elsevier Inc. All rights reserved.

vetequine.theclinics.com

Printed and bound by CPI Group (UK) Ltd, Croydon, CR0 4YY

03/10/2024

01040409-0008